TOWARD ACTIVE LIVING

PROCEEDINGS OF THE INTERNATIONAL CONFERENCE ON PHYSICAL ACTIVITY, FITNESS, AND HEALTH

H. Arthur Quinney, PhD
University of Alberta

Lise Gauvin, PhD
Concordia University

A.E. Ted Wall, PhD
McGill University

Editors

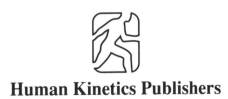

Human Kinetics Publishers

Library of Congress Cataloging-in-Publication Data

International Conference on Physical Activity, Fitness, and Health
(1992 : Toronto, Ont.)
Toward active living : proceedings of the International Conference
on Physical Activity, Fitness, and Health / H. Arthur Quinney, Lise
Gauvin, A.E. Ted Wall (editors).
p.   cm.
Selected papers from a conference held in May, 1992, at Toronto.
ISBN 0-87322-523-6
1. Exercise--Health aspects--Congresses.   2. Physical fitness-
-Congresses.   3. Physical fitness--Social aspects--Congresses.
4. Health--Congresses.   I. Quinney, H. Arthur.   II. Gauvin, Lise.
III. Wall, A.E. Ted.   IV. Title.
RA781.I485   1994
613.7--dc20   93-29972
                                                                    CIP

ISBN: 0-87322-523-6

Copyright © 1994 by Human Kinetics Publishers, Inc.

Developmental Editor: Marni Basic
Assistant Editors: Julie Lancaster and Jacqueline R. Blakley
Copyeditors: Stefani Day, Moyra Knight, and Julie Anderson
Proofreader: Karin Leszczynski
Production Director: Ernie Noa
Typesetters and Text Layout: Julie Overholt and Angie Snyder
Text Designer: Jody Boles
Cover Designer: Jack Davis
Photographer (cover): Wilmer Zehr
Printer: Braun-Brumfield

Printed in the United States of America   10   9   8   7   6   5   4   3   2   1

Human Kinetics Publishers
Box 5076, Champaign, IL 61825-5076
1-800-747-4457

Canada: Human Kinetics Publishers, Box 24040,
Windsor, ON N8Y 4Y9
1-800-465-7301 (in Canada only)

Europe: Human Kinetics Publishers (Europe) Ltd.,
P.O. Box IW14, Leeds LS16 6TR, England
0532-781708

Australia: Human Kinetics Publishers, P.O. Box 80,
Kingswood 5062, South Australia
618-374-0433

New Zealand: Human Kinetics Publishers, P.O. Box 105-231,
Auckland 1
(09) 309-2259

Contents

List of Contributors

Per-Olof Åstrand
Department of Physiology III
Karolinska Institutet
Lidingovagen 1
Box 5626
Stockholm, Sweden, S-114 86

Carolyn E. Barlow
The Cooper Institute for Aerobics Research
12330 Preston Road
Dallas, TX 75230, USA

Oded Bar-Or
Children's Exercise Nutrition Center
Chedoke Hospital
Hamilton, Ontario, Canada L8N 3Z5

Steven N. Blair
Department of Epidemiology
The Cooper Institute for Aerobics Research
12330 Preston Road
Dallas, TX 75230, USA

Claude Bouchard
Laboratoire des sciences de l'activite physique
PEPS
Universite Laval
Ste-Foy, Quebec, Canada G1K 7P4

Patricia A. Brill
The Cooper Institute for Aerobics Research
12330 Preston Road
Dallas, TX 75230, USA

Thomas L. Burton
Faculty of Physical Education and Recreation
W1-34 Van Vliet Physical Education and Recreation
    Centre
University of Alberta
Edmonton, Alberta, Canada, T6G 2H9

Warren C. Campbell
2 Muir Drive
Scarborough, Ontario, Canada M1M 3B4

Albert V. Carron
Faculty of Physical Education
The University of Western Ontario
London, Ontario, Canada N6A 3K7

Michael H. Cox
Human Performance Division
The Graduate Hospital Human Performance and Sports
    Medicine Center
200 West Lancaster Avenue
Wayne, PA 19087, USA

Peter R.E. Crocker
College of Physical Education
University of Saskatchewan
Saskatoon, Saskatchewan, Canada S7N 0W0

Rod K. Dishman
Department of Exercise Science
School of Health and Human Performance
The University of Georgia
Athens, GA 30602, USA

Barbara L. Drinkwater
Department of Medicine
Pacific Medical Center
1200 12th Avenue South
Seattle, WA 98144, USA

Joan L. Duda
Department of Health, Kinesiology,
    and Leisure Studies
1362 Lambert
Purdue University
West Lafayette, IN 47907, USA

Peggy Edwards
Chelsea Group Communications
26 Osborne Street
Ottawa, Ontario, Canada K1S 4Z9

Shannon E. Etkin
President
SEE Consulting Services
304 Essex Avenue
Richmond Hill, Ontario, Canada L4C 8M6

Jonathan E. Fielding
Johnson & Johnson Health Management, Inc.
2500 Broadway, Suite 100
Santa Monica, CA 90404, USA

Lise Gauvin
Department of Exercise Science
7141 Sherbrooke Street West
Montreal, Quebec, Canada H4B 1R6

Norman Gledhill
Bethune College, Room 343
York University
4700 Keele Street
Downsview, Ontario, Canada M3J 1P3

Benjamin H. Gottlieb
Department of Physiology, and Gerontology
    Research Center
University of Guelph
Guelph, Ontario, Canada N1G 2W1

William L. Haskell
Stanford Center for Research in Disease Prevention
Stanford University School of Medicine
730 Welch Road, Suite B
Palo Alto, CA 94304-1583, USA

Carol Hills
University of Alberta
Edmonton, Alberta, Canada T6G 2H9

Michele Hobson
Department of Health and Sport Sciences
Wake Forest University
307 Reynolds Gym
Box 7234
Winston-Salem, NC 27109, USA

Tammy Horne
Alberta Centre for Well-Being
G-110 Education South
University of Alberta
Edmonton, Alberta, Canada T6G 2H9

Don Hunter
Municipality of Saanich
770 Vernon Avenue
Victoria, British Columbia, Canada V8X 2W7

Robert T. Hyde
Division of Epidemiology
Stanford University School of Medicine
Stanford, CA 94305-5092, USA

James B. Kampert
Stanford University School of Medicine
Stanford, CA 94305-5092, USA

Norah C. Keating
Department of Family Studies
3-38 Assiniboia Hall
University of Alberta
Edmonton, Alberta, Canada T6G 2E7

Kevin K. Knight
Johnson & Johnson Health Management, Inc.
2500 Broadway, Suite 100
Santa Monica, CA 90404, USA

Ronald Labonté
Community Health Consultant
90 Coady Avenue
Toronto, Ontario, Canada M4M 2Y8

Daniel M. Landers
Exercise and Sport Science Research Institute
Department of Health and Physical Education
Arizona State University
Tempe, AZ 85287-0404, USA

I-Min Lee
Department of Epidemiology
School of Public Health
Harvard University
677 Huntington Avenue
Boston, MA 02115, USA

John Lord
Centre for Research and Education in Human
    Services
26 College Street
Kitchener, Ontario, Canada N2H 4Z9

Edward McAuley
Department of Kinesiology
University of Illinois at Urbana-Champaign
215 Freer Hall
906 S. Goodwin Ave.
Urbana, IL 61801, USA

Barry D. McPherson
Faculty of Graduate Studies
Wilfred Laurier University
75 University Avenue West
Waterloo, Ontario, Canada N2L 3C5

Lyle Makosky
Fitness and Amateur Sport
365 Laurier Avenue West
Ottawa, Ontario, Canada K1A 0X6

Robert M. Malina
Department of Kinesiology and Health Education
University of Texas at Austin
Austin, TX 78712, USA

Daniel S. Miles
The Graduate Hospital Human Performance and
    Sports Medicine Center
Human Performance Division
200 West Lancaster Ave.
Wayne, PA 19087, USA

Michelle F. Mottola
Faculty of Kinesiology
Department of Anatomy
University of Western Ontario
London, Ontario, Canada N6A 3K7

Sandra O'Brien Cousins
Faculty of Physical Education and Recreation
University of Alberta
Edmonton, Alberta, Canada T6G 2H9

William A.R. Orban
Centre de Sante
Elizabeth-Bruyere
Ottawa, Ontario, Canada K1N 5C8

Ralph S. Paffenbarger, Jr.
Department of Health Research and Policy
Stanford University School of Medicine
HRP Building, Room 113
Stanford, CA 94305-5092, USA

Steven J. Petruzzello
Department of Kinesiology
University of Illinois
Louise Freer Hall
906 S. Goodwin Ave.
Urbana, IL 61801, USA

H. Arthur Quinney
Faculty of Physical Education
    and Sports Studies
University of Alberta
Edmonton, Alberta, Canada T6G 2H9

W. Jack Rejeski
Department of Health and Sport Sciences
Wake Forest University
307 Reynolds Gymnasium, Box 7234
Winston-Salem, NC 27109, USA

Michael T. Sharratt
Faculty of Applied Health Sciences
University of Waterloo
Waterloo, Ontario, Canada N2L 3G1

Jacqueline K. Sharratt
Department of Health Studies
University of Waterloo
Waterloo, Ontario, Canada N2L 3G1

Roy J. Shephard
School of Physical and Health Education
University of Toronto
320 Huron Street
Toronto, Ontario, Canada M5S 1A1

R.D. Steadward
Faculty of Physical Education and Recreation
University of Alberta
Edmonton, Alberta, Canada T6G 2H9

A.E. Ted Wall
Faculty of Education
Department of Physical Education
McGill University
3700 Mctavish Street
Montreal, Quebec, Canada H3A 1Y2

Leonard M. Wankel
Faculty of Physical Education and Recreation
University of Alberta
E-411 Physical Education Building
Edmonton, Alberta, Canada T6G 2H9

E.J. Watkinson
Associate Dean
Faculty of Physical Education and Recreation
University of Alberta
Edmonton, Alberta, Canada T6G 2H9

Jack H. Wilmore
Department of Kinesiology and Health Education
University of Texas at Austin
Austin, TX 78712, USA

Alvin L. Wing
Stanford University School of Medicine
Stanford, CA 94305-5093, USA

Larry A. Wolfe
School of Physical and Health Education
Queen's University
Kingston, Ontario, Canada K7L 3N6

Preface

In May 1992, the Second International Consensus Symposium on Physical Activity, Fitness, and Health was held in Toronto, Ontario, Canada. For this symposium, 80 of the world's top scientists and scholars were invited to develop consensus statements in 70 specific areas. Immediately following the Consensus Symposium, the 3-day International Conference on Physical Activity, Fitness, and Health, which attracted over 950 scientists, educators, practitioners, and policymakers, was held at the Metro Toronto Convention Centre. The sequence of these two events meant that the results of the Consensus Symposium could be immediately presented to a large, receptive audience. This book contains the text of many of the conference presentations and forms one part of the trilogy of publications resulting from the combined Consensus Symposium and International Conference on Physical Activity, Fitness, and Health.

The 1992 conference, which coincided with the celebration of Canada's 125th birthday, is the most recent of a number of significant Canadian contributions to our understanding of the relationships of physical activity and fitness to health. Of particular note are the 1966 International Conference of Physical Activity and Cardiovascular Health, convened in Toronto by Dr. Roy Shephard, and the 1988 International Consensus Conference on Exercise, Fitness, and Health.

The 1992 conference provided a unique opportunity for researchers and practitioners to share knowledge and information that will lead to the promotion of physical activity through better programs and policies. The conference structure, format, and goals differed from those of the typical research-oriented or practitioner-oriented conference through the development of a bridge between our latest research findings and their application to practice and policy development.

The concept of active living was deeply embedded in the framework of the conference. This concept incorporates daily physical activity as a lifelong behavior and encourages community-based support structures to ensure that all individuals can benefit. The conference provided participants the opportunity to explore and critique the concept on the basis of the research literature, public policy, and from the perspective of practice initiatives.

Acknowledgments

The editors would like to thank the members of the organizing committees of both the Consensus Symposium and the International Conference. These individuals contributed significant time and expertise during the 3 years preceding these events. The editors are particularly grateful to Dr. Barry McPherson, Wilfrid Laurier University; Dr. Norman Gledhill, York University; Dr. Claude Bouchard, Universite Laval; and Art Salmon, ParticipACTION; all of whom contributed so much to the development and organization of these events.

The Conference Organizing Committee

The planning and organization of the conference program were the responsibility of the following:

Chair: Dr. Art Quinney
            University of Alberta
            Edmonton, Alberta

Members: Dr. Claude Bouchard
            Chair of the Consensus
                Symposium Organizing Committee
            Universite Laval
            Ste-Foy, Quebec

            Ms. Cora Craig
            Canadian Fitness and Lifestyle
                Research Institute
            Ottawa, Ontario

            Dr. Lise Gauvin
            Concordia University
            Montreal, Quebec

            Dr. Norman Gledhill
            Chair of Finance Committee
            York University
            Downsview, Ontario

            Ms. Joyce Gordon
            The Donwood Institute
            Toronto, Ontario

            Dr. Mary Keyes
            McMaster University
            Hamilton, Ontario

            Dr. Ted Wall
            McGill University
            Montreal, Quebec

Ms. Dayle Levine
Executive Assistant
York University
Downsview, Ontario

Dr. Barry McPherson
President of the Conference and
    Consensus Symposium Board
Wilfrid Laurier University
Waterloo, Ontario

Mr. Stan Murray
Ministry of Tourism and Recreation
Government of Ontario
Toronto, Ontario

Mrs. Barbara O'Brien Jewett
Fitness Canada
Government of Canada
Ottawa, Ontario

Dr. Irving Routman
University of Toronto
Toronto, Ontario

Mr. Art Salmon
Chair of the Site Committee
ParticipACTION
Toronto, Ontario

The Consensus Symposium Organizing Committee

The conference was closely integrated with and heavily dependent upon the Consensus Symposium that preceded it. The committee members responsible for this event are as follows:

Dr. Claude Bouchard
Chairperson of the Consensus Symposium
 Organizing Committee
Universite Laval
Ste-Foy, Quebec

Dr. Norman Gledhill
Chair of Finance Committee
York University
Downsview, Ontario

Ms. Dayle Levine
Executive Assistant
York University
Downsview, Ontario

Dr. Barry McPherson
President of the Conference and Consensus
 Symposium Board
Wilfrid Laurier University
Waterloo, Ontario

Dr. Art Quinney
Chairperson of Active Living
Conference Organizing Committee
University of Alberta
Edmonton, Alberta

Dr. Elizabeth Ready
University of Manitoba
Winnipeg, Manitoba

Mr. Art Salmon
Chair of the Site Committee
ParticipACTION
Toronto, Ontario

Dr. Roy J. Shephard
University of Toronto
Toronto, Ontario

Dr. Thomas Stephens
Consultant
Manotick, Ontario

Other Guests and Support Personnel

The editors are also greatly indebted to Ms. Dayle Levine, the executive assistant, for her support throughout the planning, organization, and execution of the project. She played a key role in providing administrative support for both events. We also acknowledge the contributions of Lori Wadge, who gave support and commitment throughout the project. Special thanks go to Ms. Veronica Jamnik, who so capably organized all of the hospitality and social events, and to Dr. Caroline Davis, who coordinated the conference registration. Our appreciation is also extended to Mr. Stan Murray, who coordinated on-site transportation, and Ms. Marion Reeves, who coordinated all of our volunteers.

Finally, we want to express our gratitude to all volunteers who helped us so much in the preparation of the meetings as well as with various responsibilities prior to and during the meeting time. These volunteers were Janet Bannister, Kelly Broadhurst, Debbie Childs, Michelle Dionne, Tony Doherty, Maria Gurevich, Brandon Hale, Marjorie Hammond, Lyse Jobin, Wendy Keeves, Jodi Liebsman, Denise Mercier, Partricia Murray, Helen Prlic, Joe Reischer, Sandra Sawatzky, and Ann Marie Vandire.

The conference and symposium organizers gratefully acknowledge the support of the following sponsors and patrons:

Major Sponsors

Ontario Ministry of Tourism and Recreation
Government of Canada, Fitness and Amateur Sport

Additional Sponsors

Air Canada
Canada 125
Canadian Association of Sport Sciences
Canadian Bureau for Active Living
Conners Brewery
Health and Welfare Canada—National Health Research
   and Development Program
Heart and Stroke Foundation of Canada
Heart and Stroke Foundation of Ontario
Imperial Oil Limited
McDonald's Restaurants of Canada Limited
Medical Research Council of Canada
Merck Frosst Canada Inc.
Molson Breweries of Canada

Ontario Ministry of Citizenship—Office for Seniors'
   Issues
Ontario Ministry of Health
Ontario Physical and Health Education Association
ParticipACTION
Servier Canada Inc.
Toshiba—Portable Computers and Printers

Patron Universities

Universite Laval, Ste-Foy, Quebec
University of Alberta, Edmonton, Alberta
Wilfrid Laurier University, Waterloo, Ontario
York University, Downsview, Ontario

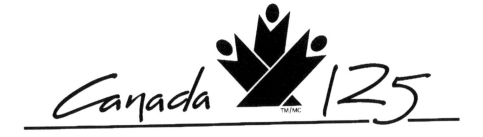

The International Consensus Symposium
and
the International Conference on Physical Activity, Fitness, and Health
were held in conjunction with the celebration of Canada's 125 years of Confederation.

Credits

Table 1.1 data from *Active Living: A Conceptual Approach*, by Fitness Canada, 1991, Ottawa: Government of Canada; and World Health Organization, 1968.

Figure 1.1 is from "The Field of the Physical Activity Sciences" by C. Bouchard. In *Physical Activity Sciences* (p. 6) by C. Bouchard, B.D. McPherson, and A.W. Taylor (Eds.), 1991, Champaign, IL: Human Kinetics. Adapted by permission.

Figure 1.3 is from "The Service Component of the Physical Activity Sciences" by P. Godbout, J. Samson, and G. Berube. In *Physical Activity Sciences* (p. 134) by C. Bouchard, B.D. McPherson, and A.W. Taylor (Eds.), 1991, Champaign, IL: Human Kinetics. Adapted by permission.

Figure 2.1 is from "Physical Activity, Fitness, and Health" by C. Bouchard and R.J. Shephard. In *Proceedings of the International Consensus Symposium on Physical Activity, Fitness, and Health*, by C. Bouchard, R.J. Shephard, and T. Stephens (Eds.), in press, Champaign, IL: Human Kinetics. Adapted by permission.

Table 2.1 is from "Physical Activity, Fitness, and Health" by C. Bouchard and R.J. Shephard. In *Proceedings of the International Consensus Symposium on Physical Activity, Fitness, and Health*, by C. Bouchard, R.J. Shephard, and T. Stephens (Eds.), in press, Champaign, IL: Human Kinetics. Adapted by permission.

Figure 3.1 data from "Women Walking for Health and Fitness" by J.J. Duncan, N.F. Gordon, and C.B. Scott, 1991, *Journal of the American Medical Association*, 66, 325-329.

Table 4.1 data from *Pilot Survey of the Fitness of Australians* by the Commonwealth Department of the Arts, Sport, the Environment, Tourism and Territories, 1991, University of Adelaide: Department of Community Medicine; and *The Well-Being of Canadians: Highlights of the 1988 Campbell's Survey*

by T. Stephens and C.L. Craig, 1990, Ottawa: Canadian Fitness and Lifestyle Research Institute.

Table 8.2 is from "The Effect of Swimming on Asthmatic Children—Participants in a Swimming Program in the City of Baltimore" by S.W. Huang, R. Veiga, U. Sila, E. Reed, and S. Hines, 1989, *Journal of Asthma*, 26 117-121. Adapted by permission from Marcel Dekker, Inc.

Table 8.3 is from "Juvenile Obesity: The Importance of Exercise—and Getting Children to Do It" by D.F. Parker and O. Bar-Or, 1991, *Physician and Sportsmedicine*, 9, 113-125, Adapted by permission from McGraw-Hill, Inc.

Figure 14.1 is from "Social Marketing and Mass Intervention" by R.J. Donovan and N. Owen. In *Exercise Adherence Volume II*, by R.K. Dishman (Ed.), in press, Champaign, IL: Human Kinetics. Adapted by permission.

Table 14.2 is from "Social Marketing and Mass Intervention" by R.J. Donovan and N. Owen. In *Exercise Adherence Volume II*, by R.K. Dishman (Ed.), in press, Champaign, IL: Human Kinetics. Adapted by permission.

Figure 15.1 is from "Stress-Related Transactions Between Person and Environment" by R.S. Lazarus and R. Launier. In *Perspectives in Interactional Psychology* (pp. 287-327), by L.A. Pervin and M. Lewis (Eds.), 1978, New York: Plenum. Adapted by permission.

Table 18.5 data from "Pregnancy and the Postnatal Period" by the American College of Obstetricians and Gynecologists, 1985, *ACOG Home Exercise Program* (pp. 1-5), Washington, DC: ACOG; *Fitness and the Childbearing Year*, by Fitness Ontario Leadership Program, 1992, Toronto: Ontario Ministry of Tourism and Recreation, Toronto; "Prescription of Aerobic Exercise in Pregnancy," by L.A. Wolfe, P. Hall, K.A. Webb, L.S. Goodman, and M.J. McGrath, 1989b, *Sports Medicine*, **8**, 273-301.

Table 18.6 data from "Pregnancy and the Postnatal Period" by the American College of Obstetricians and Gynecologists, 1985, *ACOG Home Exercise Program* (pp. 1-5), Washington, DC: ACOG.; "Prescription of Aerobic Exercise in Pregnancy," by L.A. Wolfe, P. Hall, K.A. Webb, L.S. Goodman, and M.J. McGrath, 1989b, *Sports Medicine*, **8**, 273-301.

Table 18.7 data from *Fitness and the Childbearing Year*, by Fitness Ontario Leadership Program, 1992, Toronto: Ontario Minisry of Tourism and Recreation, Toronto.; "Pregnancy," by L.A. Wolfe. In *Exercise Testing and Prescription for Special Cases: Theoretical Bases and Practical Application (2nd ed.)* by J.S. Skinner (Ed.), in press, Philadelphia: Lea & Febiger.

Table 18.8 data from Fitness Ontario Leadership Program, 1992, *Fitness and the Childbearing Year*, Toronto: Ontario Ministry of Tourism and Recreation, Toronto.; Wolfe, L.A., Hall, P. Webb, K.A., Goodman, L.S., and McGrath, M.J., 1989b, Prescription of Aerobic Exercise in Pregnancy, *Sports Medicine*, **8**, 273-301.

Figure 20.1 is from "Growth of School Children With Early, Average, and Late Ages of Peak Height Velocity" by G. Lindgren, 1978, *Annals of Human Biology*, **5** 253-267. Adapted by permission.

Figure 20.2 is from "Sports Activities Among Young People in Sweden—Trends and Changes" by L. Engström. In *Physical Activity and Life-Long Physical activity* (p. 15) by R. Telema, L. Laasko, M. Péiron, I. Ruoppila, and Vihko (Eds.), 1990, Jyväskglä: Report of Physical Culture and Health 73. Adapted by permission.

Figure 20.3 is from "Sports Activities Among Young People in Sweden—Trends and Changes" by L. Engström. In *Physical Activity and Life-Long Physical activity* (p. 19) by R. Telema, L. Laasko, M. Péiron, I. Ruoppila, and Vihko (Eds.), 1990, Jyväskglä: Report of Physical Culture and Health 73. Adapted by permission.

Figure 20.4 is from "In Search of Methusula: Estimating the Upper Limits to Human Longevity" by S.J. Olshansky, B.A. Carnes, and C. Cassel, 1990, *Science*, **250**, 143-149. Copyright 1990 by the American Association for the Advancement of Science. Adapted by permission.

Figure 21.7 is from "Physical Activity and Cardiovascular Disease" by M. Jette and F. Landry, in press, *Revue deScienie et Technique des Activities Physique et Sportive*. Adapted by permission.

Table 22.1 data from "Understanding and Changing Physical Activity Delivery Systems," by M. Smith, 1988. In *Jasper Talks Proceedings: Strategies for Change in Adapted Physical Activity in Canada* (pp. 32-35) October 9-12, 1986, Jasper, Alberta: CAHPER/ACSEPC.

Figure 23.1 is from "The Seven Dynamics of Implementation" by D.H. Daisey, 1990, *Total Quality Dynamics*, **1**(2), 4-5. Reprinted by permission from METAPRO Excellence Institute.

Figure 25.1 is from *Evaluation: A Systematic Approach, 2nd ed.* by P.H. Rossi and H.E. Freeman, 1982, Beverly Hills, CA: Sage Publications. Reprinted by permission.

Table 28.1 is from *Lives in Transition: The Process of Personal Empowerment* by J. Lord, 1991, Kitchener, ON: Centre for Research & Education in Human Services. Reprinted by permission.

Table 29.2 data from Kindervattner, as cited in Quinney, H.A., Wall, A.E., and Gauvin, L., 1992. *Physical Activity, Fitness and Health: Policy and Practice*, unpublished manuscript.

1

Physical Activity, Fitness, and Health: Research and Practice

Lise Gauvin
A.E. Ted Wall
H. Arthur Quinney

The International Conference on Physical Activity, Fitness, and Health (ICPAFH) presented a unique opportunity for researchers and practitioners to share knowledge and information that can best promote physical activity and health in the population. The ICPAFH differed from the typical research-oriented or practitioner-oriented conference in that presenters actively sought a bridge between research and practice as opposed to simply presenting research findings or practice strategies. In this chapter we describe the conceptual framework of the ICPAFH program and proceedings and introduce the different sections of the proceedings. We trust that this effort will show how the vastly different contents and formats of the chapters contribute to our understanding of physical activity, fitness, health, and active living.

Physical Activity, Fitness, and Health: Definitions and Distinctions

As a framework for program development, the program committee adopted a series of definitions that would clearly identify the focus of the ICPAFH. These definitions are, for obvious reasons, similar to those employed by the International Consensus Symposium on Physical Activity, Fitness, and Health (see Bouchard, chapter 2).

According to Bouchard and Shephard (1991), physical activity can be defined as ''any body movement produced by skeletal muscles and resulting in a substantial increase over the resting energy expenditure'' (p. 3). According to this definition, physical activity encompasses leisure physical activity, exercise, sport, occupational work, and other chores. The focus of the ICPAFH

was limited to leisure physical activity, exercise, and sport; in addition, the consequences of physical activity were seen to comprise both fitness and health. Two types of fitness can be distinguished: performance-related fitness and health-related fitness. Performance-related fitness refers to components of fitness, including motor skills, cardiorespiratory power and capacity, muscular strength, and endurance, that are necessary for optimal work or sport performance. Health-related fitness refers to the capacity to perform daily activities with vigor and to demonstrate low risk of development of hypokinetic disease. The ICPAFH focused mainly on health-related fitness, although issues pertinent to performance-related fitness were broached in selected instances. The definitions of these concepts are included in Table 1.1.

The concept of active living, developed by Fitness Canada, was also deeply embedded in the framework of the conference. Active living is defined as ''a way of life in which physical activity is valued and integrated into daily life'' (Fitness Canada, 1991, p. 4). Although active living has not yet become the norm in Canada or other countries, the concept appears to be gaining widespread recognition as a concept that may have theoretical and practical relevance. As implied by the definition, active living incorporates the concepts of physical activity, total life experience, relevance of physical activity to daily life, and its facilitation with communities. The ICPAFH served as a vehicle for examining (a) the value and relevance of the concept of active living in public policy and practice initiatives and (b) the ties between active living and the concepts of physical activity, fitness, and health.

Table 1.1 Definitions of Key Concepts

Concept	Definition
Physical activity[a]	Any body movement produced by skeletal muscles and resulting in a substantial increase over the resting energy expenditure
Leisure physical activity[a]	Activity undertaken in the individual's discretionary time that leads to a significant increase in the total daily expenditure
Exercise[a]	Form of leisure physical activity undertaken with a specific external objective such as the improvement of fitness, physical performance, or health, in which the participant is advised to conform to recommended mode intensity, frequency, and duration of such activity
Sport[a]	Form of physical activity that involves competition and games
Fitness[b]	Ability to perform work satisfactorily
Performance-related fitness[a]	Fitness necessary for optimal work or sport performance that depends heavily upon motor skills, cardiorespiratory power and capacity, muscular strength, power or endurance, body size, body composition, motivation, and nutritional status
Health-related fitness[a]	Fitness characterized by a person's ability to perform daily activities with vigor and to demonstrate traits and capacities that are associated with low risk of premature development of hypokinetic diseases and conditions
Health[a]	Human condition with physical, social, and psychological dimensions, each characterized on a continuum with positive and negative poles; positive health is associated with a capacity to enjoy life and to withstand challenges; negative health is associated with morbidity and premature mortality
Active Living[c]	Way of life in which physical activity is valued and integrated into daily life

[a]From Bouchard and Shephard (1991). [b]From World Health Organization (1968). [c]From Fitness Canada (1991).

Sources of Knowledge on Physical Activity, Fitness, and Health

In 1991, Bouchard proposed a conceptual model that defines the relationships between different subdisciplines of the physical activity sciences and their areas of professional involvement and scientific knowledge. This model is presented in Figure 1.1.

Bouchard defined the physical activity sciences as ''the field of study devoted to the understanding of all aspects of human physical activity (biological, physical, behavioral, and social) and the application of this understanding to meet the needs of the entire population (male or female; disabled or gifted; child, adult or senior)'' (1991, p. 5). The model suggests that knowledge in the physical activity sciences accrues from two sources, scientific research and professional practice.

The ICPAFH program committee espoused this view of the physical activity sciences and developed a program that highlighted the value and relevance of this model. The ICPAFH was therefore developed with the aim of delivering knowledge in the physical activity sciences mainly for the benefit of those involved in professional practice. In the following paragraphs, we will outline how the scientific and professional practice areas of knowledge were meshed within the conference program and the proceedings.

Model of Scientific Knowledge

The program committee sought to identify the areas of scientific knowledge that would be of greatest interest to practitioners and policymakers. After much deliberation, the Committee agreed to focus mainly on *outcomes* and *determinants* of physical activity, fitness, and health. The outcomes of physical activity were defined as biological or psychological/sociological changes which would be associated with the adoption, maintenance, or cessation of physical activity. In other words, the outcomes of physical activity are the consequences of physical activity/inactivity. Determinants of physical activity were defined as those biological and psychological/sociological factors that promote the initiation of, maintenance of, or disengagement from physical activity as a lifestyle behavior. In other words, the determinants of physical activity are the antecedents of physical activity. In subsequent refinements to the program,

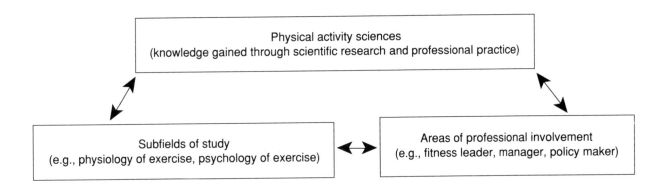

Figure 1.1 The interaction between the physical activity sciences and their research and service components (adapted from Bouchard, 1991, p. 6).

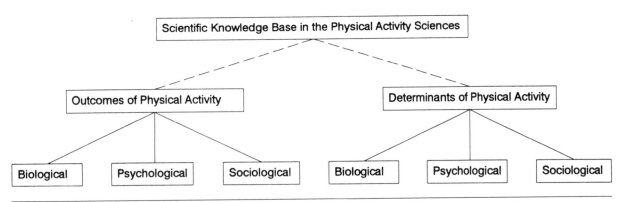

Figure 1.2 Model of the topics of scientific knowledge of greatest interest to practitioners and policymakers.

the committee sought to create a balance between issues pertaining to biological and psychological/sociological aspects as well as between individual and societal concerns. The previously described blueprint to the program is hierarchically illustrated in Figure 1.2.

In the end, researchers who participated in the ICPAFH presented scientifically-derived knowledge about the outcomes and determinants of physical activity and underscored some of the policy and practice implications of this knowledge. In so doing, the Committee believed that a significant portion of the professionally-relevant knowledge-base would be conveyed to delegates.

Model of Knowledge Evolving From Practice Initiatives

Understanding that practice and policy in the physical activity sciences do not develop solely from scientific research, the program committee included sessions that dealt with knowledge gained through field initiatives. The assumption was that the illustration of a successful program would do a great deal to highlight knowledge, to stimulate discussions and interactions among ICPAFH delegates, and to underscore knowledge derived from sources other than scientific research.

Although the committee did not develop a model of knowledge evolving from practice initiatives, a model of the role of physical activity specialists, which was elaborated upon by Godbout, Samson and Bérubé (1991), was employed (see Figure 1.3). Godbout et al.'s model identifies categories of specialists and focuses of intervention of different practitioners in our field.

Sessions in the ICPAFH therefore featured speakers who were practitioners, program executives, supervisors, policymakers, and consultants, as well as researchers. We thought that by presenting a good balance of speakers from each area of professional responsibility in our field, we could make available to delegates a substantial and relevant portion of the knowledge that is derived from practice initiatives. Thus, within the context of the ICPAFH, selected speakers were charged with introducing the audience to specific practice initiatives and highlighting the knowledge of the physical activity sciences contained therein.

An Opportunity to Have an Impact

The program committee sought to include opportunities for critical thought and discussions of topics of current concern. For example, one session dealt with critically

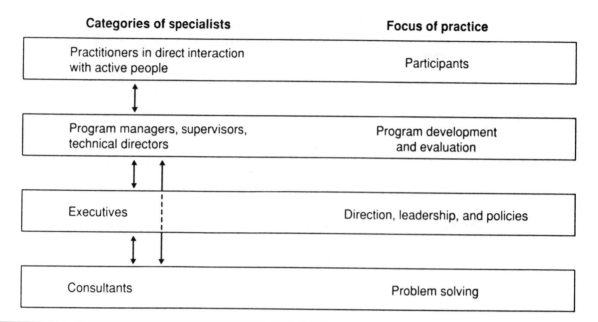

Figure 1.3 Model of the different roles of physical activity professionals (adapted from Godbout, Samson, & Bérubé, 1991, p. 134).

examining the concept of active living and providing opportunities to impact policy. Similarly, on the last day of the ICPAFH, limitations with the extant knowledge base and issues for the future were discussed. Our hope was that such sessions would allow participants to identify areas where a comprehensive knowledge base is still unavailable and to discuss what the movement toward physical activity, fitness, health, and active living could eventually represent for society.

Organization of This Book

In accordance with this framework, we organized the proceedings of the ICPAFH into five parts, including two that deal with scientific information, two that present information yielded mostly from practice initiatives, and one that provides critical thought. As a prelude to the presentation of scientific knowledge and as a complement to our chapter, Bouchard (chapter 2) describes the International Consensus Symposium on Physical Activity, Fitness, and Health and summarizes selected findings of the emerging Consensus Statement. Parts I and II of the proceedings focus on scientific information yielded from the biological and sociopsychological sciences, respectively. Part III presents contributions from practitioners and researchers relevant to the promotion of physical activity, fitness, health, and active living in specific populations and settings. Part IV addresses the role of community determinants of physical activity and active living, again providing a blend of knowledge from applied and scientific traditions. Part V presents an in-depth discussion of the concept of active living

accompanied by several critical examinations of the concept from biological, sociopsychological, and public health perspectives. Finally, the last chapter explores the limitations of the knowledge of physical activity, fitness, health, and active living.

Closing Comments and Reflections

In closing this chapter, we would like to place the themes and activities of the ICPAFH into a broader perspective. Each contribution in the proceedings clearly supports the fact that our field has progressed in its scientific understanding of physical activity and its capacity to generate a variety of programs designed to meet the needs of a wide spectrum of individuals and communities. The ICPAFH celebrated the fact that physical activity is a central feature of our identity. In this regard, the recent emergence of the concept of active living reflects just how central physical activity is in the lives of many individuals.

Ironically, because physical activity is a central feature of our identity, we clearly need to examine our field, assessing where we have come from, where we are now, and, most importantly, where we should be going. Much more needs to be done to facilitate communication between researchers and practitioners, between policymakers and programmers; there are still challenging questions related to equity for women, persons with disabilities, the socioeconomically disadvantaged, and different ethnic groups within the community, including aboriginal peoples.

One viable means of achieving this end is to maintain an ongoing examination of the relationship between scientific, rationally based research and more subjective descriptions and appreciations of active living. More crucial still is to ensure that the values underlying our modern identity are recognized, respected, and understood within our field. All the ICPAFH presenters and proceedings contributors significantly enhanced the ongoing examination of the interface between research, practice, and the values that underlie both. We trust that the physical activity professionals who peruse these proceedings will perpetuate this trend.

References

Bouchard, C. (1991). The field of the physical activity sciences. In C. Bouchard, B.D. McPherson, & A.W. Taylor (Eds.), *Physical activity sciences*. (pp. 1-8). Champaign, IL: Human Kinetics.

Bouchard, C., & Shephard, R. (1991). *Physical activity, fitness and health: A model and key concepts*. Consensus Doc-017, August 22, document prepared for the International Consensus Symposium on Physical Activity, Fitness and Health.

Fitness Canada. (1991). *Active living: A conceptual overview*. Ottawa: Government of Canada.

Godbout, P., Samson, J., & Bérubé, G. (1991). The service component of the physical activity sciences. In C. Bouchard, B.D. McPherson, & A.W. Taylor (Eds.), *Physical activity sciences*. (pp. 131-138). Champaign, IL: Human Kinetics.

2

Physical Activity, Fitness, and Health: Overview of the Consensus Symposium

Claude Bouchard

The International Conference on Physical Activity, Fitness, and Health, held in May 1992 in Toronto, was preceded by a Consensus Symposium known under the label of the 1992 International Consensus Symposium on Physical Activity, Fitness, and Health (ICSPAFH). The city of Toronto has a tradition of being host to major consensus activities pertaining to physical activity and health. Thus, a landmark conference on physical activity and cardiovascular health was organized in Toronto in 1966 by Professor Roy J. Shephard and his associates (Proceedings of the International Symposium on Physical Activity and Cardiovascular Health, 1967). More recently, in 1988, a first consensus conference on physical activity, fitness, and health took place and the sessions were opened to all registered participants (Bouchard, Shephard, Stephens, Sutton, & McPherson, 1990). The 1988 consensus activities revolved around 33 topics. The 1992 ICSPAFH was quite different both in scope and in the manner it was approached and organized. Thus, only the invited experts and the support personnel were involved in the 4-day, 1992 ICSPAFH meeting, for a total of about 100 persons. Seventy-two different topics were considered and the experts confronted their views in eight different groups that met for about 6 to 10 hours per day in addition to several plenary sessions.

Prior to the ICSPAFH meeting time in Toronto, each invited participant prepared a draft of a review paper summarizing the evidence available on his or her assigned topic, assessing the quality of the evidence, and defining the most pressing research questions to be addressed in his or her particular area. Also, each participant prepared a draft of a consensus text on their topic which was reviewed by the editors of the final consensus document, C. Bouchard, R.J. Shephard, and T. Stephens. A 300-page draft of the consensus proposal was available to participants 6 weeks before the meeting time in Toronto. It is impossible to review here all the procedures followed during the 1992 ICSPAFH and all the

conclusions reached by the participants. However, all relevant details will be given in two publications that will emanate from the Consensus Symposium, one containing only the final consensus text (C. Bouchard, R.J. Shephard, & T. Stephens, Eds., *Physical Activity, Fitness, and Health: Consensus Statement*) and the other including the consensus text plus all 72 chapters reviewing the evidence and the views of each author (C. Bouchard, R.J. Shephard, & T. Stephens, Eds., *Physical Activity, Fitness, and Health: International Proceedings and Consensus Statement*).

Objectives

The objectives of the 1992 ICSPAFH were as follows:

- To revise and expand the 1988 consensus statement from the perspective of the biological, social, and behavioral sciences.
- To achieve a better integration of the evidence regarding the role of regular physical activity, fitness, and their respective and interactive contributions to health.
- To identify the type (experimental, epidemiological, clinical), quality and extent of the evidence in support of the conclusions reached.
- To identify the areas of needed research and the most pressing questions to be addressed.

Physical Activity, Fitness, and Health

There is no doubt that the relationships between physical activity, fitness, and health are highly complex. One approach to make these relationships amenable to discussion is to cast them into a format that specifies the hierarchical relations among the major elements. Figure 2.1 is the result of such an attempt. It was put together

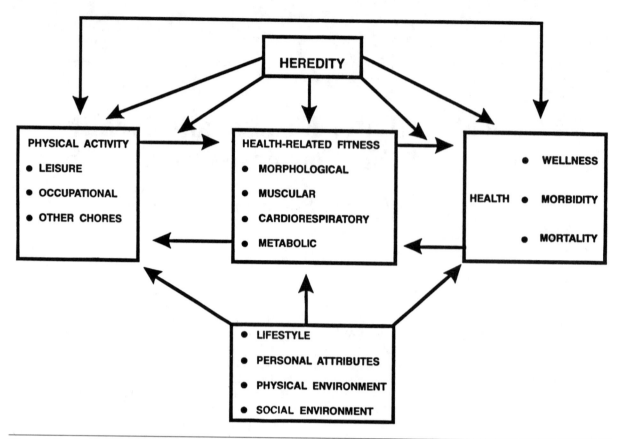

Figure 2.1 A model describing the complex relationships among habitual physical activity, health-related fitness and health status (adapted from Bouchard & Shephard, in press).

for the 1988 International Consensus Conference on Physical Activity, Fitness, and Health, held in Toronto (Bouchard et al., 1990), and has been modified for the 1992 Consensus Symposium on the same topic (Bouchard & Shephard, in press). The model defines how the components are related to one another, the causal relationships, the feedback loops, and the endogenous and exogenous affectors of the various components.

The model specifies that habitual physical activity can influence fitness, which in turn may modify the level of habitual physical activity of the individual. For instance, the fittest individuals tend to be the most active and, with increasing fitness, people tend to become more active. The model also specifies that fitness is related to health in a reciprocal manner. That is, fitness not only influences health, but health status also influences both habitual physical activity and fitness levels. In reality, the relationships between the level of habitual physical activity, fitness, and health are more complex. Other factors are associated with individual differences in health status. Likewise, the levels of fitness are not determined entirely by an individual's level of habitual physical activity. Thus, other lifestyle components, physical and social environmental conditions, personal attributes, and genetic characteristics also affect the major components of the basic model and their interrelationships.

Physical Activity

In the context of the model, physical activity comprises any body movement produced by the skeletal muscles and resulting in an increase in energy expenditure. We are particularly interested in leisure time physical activity such as exercise, sport, and a variety of outdoor activities, and by occupational work and other chores. That is, all the activities that may impact on the total daily energy expenditure. Physical activity is clearly the most variable component of the total daily energy expenditure. Depending on the age, health status, and fitness level of the individual, it is not uncommon to observe that a three- to twentyfold increase of resting metabolic rate associated with the demands of physical activity can be sustained for a few minutes.

The concept of habitual physical activity is one that has been present in the exercise and epidemiology literature for decades. By definition, it encompasses information on leisure physical activity, exercise, sports, occupational work, and other chores to assess the overall level of regular engagement in physical activity. This is not easily achieved, however, as there are methodological difficulties in assessing the pattern of activity over defined periods of time. Nonetheless, the concept of habitual physical activity, as an integrator of the amount of energy expended for activity, is a very useful one.

Health-Related Fitness

There is no universally agreed upon definition of fitness and of its components. In the present context, we are particularly interested by what is now referred to as health-related fitness, that is, by the physical and physiological components of fitness that impact more directly on health status. The World Health Organization (1968) defined fitness as "the ability to perform muscular work satisfactorily." The definition is relevant to health but was not specific enough for our purpose.

Health-related fitness refers to those components of fitness that are favorably influenced by habitual physical activity and relate to health status. It is defined as the state of physical and physiological characteristics that influence the risk levels for the premature development of diseases or morbid conditions presenting a relationship with a sedentary mode of life. Important determinants of health-related fitness include body mass for height, body composition, subcutaneous fat distribution, abdominal visceral fat, bone density, strength and endurance of the abdominal and dorso-lumbar musculature, heart and lung functions, blood pressure, maximal aerobic power and tolerance to submaximal exercise, glucose and insulin metabolism, blood lipid and lipoprotein profile, and the ratio of lipid to carbohydrate oxidized in a variety of situations. A favorable profile for these various factors presents a clear advantage in terms of health outcomes as assessed by morbidity and mortality statistics.

In contrast, performance-related fitness refers to those components of fitness that are necessary for optimal work or sport performance. It is defined in terms of the ability in athletic competition, performance tests, or occupational work. Performance-related fitness depends heavily upon motor skills, cardiorespiratory power and capacity, muscular strength, power and endurance, body size, body composition, motivation, and nutritional status.

The components of health-related fitness are numerous and are determined by several variables, including the level and pattern of habitual physical activity, diet, and heredity. There are various ways of defining and classifying the components of fitness, and one such proposition (by Bouchard & Shephard, 1992) is summarized in Table 2.1. It includes morphological, muscular, motor, cardiorespiratory, and metabolic fitness components.

Health

Defining health remains a major challenge, despite the progress made in treating diseases and increasing the average life duration in Western societies. At the 1988 consensus conference, health was defined as a human

Table 2.1 The Components and Factors of Fitness

Morphological component
  Body mass for height
  Body composition
  Subcutaneous fat distribution
  Abdominal visceral fat
  Bone density
  Flexibility

Muscular component
  Strength and power
  Endurance

Motor component
  Speed
  Agility
  Balance
  Coordination

Cardiorespiratory component
  Submaximal exercise capacity
  Maximal aerobic power
  Heart functions
  Lung functions
  Blood pressure

Metabolic component
  Glucose tolerance
  Insulin sensitivity
  Blood lipids and lipoproteins
  Ratio of lipid to carbohydrate oxidized

(Adapted from Bouchard & Shephard, in press)

condition with physical, social, and psychological dimensions, each characterized on a continuum with positive and negative poles. Positive health is associated with a capacity to enjoy life and to withstand challenges; it is not merely the absence of disease. Negative health is associated with morbidity and, in the extreme, with premature mortality. Morbidity can be defined as any departure, subjective or objective, from a state of physical or psychological well-being, short of death. On the other hand, wellness is a holistic concept, describing a state of positive health in the individual, and comprising physical, social, and psychological well-being.

Traditional illness and mortality statistics do not provide a full assessment of health. A more comprehensive approach requires that the profile of the individual be established in terms of common health endpoints, an assessment of health-related fitness status, information on temporary and chronic disabilities, absenteeism, overall productivity, and use of all forms of medical services, including prescribed and non-prescribed drugs.

Factors Affecting Physical Activity, Fitness, and Health

Other affectors are important to consider in the relationships between physical activity, fitness, and health.

They include the lifestyle factors other than habitual activity level, physical and social environment, personal attributes, and inherited differences.

Lifestyle comprises the aggregate of behaviors, actions, and habits that can affect health-related fitness and health status. Habitual physical activity is one such behavior. In addition, we are particularly concerned by smoking, diet (energy intake and dietary composition), and alcohol intake as they impact on health-related fitness and on health in general. An understanding of the role of lifestyle on fitness and health should also include an assessment of sleeping patterns, perceived stresses, drug addiction, and the general avoidance of hazardous behaviour.

In the present context, the social environment may be defined as the combination of social, cultural, political, and economic conditions that affect participation in physical activity, health-related fitness, and health status. Social networks may have a positive influence on attitudes toward physical activity and other healthy behaviors. Friends, members of the family, other relatives, social clubs, church organizations, and other groups are all part of the social milieu that can affect both health and the sense of well-being of an individual. All these elements of the social network can exert powerful influences. Several personal attributes shape the lifestyle pattern of a person, including the attitude towards physical activity and other healthy habits. These attributes include the age, sex of the person, socioeconomic status, personality characteristics, and motivation.

Participation in leisure time physical activity, fitness level, and health status are all influenced by environmental conditions such as temperature, humidity, air quality, altitude, and climatic changes. Such conditions influence not only the ability to exercise, but also the physiological response to the demands of exercise. Certain types of physical activity may be hazardous to health because of prevailing environmental conditions.

Heredity and Individual Differences

A comprehensive evaluation of the relationships between physical activity, fitness, and health must include considerations about the role of inherited differences. Humans are genetically quite diverse. Variations in DNA sequence constitute the molecular basis of genetic individuality and of human genetic variation. Given these circumstances, an equal state of health and of physical and mental well-being is unlikely to be achieved for all. Some will thrive better and will remain free from disabilities for a longer period of time than others.

Genetic differences do not operate in a vacuum. They interact constantly with existing cellular and tissue conditions to provide a biological response commensurate with environmental demands. In that sense, the genes are constantly interacting with everything in the physical and social environment, as well as with lifestyle characteristics of the individual that translate into a signal capable of affecting the cells of the body. Thus, overfeeding, a high fat diet, smoking, and regular endurance exercise are all powerful stimuli that may elicit strong biological responses. However, because of inherited differences at specific genes, the amplitude of adaptive responses varies from one individual to the other. Inheritance is one of the important reasons why we are not equally prone to diabetes, hypertension, or heart attacks. It is also one major explanation for individual differences in the response to dietary intervention or exercise training. A recognition of the critical role of DNA sequence variation in human response to a variety of challenges and environmental conditions is essential to all those interested in the physical activity, fitness, and health paradigm.

Selected Highlights From the Consensus Symposium

In spite of all the limitations inherent to such a complex process, a consensus was reached on a large number of issues. Obviously, they cannot be summarized adequately in a few paragraphs. The interested reader should consult the full proceedings of the Consensus Symposium meeting to get all the details. While acknowledging that any attempt to identify the highlights of the consensus text is bound to be subjective and reflects personal biases of the author, I shall yield under the pressure of the chairman and present a brief exposé of my views on the subject matter.

One common observation across the eight working groups of the Consensus Symposium applicable to all 72 program topics was that not only do we need research, but we need more research of the highest possible quality. Indeed, we have reached the point where more descriptive or cross-sectional association studies, or in general more research with low statistical power or low generalizability, will not contribute to the knowledge base in a meaningful manner. This has a lot of implications for the scientists who are trying to decide on the nature of the question of what to investigate next, and the study design best suited to address the problem. But, it is also of great importance for the planners, policy makers, and scientific officers who have to make recommendations on how to best spend the research dollars. Their attitudes regarding these questions will impact enormously on the progress we can really make in our knowledge base, given the limited research budget available in the biological sciences as well as in the behavioral and social sciences. We must not be afraid of tackling important research questions on a grand scale as it is likely the most reasonable way to come up with solid, credible, and reliable evidence. Incidentally, more than 300 important research questions were identified by the experts who took part in the 1992 Consensus Symposium and are listed in *Physical Activity, Fitness, and Health: Consensus Statement* (Bouchard, Shephard, & Stephens, 1993).

One important observation which is constantly gaining strength is that, even among the most blessed of the industrialized countries, individual differences in lifestyle are significantly related to the mortality and morbidity statistics. A striking example along these lines comes from the North Korelia Coronary Heart Disease (CHD) Prevention Study in Finland. Around 1970, the death rate from CHD reached about 720 per 100,000 in this population. Over a 20 year period, a prevention program emphasizing reduction of dietary fat, cessation of smoking and other lifestyle changes was promoted in the community. By 1990, mean plasma cholesterol had decreased from 7.0 to 6.2 mmol/L and death rate from CHD was down to about 360 per 100,000, a reduction of 50%. This is a very important observation.

In this context, it is appropriate to remember that there are currently about 9 million days of hospitalization per year as a result of the debilatating consequences of cardiovascular diseases in Canada. Among the adult Canadians over 35 years of age, approximately 45,000 will die from a heart attack this year and 14,000 from stroke. These numbers are not that surprising when seen in light of the data on the risk profile of the Canadian adults (Table 2.2). The table is based on several national surveys and it indicates that Canadians have a risk profile commensurate with their death rate from vascular diseases: There are notable numbers of adults who have elevated blood cholesterol levels, smoke, and are hypertensive, overweight, and sedentary.

National surveys conducted in several countries of the industrialized world reveal that only about 10% to 15% of the adults are active to the point that an augmentation of maximal aerobic power can be expected. Almost 50% of these populations can be classified as moderately or occasionally active. If the most important point is to become active, we must recognize that our knowledge base about the determinants of participation in physical activity is very deficient. Since the 1988 consensus meeting, about 30 new studies have dealt with this topic but only half of them were based

Table 2.2 National Surveys of Canadian Adults

46% with elevated blood cholesterol (≥ 5.2 mmol/l)

15% with high blood pressure (diastolic ≥ 90 mmHg or on treatment)

35% with BMI ≥ 27

29% smoke regularly

40% are totally sedentary

on a longitudinal or a prospective design. Interestingly, these studies suggest that participation in moderate and vigorous activities appears to be determined by different factors.

There are new data indicating that participation in physical activity may impact on health in a manner analogous to cessation of smoking. Past activity level may be less important than current activity status. Thus, cessation of participation in physical activity seems to be associated with the progressive loss of the protective effect against premature death. On the other hand, becoming active after having been sedentary for many years appears to be related to a reduction in the relative risk of death. Continuous adherence would therefore be the most favorable course. More research is clearly needed on this important but highly complex topic.

So far, most of the research pertaining to the relationship between physical activity and vascular diseases has been epidemiological and associative. There is a strong belief that more should be done on vascular wall biology and on the cellular and molecular basis of atherosclerosis. If we are to truly understand how regular physical activity may alter the course of the atherosclerotic diseases (the number one killer in our societies), strong research programs should be developed about the effects of the metabolic and mechanical demands of various types of physical activity regimens on the vessel wall, proper controls over diet, modification of the lipoprotein particles, endothelium properties, macrophage and platelet functions, smooth muscle cells, activators and inhibitors of thrombus formation, growth factors, and immune response components involved in the atherosclerotic process.

It is estimated that about 2 to 3 adults per 1,000 suffer from peripheral vascular disease. Even though the exact mechanisms are still not fully understood, regular walking and other forms of physical activity are associated with a reduction of the typical pain in the legs, and an increase in the walking performance before the onset of the claudicating pain. The improvement is generally quite dramatic and of the order of 60% to 100% after at least 3 months of therapeutic physical activity. However, less is known about the potential of regular physical activity to prevent the advent of peripheral vascular disease.

One can find about 50 studies that have dealt with the role of regular physical activity on blood pressure. The trends in the results are quite informative:

- When subjects were normotensive, the changes in blood pressure were negligible.
- When subjects were borderline hypertensive, the reduction reached a mean of about 6 mmHg for systolic and diastolic blood pressures.
- When the studies were undertaken with hypertensive patients, regular physical activity was associated with a mean decrease of about 10 mmHg for systolic and 8 mmHg for diastolic blood pressure.

It should also be noted that programs of moderate intensity seemed to fare better than those of high and very high intensities.

An exciting finding emerging from the scientific and clinical research of about the last 20 years is that regular physical activity engenders pervasive and favorable effects on lipid metabolism. For instance, in most people, regular physical activity decreases blood triglycerides and very low density lipoprotein (VLDL) cholesterol, but increases high density lipoprotein (HDL) cholesterol, particularly the HDL_2 fraction. Regular physical activity is also associated with a reduction of the activity of hepatic lipase and a decrease in the hepatic production of VLDL and ketone bodies. Lipid metabolism in skeletal muscle and cardiac muscle is dramatically altered by regular physical activity. Thus, it elevates the activity of key enzymes of the lipid oxidation pathways and effectively augments the capacity to oxidize lipid substrates in these tissues. It is also accompanied by an increase in lipoprotein lipase (LPL) activity and an enlargment of the lipid stores in muscle. Adipose tissue lipid metabolism is influenced to a considerable extent by regular physical activity. Adipose tissue lipolysis is increased along with LPL activity. The adipose cell becomes more sensitive to the antilipolytic effect of insulin. Local adipose tissue blood flow is augmented, and free fatty acids re-esterification is decreased. All these changes, and undoubtedly others, are favorable in the sense that they translate into

- a greater rate of lipid oxidation,
- improved conditions to achieve a balance between the lipid content of the diet and the amount of lipid oxidized, and
- a less atherogenic blood lipid and lipoprotein profile.

In spite of more than two decades of research on physical activity and non insulin dependent diabetes mellitus (NIDDM), our knowledge base regarding the prevention and the treatment of this disease is still quite limited. The research is generally inconclusive primarily because it is of a low power and low generalizability type. An important observation is that regular physical activity may be effective in the primary prevention of NIDDM and perhaps more so in the high risk cases, such as those who are overweight, or have a familial history of the disease. There are reasons to believe that it may also lead to marked improvement in patients with impaired glucose tolerance. However, in well established cases of NIDDM, regular physical activity does not seem to have a major impact on the disease, although it can significantly improve the cardiovascular risk profile of these patients.

The proportion of the North American citizenry over 65 years of age was about 1 in 10 around 1980 and it should reach 1 in 6 by about 2020. This change in the age composition of the population has enormous impact for those interested by the physical activity, fitness, and health paradigm. To age with a reasonable fitness level, complete autonomy, and free from any disability or impairment is one of the greatest assets that we all wish for our personal life. It is becoming increasingly recognized that regular physical activity, in otherwise healthy individuals, is a cornerstone of successful aging. Older persons respond just as well as younger adults to regular physical activity when the results are considered relative to the current level of fitness of the subject. This is true not only for performance phenotypes such as maximal oxygen uptake and exercise tolerance, but also for important clinical markers such as plasma triglycerides and HDL cholesterol, body fat content, blood pressure, glucose tolerance, and insulin sensitivity.

As a result, dose-response issues become particularly important. It is essential to understand the mechanisms involved in the relation among physical activity and each specific morphological, physiological, metabolic, and psychosocial outcome in order to define the nature of the dose-response circumstances. This is of particular interest to all those involved in the promotion of physical activity for the purpose of protecting and enhancing health and well being. Recommendations about the specific circumstances of regular physical activity should be designed to impact as favorably as possible on the targeted health outcome. For instance, if the prevention of obesity or the treatment of excess body fat is the aim, the most important characteristic will then be the total amount of energy expended through daily physical activity. If bone density is the focus of the activity program, weight bearing activities and moderate to high resistance exercise should be recommended. When the emphasis is on blood pressure and the metabolic profile (insulin action, plasma lipids, and lipoproteins), favorable effects can be expected over a wide range of activities undertaken in a variety of circumstances. But, locomotor activities of moderate intensity, about 4 times a week for about 1 hour per session, are believed to generate an adequate stimulus. If prevention of injuries and minimal risk is a major concern, recommendations should then emphasize the benefits derived from low to moderate intensity exercise. When continuous adherence is a major objective, it would be advisable to avoid high to very high intensity activities and to introduce variety in the program. These suggestions are presented only to illustrate that increasing knowledge about the effects of regular physical activity, and of the mechanisms implicated, should eventually be more precise regarding the details of the dose-response circumstances.

One of the most important advances of the last few years has to do with the understanding that it is not always essential to exercise at high intensities to benefit from a fitness and health point of view. It seems to apply even to the risk of death. Indeed, at levels of regular physical activity slightly above a sedentary mode of life, mortality rate from all causes, or from cardiovascular diseases, is reduced in both men and women. Clearly, maximal oxygen uptake is best improved with a high intensity physical activity regimen. However, favorable morphological, physiological, and metabolic changes are engendered by moderate intensity physical activity, particularly when sessions are frequent and of long duration. Dramatic reduction in the risk profile, and improvement in the general health of most adults can be expected with, for instance, a daily one-hour walk at about 50% of maximum walking speed. Also, a less demanding physical activity regimen will likely improve the general health status of most people, albeit to a lesser extent. These are major advances in our knowledge on physical activity and have enormous implications for public health policy.

However, it is obvious that it is impossible to define a single set of intensity, frequency, and duration conditions that would optimally impact on all the health outcomes. In other words, recommendations about regular physical activity have to be adjusted to the individual or group and the desired outcome if maximal benefit is of concern. It should also be kept in mind that the response to regular physical activity may be blunted or even enhanced by factors that cannot always be controlled. For instance, smoking may attenuate the gains expected from the program. A cold environment may augment energy expenditure beyond the anticipated cost of the exercise regimen. Perhaps more importantly, there are considerable interindividual differences in response to regular physical activity that are determined by inherited factors. Thus, genetic individuality accounts for a three- to tenfold range in the response of morphological, physiological, and metabolic phenotypes to regular physical activity. We have become accustomed to describing the effects of regular physical activity in terms of the mean changes observed in a group of individuals. However, the mean value can be quite misleading as there are nonresponders, lowresponders, and highresponders with many others in between these categories.

An important issue is whether there are adjuvants to physical activity that can enhance the benefits associated with regular physical activity. The topic was addressed in the 1992 ICSPAFH, and the overall picture is not a very optimistic one for all those who have faith and invest time and money into these practices thinking that they help. Some of these adjuvants may indeed have positive influences, particularly in terms of relaxation and recovery from fatigue. There are reasons to believe that it may be beneficial to use massage and sauna. Other adjuvants appear to be devoid of any apparent benefit. Included in this category one would find things such as sudation garments, passive exercise devices, spot reducing devices, bust developers, and most nutritional supplementations. We found that most of the claims made by the proponents of these practices or devices were unsubstantiated and scientifically misleading.

Conclusion

The 1992 ICSPAFH was organized and designed to review, in a critical manner, the present knowledge base regarding the relationships between physical activity, fitness, and health, and to identify the most pressing research questions to be addressed. We believe that the issues highlighted here provide support for the contention that regular physical activity is almost universally accepted as relevant to health. However, there are still many unanswered questions and several issues are only partially resolved. For instance, we still do not know enough about the optimum combination of mode, intensity, frequency, and duration of activity with respect to health and wellness, or specific health objectives. The cumulative impact of many years of participation remains to be elucidated. The interactions between regular physical activity and other lifestyle components such as nutrition, sleeping habits, smoking, and alcohol consumption are largely unknown. We are even more ignorant about the individual differences in the sensitivity to an active mode of life in terms of health outcomes.

We still have a long way to go before a complete understanding of all the effects of regular physical activity or a persistent sedentary lifestyle is achieved. Thus, at present, an evaluation of the benefits and risks of regular physical activity or of an inactive lifestyle can be based only on partial evidence. Moreover, the small body of knowledge accumulated to date, although impressive by some standards, pertains only to mean effects seen in limited samples of a population. It does not even begin to seriously address the issue of individual differences in host susceptibility to benefits and risks. It is important for all those involved in the areas of physical activity, fitness, and health to be neither overly optimistic about the role of regular physical activity on health outcomes nor unduly pessimistic about the consequences of a sedentary mode of life. A missionary or crusading attitude cannot replace solid scientific evidence. Further progress in this field, as in any other areas pertaining to health and well-being of humans, will come about only as a result of long-term, excellent programs of basic and clinical research. There is no reasonable and credible alternative.

References

Bouchard, C., Shephard, R.J., Stephens, T., Sutton, J.R., & McPherson, B.D. (Eds.) (1990). *Exercise, fitness and health: A consensus of current knowledge*. Champaign, IL: Human Kinetics.

Bouchard, C., & Shephard, R.J. (in press). Physical activity, fitness and health. In C. Bouchard, R.J.

Shephard, & T. Stephens (Eds.), *Physical activity, fitness, and health: International proceedings and consensus statement*. Champaign, IL: Human Kinetics.

Bouchard, C., Shephard, R.J., & Stephens, T. (Eds.) (1993). *Physical activity, fitness, and health: Consensus statement*. Champaign, IL: Human Kinetics.

Bouchard, C., Shephard, R.J., & Stephens, T. (Eds.) (in press). *Physical activity, fitness, and health: International proceedings and consensus statement*. Champaign, IL: Human Kinetics.

Proceedings of the International Symposium on Physical Activity and Cardiovascular Health (1967). *Canadian Medical Association Journal*, **96**(12), 695-915.

World Health Organization. (1968). *Meeting of investigators on exercise tests in relation to cardiovascular function*. (WHO Technical Report 388). Geneva: WHO.

Part I

Biological Aspects of Physical Activity, Fitness, and Health

The Campbell Survey on Well-Being (T. Stevens & C.L. Craig, *The Well-Being of Canadians: Highlights of the 1988 Campbell's Survey*, 1990), indicates that the public at large rates physical activity as an important contributor to physical health. However, the public is probably far less knowledgeable about the specific biological outcomes of exercise and the impact that these outcomes may have on specific health conditions. Part I of the proceedings addresses this important base of scientific knowledge.

Specifically, Haskell outlines the health-related biological outcomes of physical activity and addresses the issue of the exercise dose required to achieve selected outcomes. Haskell also pinpoints the role of exercise in different health-related outcomes such as osteoporosis and glucose metabolism. Blair, Brill, and Barlow focus on the role of physical activity in disease prevention through an examination of different epidemiological data relating inactivity to cardiovascular diseases and diabetes. Blair and colleagues build a strong case for the idea that sedentariness is a major risk factor for health.

Drinkwater deals with the role of exercise and physical activity in the health of women through a comprehensive examination of issues including pregnancy, obesity, eating disorders, menopause, osteoporosis, and rehabilitation from diseases of cardiovascular origin. Drinkwater eloquently underscores how gender and physical activity interact in producing specific outcomes. Sharratt and Sharratt examine the role of active living for persons with chronic conditions ranging from osteoarthritis and cardiovascular disease to chronic obstructive pulmonary disease and diabetes. An examination of selected data on quality of life leads Sharratt and Sharratt to conclude that active living could be a useful strategy in the promotion of health for persons with chronic conditions. Malina addresses the effects of exercise and physical activity on growth and maturation throughout the life span by concisely surveying relevant research. Malina encourages a broader view of the promotion of physical activity that includes the learning and mastering of a breadth of motor skills, the internalization of positive attitudes toward physical activity, and the benefits of sustained physical activity throughout the adult and senior years.

Bar-Or examines the effects of exercise and physical activity on children who suffer from specific conditions including asthma, cerebral palsy, cystic fibrosis, hypertension, myopathies, and obesity. Importantly, Bar-Or deals with both the benefits and contraindications of exercise and physical activity in these children and concludes that clinicians and researchers should carefully prescribe exercise to children with such conditions in order to maximize benefits and minimize negative outcomes.

Paffenbarger, Hyde, Wing, Lee, and Kampert examine the role of exercise in longevity through a detailed review of relevant research, focusing on the ongoing study of Harvard alumni. Paffenbarger and colleagues conclude that the risk of premature death can be reduced by an active lifestyle. Finally, Wilmore, Gledhill, and Quinney examine whether some of the popular practices in the fitness industry, including massage, electrical stimulation, and sudation garments, have a positive or negative impact on the biological outcomes of exercise and physical activity. Wilmore and colleagues provide concise and up-to-date information that will be of use to practitioners who must dispel the myths perpetuated by some product manufacturers.

3

Physical/Physiological/Biological Outcomes of Physical Activity

William L. Haskell

People who are more physically active throughout life generally benefit from a higher level of health and functional capacity than their sedentary counterparts. These health and performance benefits are the integrated outcome of a wide variety of physical and biological changes produced by being more physically active. In response to the increased energy demands of the exercising muscle, many of the systems of the body are activated and their responses are the stimuli that produce most of the biological and physical adaptations referred to as the training response. Also, the physical stress of contracting muscle and the effects of gravity during movement on muscle, bone, and connective tissue cause adaptive responses. Exercise, depending on its type, intensity, duration, and frequency, will activate many of the body's systems (e.g., muscle, skeletal, cardiorespiratory, metabolic, neuro-endocrine, gastrointestinal, immune) and produce health-related benefits. Some of these changes are well established while others still need further investigation.

To design effective health-oriented physical activity regimens, we not only need to know what benefits can be achieved, but also the characteristics of the physical activity that will most effectively produce these benefits. For example, in some cases such as the reduction in blood pressure, lower intensity exercise may be more effective than exercise at a higher intensity. Or, it may be that short bouts of activity spread throughout each day may be more effective at producing some health-related benefits than a longer bout of activity performed every other day. As with physical performance outcomes of exercise training, the physical activity dose appears quite specific for each of the biological changes that contribute to improved health.

The primary focus of this presentation is a general review of selected health-related biological and physical changes produced by frequent participation in physical activity. The presentation will also discuss some of the issues involved in the physical activity dose-response relationship for these changes.

Optimal Versus Adequate Versus Minimal Dose

Currently we know a substantial amount about what the *adequate* dose of exercise is to achieve many health-related biological or physical outcomes, but we still know very little about the *optimal* or *minimal* dose of activity necessary to achieve these benefits as effectively as possible. For exercise prescriptions or guidelines to be scientifically sound and produce the desired effects, it is important to develop the data required to understand what the optimal dose of exercise is to achieve a desired otucome. This optimal dose would maximize benefit and minimize risk and cost. What the minimal dose is for a specific benefit is what much of the general public would like to know (not how much do I have to do, but how little can I get away with). While information for many health-related biological and physical changes is still incomplete, it is adequate for use in the design and implementation of specific physical activity regimens directed at improving health outcomes.

For many of the favorable biological responses attributed to physical activity, very little is known about the response to a specific dose of activity. Data are available that describe reasonably well the type, intensity, and amount of activity that improves maximal oxygen uptake of a group (American College of Sports Medicine, 1990) and an adqute prescription probably can be constructed for other health related outcomes such as weight loss or improvement in insulin resistance. However, even for these responses, very little is known about why there is a substantial variation in the response to the same dose of physical activity among individuals who

17

appear to have relatively homogeneous key characteristics. For example, Dionne et al. (1991) reported the individual changes in maximal oxygen uptake of sedentary men aged 24 to 29 years to a highly standardized endurance training program (20 minutes per session at the onset of blood lactic acid, 3 times a week for 12 weeks). Among the 29 men training at Arizona State University, the increase in maximal oxygen uptake ranged from 0.07 to 0.96 l/min, a fourteenfold difference. Interindividual variations in the responses to other biologic variables have been reported by other investigators (Bouchard, 1988), but so far little attention has been paid to this important issue. Why such variations exist are not well understood and require substantial investigation.

Health-Related Biological Outcomes of Physical Activity

The health-related biological outcomes derived from performing frequent bouts of physical activity appear to be numerous and highly diverse (see Table 3.1). These changes range from increases in bone mineral density, to enhanced activity of metabolic enzymes in skeletal and cardiac muscle, to decreases in the sympathetic activity of the nervous system. Some of these changes are scientifically proven to occur to some degree in all people who perform the appropriate physical activity regimen. Other outcomes listed in Table 3.1 have been indicated as possible beneficial outcomes, but either the data are too preliminary, the results from different studies are not consistent, or other measurement issues exist thus the outcomes require further scientific documentation.

It is important to understand that these biological outcomes of activity, while possibly the "mechanism" by which physical activity enhances health, still are not adequate evidence by themselves to prove that physical activity improves clinical outcomes, that is, reduces morbidity or mortality (Haskell, 1984). For example, there is increasing evidence that physical activity, especially heavy resistance exercise, increases bone mineral density (Dalsky, Stocke, & Ehsani, 1988). But so far no study has been reported that determined if more physically active older women have fewer osteoporotic fractures.

Dose-Response for Selected Health-Related Biological Outcomes

Over the past several decades there have been hundreds, if not thousands, of studies that have evaluated the relationship between physical activity and biological and physical status. These include cross-sectional and longitudinal observational studies and exercise training studies. These studies have included a wide

Table 3.1   Major Health and Performance Outcomes as a Result of Frequent Physical Activity

Adapted From ...

Skeletal muscle
 Hypertrophy
 Increased capillarization and maximal blood flow
 Increased substrate availability and metabolic capacity
 Increased strength and endurance

Cardiovascular
 Increased stroke volume and cardiac output at rest and exercise
 Lower heart rate and blood pressure at rest and submaximal exercise
 Increased cardiac mass
 Possible increased cardiac vascularization
 Decreased peripheral vascular resistance
 Increased fibrinolysis
 Decreased tendency for blood clotting

Metabolic
 Improved lipoprotein profile (decreased triglycerides and increased high density cholesterol)
 Increased insulin mediated glucose uptake
 Decreased adiposity
 Possible increased resting metabolism

Respiratory
 Increased ventiallatory-diffusion efficiency during exercise
 Possible decreased work of breathing

Neuro-endocrine
 Decreased sympathetic tone at rest and during submaximal exercise
 Possible decreased beta receptor activity

Skeletal
 Increased bone mineral density in youth
 Possible retention of bone mineral density in older adults

Note. There are inadequate data to support claims that exercise has clinically meaningful effects on digestive or immune functions.

variety of exercise types, intensities, durations, and frequencies, but only a limited number of studies have systematically studied the dose-response relationship between physical activity and health-related outcomes using a randomized, controlled design. Because individual characteristics (age, gender, health status, prior training), measurement procedures, specifics of the activity regimen, and the physical environment all can influence the dose-response relationship, comparison of data from one study to another is fraught with hazards. For example, extreme care should be taken in combining data from different studies to establish an activity threshold for a specific benefit. Presented in this section is a brief review of the dose-response relationship for exercise and several major health-related biological outcomes.

Physical Activity and Obesity

In theory, there should be a linear dose-response relationship between changes in adiposity and changes in physical activity as defined by energy expenditure when caloric intake is held constant. However, such a relationship usually has not been demonstrated in physical activity training studies in the general population or overweight individuals. Highly active endurance athletes are substantially leaner than sedentary persons at all ages (Martin, Haskell, & Wood, 1977) for both men and women. Cross-sectional studies have observed that more active or fit persons tend to be leaner (Cooper et al., 1976). Changes in physical activity are often accompanied by spontaneous changes in caloric intake so that weight stays constant, or the changes are much less than expected. There is increasing evidence that under some weight loss circumstances, there is a decrease in metabolic rate during rest, or exercise that reduces the amount of negative caloric balance and the weight loss is less than expected (Donohoe, Lin, Kirschenbaum, & Keesey, 1984). Also, large interindividual variations in magnitude of weight change, with either a standard caloric intake or caloric expenditure, have been identified during the study of identical twins (Bouchard, 1988).

Usually relatively small increases in physical activity (≤ 200 calories burned per day, 3 times a week), are not associated with significant changes in adiposity over 12 to 24 weeks of observation. Above this amount of moderate intensity activity, there tends to be a quite consistent reduction in adiposity with greater amounts of exercise associated with greater weight loss; especially when individuals are in the range of 5 to 20 kg overweight at the start of exercise (Wood et al., 1988). How much of the decrease in adiposity from physical activity is the result of an increase in resting metabolic rate has not been established (Poehlman, 1989). Since a greater portion of the substrate used for the energy of muscle contraction is derived from fat at moderate versus near maximal exercise intensity, it has been proposed that greater weight loss is achieved by the same total caloric expenditure if the exercise intensity is moderate (50% to 75% of capacity) compared to high intensity (> 75% of capacity). There is no good evidence that this is the case, but for practical purposes for weight loss using exercise, this issue probably is not important.

Physical Activity and Lipoprotein Metabolism

Endurance trained athletes and generally more physically active persons have a more favorable plasma lipoprotein profile than less active persons (Haskell, 1986). Endurance-type activity decreases plasma triglyceride concentrations; increases high density lipoprotein cholesterol (HDL-C), apolipoprotein AI, and the high density to low density cholesterol ratio; and is, in some cases, associated with relatively small decreases in low density lipoprotein cholesterol. In cross-sectional studies, plasma triglyceride concentrations are negatively related to the level of fitness or activity status throughout their full range. Lowest values are measured in lean, highly trained endurance athletes, joggers, tennis players, soccer players, and people who regularly participate in similar aerobic-based activities (Haskell, 1986). The typical rise in triglyceride concentration with age, seen in the general population, is not observed in endurance trained, lean persons (Martin, Haskell, & Wood, 1977).

If baseline triglyceride concentrations are above 1.25 mmol/l (120 mg/dl), endurance exercise training usually lowers their concentration, with both acute and chronic effects taking place. Below this concentration, exercise induced decreases are usually not observed. The dose of exercise required to reduce triglyceride concentrations is not great, with endurance exercise performed at 65% of VO₂max for 30 minutes, 3 times a week having a significant effect (Oscai, Patterson, Bogard, Beck, & Rothermel, 1972). It has been demonstrated that in hypertriglyceridemic men, fasting plasma triglyceride concentration the morning after a 45-minute bout of exercise at approximately 75% of aerobic capacity is lower than when such exercise is not performed (Oscai et al., 1972). Over a five day period, if exercise is performed every day, triglyceride concentration decreases further the following day. Thus, this acute response is augmented by repeated bouts of exercise. The reduced triglyceride concentration is rapidly reversed if the exercise is not performed. This effect occurs even if the increased caloric expenditure is compensated for by increased caloric intake (Gyntelberg et al., 1977), it is likely the effect will occur due to an increase in lipoprotein lipase activity in response to the exercise (Lithell, Hellsing, Lundqvist, & Malmberg, 1979). This could be called an augmented acute response in that there is no further decrease even after weeks of exercise training on a regular basis.

Originally it appeared that a large dose of exercise was required to produce significant increases in HDL-C concentrations in ambulatory healthy adults. The volume of exercise may be more important than the relative intensity, with more than 1,200 to 1,500 calories per week of moderate intensity exercise for 12 weeks or more required by healthy ambulatory men and women to obtain significant increases in HDL-C concentration (Wood, Williams, & Haskell, 1984). The volume of activity required to get consistent increases in HDL-C in women also appeared to be greater than that observed for men. It has been speculated that this difference is due to some role played by sex hormones in the exercise mediated changes in HDL-C. However, recently Dunan, Gordon, and Scott (1991) reported that walking 4.8 km per day, 5 days a week at 4.8 km/hour for 24 weeks significantly increased plasma HDL-C concentrations in sedentary, healthy, premenopausal women (Figure

3.1). At a faster walking pace of 8.0 km/hour, the increase in HDL-C was not any greater. Another interesting aspect of these results was the lack of association between the increase in aerobic capacity and HDL-C among the different walking groups. It also should be pointed out that observational studies have shown HDL-C to be lower in bed-rested patients (Nikkila, Kuusi, & Myllynen, 1980) and higher in postal carriers than sedentary controls (LaPorte et al., 1983). These data suggest that dose-response for HDL-C may exist throughout much of the range of physical activity.

Exercise and Resting Blood Pressure

It appears that exercise may have both acute and chronic beneficial effects on resting blood pressure in people with mild to moderate hypertension. The reduction in systolic blood pressure after a single bout of exercise occurs with exercise at 50% of VO_2max for 30 minutes, but exercise at 75% of capacity for 45 minutes produces even a greater reduction for at least 3 hours (Hagberg, Montain, & Martin, 1987). This acute reduction occurs primarily in systolic pressure, not diastolic pressure, and is the result of a decrease in cardiac output due to a decrease in stroke volume. What the blood pressure profile looks like for the remainder of the day after bouts of exercise of various types, intensities, and durations have not been adequately investigated to define this acute response. What would happen to average blood pressure throughout the day if a person was to perform short bouts of exercise (5 to 10 minutes) every hour or so has not been determined.

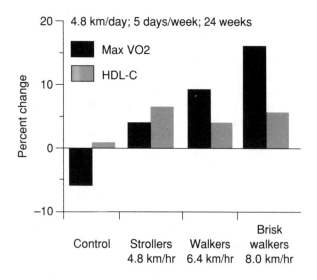

Figure 3.1 Percent changes in maximal oxygen uptake and high density lipoprotein cholesterol in response to walking programs of various speeds in premenopausal women (data from Duncan, Gordon, & Scott, 1991).

In cross-sectional studies of the general population, more physically active and physically fit adults generally have lower blood pressure and less hypertension (Paffenbarger, Wing, Hyde, & Hsieh, 1983; Reaven, Barrett-Conner, & Edelstein, 1991) than inactive or low fit persons with the relationship generally existing across all levels of activity and fitness (Blair, Goodyear, Gibbons, & Cooper, 1984; Jennings et al., 1986; Reaven et al., 1991). In a study of the relationship of blood pressure to physical activity status in older women (Reaven et al., 1991), it is important to note that a relatively small difference in mean blood pressure in more active women was associated with a quite large difference in the prevalence of hypertension. This is very important from a public health perspective given the possible role of physical activity in the prevention of hypertension as compared to its role in the treatment of hypertensives. This inverse relationship between activity and blood pressure or hypertension appears to be the case for endurance exercise and aerobic capacity, but not necessarily for heavy resistance exercise or measures of strength. Some of the association between activity and fitness and lower blood pressure can be accounted for by less adiposity in the more active.

Reduction of both systolic and diastolic blood pressure as the result of endurance training has been reported for patients with mild hypertension (Kiyonga, Arakawa, Tanaka, & Shindo, 1985). Moderate intensity exercise (50% to 65% of aerobic capacity) appears to be more effective in lowering blood pressure than higher intensity exercise (Jennings et al., 1986). Also, more frequent moderate intensity endurance activity (7 times a week versus 3 times a week) was found to produce slightly greater blood pressure lowering in sedentary, healthy adults.

The effects of exercise training on resting blood pressure are highly dependent on the baseline pressure, with most of the reduction occurring in patients with moderate hypertension. In a summary of the effects of endurance exercise on blood pressure presented as a part of this symposium (Fagard & Tipton, in press) it was concluded that exercise training reduced both the systolic and diastolic blood pressure in normotensive persons by 3 mmHg, in borderline hypertensive patients by 6 mmHg and in hypertensive patients by 6 to 9 mmHg. Data from prospective observational studies support the idea that regular exercise may help prevent the development of hypertension but data are not adequate to define an optimal dose for such an effect.

Insulin Mediated Glucose Uptake

Endurance exercise generally enhances insulin mediated glucose uptake or insulin sensitivity. That is, less insulin is required for removing a similar amount of glucose from the blood following an oral glucose challenge.

Initially, this effect was considered a response to endurance training (Hollenbeck, Haskell, Rosenthal, & Reaven, 1984), but more recently it has been demonstrated to be a response to the last exercise training session (Heath et al., 1983). However, it might be more accurate to consider the improvement in insulin action to be an interaction between an acute response to exercise and the increased exercise capacity produced by endurance exercise training. The very sedentary person with a low exercise capacity may not be able to expend sufficient energy during a single exercise bout to increase insulin sensitivity. After weeks or months of endurance training, the volume of exercise performed in a single training session has increased so that it now is adequate to stimulate a short term (24 to 72 hours) improvement in insulin sensitivity. Also, at the beginning of training, there may be an "augmented acute response," in that if the person exercises daily, after several sessions insulin action is improved, but that such an effect is not seen after one or two exercise sessions. This augmented acute response may explain the improved insulin sensitivity seen after seven consecutive days of training (Rogers et al., 1986).

Bone Density and Osteoporosis

During youth, vigorous exercise increases bone density and cross-sectional area. For example, the diameter of the distal radius of the dominant arm of tennis players is significantly larger than their non-dominant arm (Huddleston, Rockwell, Kulund, & Harrison, 1980). Such a comparison eliminates the possibility that this increase in bone mass is due to a difference either in heredity or nutrition.

In cross-sectional studies of older athletes versus non-athletes, more active persons have greater bone mineral density in the spine, legs, arms, hands, and feet than sedentary controls (Brewer, Meyer, Keele, Upton, & Hagan, 1983; Lane et al., 1986). A rapid decrease in activity or gravity via bed rest or space flight results in a rapid loss of bone calcium and bone mineral density. However, it has been more difficult to demonstrate that initiation of exercise training by ambulatory adults produces significant increases in bone mineral density (Marcus et al., 1992). One of the issues in some of these studies is that the exercise regimen was designed more to increase muscular endurance and aerobic capacity than to maximize loading of the bone either by gravity or forceful muscle contraction using heavy resistance exercise.

For maximizing bone mineral density development in youth, activities that repeatedly put physical stress on the bone will help to increase peak bone density (usually achieved by late teens or early twenties). Since most of the benefit appears to be due to a direct effect on the bone, activities that involve the upper as well as the lower body should be included. Also, to ensure maximum benefit, a well designed program that includes heavy resistance exercise should be performed. Nine months of weight-bearing and nonweight-bearing exercise with resistance produced a 5.2% increase in spinal bone content in postmenopausal women. After 13 months the increase was 6.1% (Dalsky, Stocke, & Ehsani, 1988). Such exercise not only enhances bone mineral density, but also increases skeletal muscle strength (Fiatarone et al., 1990), which also appears to be important in reducing fracture risk in older persons, especially osteoporotic fractures in women. Light to moderate intensity exercise in older women has been shown to reduce the loss of bone mineral density in some studies (Smith, Gilligan, McAdam, Ensign, & Smith, 1989), but not others (White, Martin, Yeater, Butcher, & Radin, 1984).

It now appears that frequent exercise may be most effective in helping to reduce the risk of osteoporotic fractures by helping to maximize peak bone density during youth rather than by actually increasing bone density in postmenopausal women and older men. The greater value of exericse in older persons may be to decrease the risk of falling by enhancing muscle strength and possibly balance. In either case, resistance-type exercise using both the lower and upper body appear to be of greatest value.

Discussion

Since the exact exercise stimulus required for producing a change in any of the health-related biological factors other than for possibly VO$_2$max and body weight is not known, it is only by trial and error type research that the dose-response relationship can be established. For example, we do not know the relative role changes in intensity, duration, or volume of exercise play in producing beneficial changes. It may be that for some benefits, intensity is not critical, and only volume of exercise influences the response. On the other hand, if beneficial changes are related to the amount of fat metabolism that occurs during exercise, then lower intensity exercise will be of greater value. But, if the changes are related to the magnitude of sympathetic drive stimulated by the exercise, then time spent at a higher intensity of exercise would be most effective.

While it generally appears that for most health-related biological changes there is a dose relationship throughout nearly the full range of exercise, in some cases there may be an upper threshold where greater intensity or volume may actually be less beneficial than a lower dose. Several studies suggest this may be the case for blood pressure (Jennings et al., 1986; Nelsen, Jennings, Elser, & Kover, 1986).

Since the risk of orthopedic and cardiac injury and the acceptability by many persons is closely linked to exercise intensity, establishing dose-response data for intensity and specific health benefits is a high priority.

In middle-age and older men and women, some data demonstrate that moderate intensity (40% to 60% of aerobic capacity) exercise provides significant health-related benefits at low risk and good adherence. The trade off of longer exercise duration, or more frequent sessions at lower intensity, for higher intensity shorter exercise sessions needs further evaluation (King, Haskell, Taylor, Kraemer, & DeBusk, 1991). Also, the health benefits of multiple short bouts of exercise per day versus a single longer bout needs to be investigated further (DeBusk, Hakansson, Sheehan, & Haskell, 1990). A brief, but more frequent stimulus, especially for some functions like platelet aggregation or fibrinolysis, might be more effective than one longer bout every day or two.

The greatest health benefits from exercise appear to occur when very sedentary persons begin a regular program of moderate intensity, endurance type exercise. Further increases in intensity or amount of exercise produce further benefits in some, but not all, biological responses. The primary stimulus for many of these changes is a sustained, repeated increase in metabolic rate and any way this can be achieved during physical activity appears to be of benefit.

Standard exercise recommendations, based on the stimulus required to produce a significant increase in aerobic capacity have been incorporated as part of the usual exercise prescription for health (aerobic activity at moderate intensity for 30 minutes or 4 kcal/kg body weight, 3 times or more per week). While such a prescription is probably adequate, it may not be optimal or minimal and selected health benefits will require more specificity. At present, it may be best to take the same approach to exercise as is recommended for diet. Exercise should be considered as a group of ''essential nutrients'' required for optimal health and that if we develop a relatively diverse program of exercise we will reap all the various benefits: A diverse diet increases the likelihood of an adequate intake of various micronutrients, but the required dose and specific mechanisms of action remain unspecified.

References

American College of Sports Medicine (1990). The recommended quality and quantity of exercise for developing and maintaining fitness in healthy adults. *Medicine and Science in Sports and Exercise*, **22**, 265-274.

Blair, S.N., Goodyear, N.M., Gibbons, L.W., & Cooper, K.H. (1984). Physical fitness and incidence of hypertension in healthy and normotensive men and women. *Journal of the American Medical Association*, **252**, 487-490.

Bouchard, C. (1988). Discussion: Heredity, fitness and health. In C. Bouchard, R.J. Shephard, T. Stephens, J.R. Sutton, B.D. McPherson (Eds.), *Exercise, fitness and health: A consensus of current knowledge* (pp. 147-153). Champaign, IL: Human Kinetics.

Brewer, V., Meyer, B.M., Keele, M.S., Upton, S.J., & Hagan, R.D. (1983). Role of exercise in prevention of involutional bone loss. *Medicine and Science in Sports and Exercise*, **15**, 445-449.

Cooper, K.H., Pollock, M.L., Martin, R.P., White, S.R., Linnerud, A.C., & Jackson, A. (1976). Physical fitness versus selected coronary risk factors. *Journal of the American Medical Association*, **236**, 116-119.

Dalsky, G., Stocke, K.S., & Ehsani, A.A. (1988). Weight-bearing exercise training and lumbar bone mineral content in postmenopausal women. *Annals of Internal Medicine*, **108**, 824-828.

DeBusk, R.F., Hakansson, U., Sheehan, M., & Haskell, W.L. (1990). Training effects of long versus short bouts of exercise. *American Journal of Cardiology*, **65**, 1010-1013.

Dionne, F.T., Turcotte, L., Thibault, C., Bonlay, M.R., Skinner, J.S., & Bouchard, C. (1991). Mitochondrial DNA sequence polymorphism, VO$_2$ max and response to endurance training. *Medicine and Science in Sports and Exercise*, **23**, 177-185.

Donohoe, C.P., Lin, D.H., Kirschenbaum, D.D., & Keesey, R.E. (1984). Metabolic consequences of dieting and exercise in the treatment of obesity. *Journal of Consulting and Clincal Psychology*, **52**, 827-836.

Duncan, J.J., Gordon, N.F., & Scott, C.B. (1991). Women walking for health and fitness. *Journal of the American Medical Association*, **66**, 3295-3299.

Fagard, R.H., & Tipton, C.M. (in press). Physical activity, fitness and hypertension. In C. Bouchard, R.J. Shephard, and T. Stephens (Eds.), *Physical activity, fitness and health: International proceedings and consensus statement*. Champaign, IL: Human Kinetics.

Fiatarone, M.A., Marks, E.C., Ryan, N.D., Meredith, C.N., Lipsitz, L.A., & Evans, W.J. (1990). High-intensity strength training in nonagenarians: Effects on skeletal muscle. *Journal of the American Medical Association*, **263**, 3209-3034.

Gyntelberg, F., Brennan, R., Holloszy, J., Schonfeld, G., Rennie, M., & Weidman, S. (1977). Plasma triglyceride lowering by exercise despite increased food intake in patients with Type IV hyperlipoproteinemia. *American Journal of Clinical Nutrition*, **30**, 716-720.

Hagberg, J.M., Montain, S.J., & Martin, W.H. (1987). Blood pressure and hemodynamic responses after exercise in older hypertensives. *Journal of Applied Physiology*, **63**, 270-276.

Haskell, W.L. (1984). Physical activity and health: The need to define the required stimulus. *American Journal of Cardiology*, **55**, 4D-9D.

Haskell, W.L. (1986). The influence of exercise training on plasma lipids and lipoproteins in health and disease. *Acta Medica Scandinavica*, (Suppl. 711), 25-37.

Heath, G.W., Gavin, J.R., Hinderlith, J.M., Hagberg, J.M., Bloomfield, S.A. & Holloszy, J.O. (1983). Effects of exercise and lack of exercise on glucose tolerance and insulin sensitivity. *Journal of Applied Physiology*, **55**, 512-517.

Hollenbeck, C., Haskell, W.L., Rosenthal, M., & Reaven, G.M. (1984). Effect of habitual physical activity on regulation of insulin-stimulated glucose disposal in older males. *Journal of the American Geriatrics Society*, **33**, 273-277.

Huddleston, A.L., Rockwell, D., Kulund, D.N., & Harrison, B. (1980). Bone mass in lifetime tennis players. *Journal of the American Medical Association*, **244**, 1107-1109.

Jennings, G., Nelson, L., Nestel, P., Esler, M., Korner, P., Burton, D., & Bazelmans, J. (1986). The effects of changes in physical activity on major cardiovascular risk factors, hemodynamics, sympathetic function, and glucose utilization in man: A controlled study of four levels of activity. *Circulation*, **73**, 30-40.

King, A.C., Haskell, W.L., Taylor, C.B., Kraemer, H.C., & DeBusk, R.F. (1991). Group- vs. home-based exercise training in healthy older men and women: A community-based clinical trials. *Journal of the American Medical Association*, **266**, 1535-1542.

Kiyonaga, A., Arakawa, K., Tanaka, H., & Shindo, M. (1985). Blood pressure and hormonal responses to aerobic exercise. *Hypertension*, **7**, 125-131.

Lane, N.E., Block, D., Jones, H., Marshall, W.H., Wood, P.D., & Fries, J.F. (1986). Long-distance running, osteoporosis and osteoarthritis. *Journal of the American Medical Association*, **255**, 1147-1151.

La Porte, R.E., Brenes, G., Dearwater, S., Murphy, M.A., Cauley, J.A., Dietrick, R., & Robertson, R. (1983). HDL-cholesterol across a spectrum of physical activity from quadraplegia to marathon running. *Lancet*, **1**, 1212-1213.

Lithell, H., Hellsing, K., Lundqvist, G., & Malmberg, P. (1979). Lipoprotein lipase activity of human skeletal muscle and adipose tissue after intense physical exercise. *Acta Physiologica Scandinavica*, **105**, 312-315.

Marcus, R., Drinkwater, B.L., Dalsky, G., Dufek, J., Raab, D., Slemenda, C., & Snow-Harter, C. (1992). Osteoporosis and exercise in women. *Medicine and Science in Sports and Exercise*, **24**(Suppl.), S301-S307.

Martin, R., Haskell, W.L., & Wood, P.D. (1977). Blood density and lipid profile of elite distance runners.

The Marathon: Phsyiological, Medical, Epidermiological and Psychological Studies (Monograph No. 301, pp. 346-360). New York: New York Academy of Sciences.

Nelson, L., Jennings, G.L., Elser, M.D., & Kover, P.I. (1986). Effects of changing levels of physical activity on blood pressure and haemodynamics in essential hypertension. *Lancet*, **8505**, 473-476.

Nikkila, E.A., Kuusi, T., & Myllynen, P. (1980). High-density lipoprotein and apolipoprotein A-I during physical inactivity. *Atherosclerosis*, **37**, 457-462.

Oscai, L.B., Patterson, J.A., Bogard, D.L., Beck, R.J., & Rothermel, B.L. (1972). Normalization of serum triglycerides and lipoprotein electrophoretic patterns by exercise. *American Journal of Cardiology*, **30**, 775-780.

Paffenbarger, R.S., Wing, A.L., Hyde, R.T., & Hsieh, C. (1983). Physical activity and incidence of hypertension in college alumni. *American Journal of Epidemiology*, **117**, 245-257.

Poehlman, E.T. (1989). A review: Exercise and its influence on resting energy metabolism in man. *Medicine and Science in Sports and Exercise*, **21**, 515-525.

Reaven, P.D., Barrett-Conner, E., & Edelstein, S. (1991). Relation between leisure-time physical activity and blood pressure in older women. *Circulation*, **83**, 559-565.

Rogers, M.A., Yamamoto, C., King, D.S., Hagberg, J.M., Ehsani, A.A., & Holloszy, J.O. (1986). Improvement in glucose tolerance after one week of exercise in patients with mild NIDDM. *Diabetes Care*, **1**, 613-618.

Smith, E.L., Gilligan, G., McAdam, M., Ensign, C.P., & Smith, P.E. (1989). Deterring bone loss by exercise intervention in premenopausal and postmenopausal women. *Calcified Tissue International*, **44**, 312-321.

White, M.K., Martin, R.B., Yeater, R.A., Butcher, R.L., & Radin, E.L. (1984). The effects of exercise on the bones of postmenopausal women. *International Orthopaedics*, **7**, 209-214.

Wood, P.D., Stefanick, M.L., Dreon, D., Hewitt-Frey, G., Garay, S., Williams, P.T., Superko, H.R., Fortmann, S.P., Albers, J.J., Vranizan, K., Ellsworth, N.M., Terry, R., & Haskell, W.L. (1988). Changes in plasma lipids and lipoproteins in overweight men during weight loss through dieting as compared with exercise. *New England Journal of Medicine*, **319**, 1173-1179.

Wood, P.D., Williams, P., & Haskell, W.L. (1984). Physical activity and high density lipoproteins. In N.E. Miller & G.J. Miller (Eds.), *Clinical and metabolic aspects of high-density lipoproteins* (pp. 133-165). London: Elsevier Science Publishers.

4

Physical Activity and Disease Prevention

Steven N. Blair
Patricia A. Brill
Carolyn E. Barlow

This chapter reviews the scientific evidence on the relation of physical activity or physical fitness to health status. The prevalence of sedentary habits will be discussed and the public health burden of inactivity estimated. Recommendations for promotion of physical activity are presented.

Physical Activity From Prehistory to the Present

Our human-like ancestors first appeared on this planet about 3.8 million years ago. For the past 1 million years we have existed as hunters and gatherers. Millennia of evolution produced our species, *Homo sapiens*, by approximately 35,000 years ago. Humans continued to survive by hunting and gathering to obtain food. This lifestyle obviously required a high total energy expenditure, with some periods of vigorous intensity. Moving camp, returning from the hunt, carrying food that has been gathered—all required high levels of exertion. Thus, our species evolved to lead a nomadic existence, and as physically active animals. With an abundance of muscle fibers with a high oxidative capacity, and little body hair and numerous sweat glands to allow efficient dissipation of heat from the body, we are well suited to endurance exercise.

Development of Agriculture

Domestication of plants and animals began about 10,000 years ago. The early agriculturalists undoubtedly had a high level of energy expenditure. Indeed, they may well have had to work harder than the hunter-gatherers, because subsistence farmers typically work long hours each day. The development of agriculture may have provided a more consistent food supply, enabled the development of settlements, and given some advantages over the nomadic way of life. This led to division of labor and, ultimately, to the establishment of towns and cities. But for most individuals, everyday existence still required reasonably high levels of physical activity. Therefore, from an energy-expending perspective, our ancestors were still living the type of lifestyle for which their evolutionary history had prepared them.

The Industrial Revolution

Division of labor continued with the rise of skilled tradesmen and artisans. Over many centuries, trade—and the merchant class—developed. Most of the power needed for manufacturing and farming was supplied by humans and other animals. Transportation was by walking or by horses. Energy expenditure for the masses remained high, although for some of the wealthier members of society a more sedentary lifestyle began to develop. Massive changes in society occurred with the development of the steam engine, which rapidly began to supply most of the energy for manufacturing and became more common for transportation. This major change occurred only about 250 years ago. The energy expenditure requirement for many people declined with further advances in modes of transportation and labor-saving devices at home and at work, and with increased urbanization. It was not until the middle third of the 20th century that these trends culminated in a reasonably sedentary life for a majority of citizens in developed societies. Throughout most of the Industrial Revolution, most individuals probably were active enough on the job and with the daily requirements of living that they got an adequate amount of activity to maintain health and function.

The Electronic Age

Scientific and technological progress has been rapid and extensive since World War II. These changes have impacted virtually all areas of human endeavor, from the ability to make war, to art and music, and experiences of daily living. Labor-saving devices are ubiquitous, and have altered, probably forever, our work lives and home activities. High levels of job-related exertion have nearly disappeared. Many formerly vigorous occupations now require no more than moderate energy expenditures, due to machines performing work once done by humans. Dr. Ralph Paffenbarger has stated that his classical study on the physical activity and health of San Francisco longshoremen (Paffenbarger & Hale, 1975) could not be conducted today, due to increased containerization and mechanization (personal communication, 1984). Most suburban North Americans have a power lawn mower; some people in our neighborhoods, whose lawns are less than one acre, have riding mowers. Automotive power steering and brakes, electronic word processors, television remote controls, moving sidewalks, restaurants and banks with drive-throughs, and a long list of other factors have gradually ratcheted downward the energy expenditure of many. It is possible for a middle-class individual in the industrialized world to live day after day and never exceed 2 or 3 METs of energy expenditure.

The conclusion of this brief examination of the history of human energy expenditure is that there are tens of millions of men and women in industrialized societies who are living a sedentary lifestyle, compared to their ancestors. We evolved to be active animals who ate a diet high in fiber and carbohydrates and low in fat, and we have no evolutionary experience with exposure to toxins such as cigarette smoke. These lifestyle insults appear to be largely responsible for the epidemic of chronic diseases in the modern world.

Definitions

It will be useful at the outset to define a few terms that will be used throughout this chapter. These are common terms and everyone has an understanding of what they mean. There are subtle differences in the way some of them are used here, so it is best to state precisely what is meant. For example, exercise is a simple word that is understood by all and is generally understood to refer to participation in sports, conditioning activities, or physical recreation. Our concern is that if people think of exercise as something that is done in an exercise facility, while they are wearing special clothing and sweating profusely, they will find it easier to avoid participating than if they have a more comprehensive view of the behavior. The following definitions for physical activity, exercise, and physical fitness are taken from Caspersen, Powell, and Christenson (1985).

- "*Physical activity* is any bodily movement produced by skeletal muscles that results in energy expenditure." (p. 127)

- "*Exercise* is planned, structured, and repetitive bodily movement done to improve or maintain one or more components of physical fitness." (p. 127)
- "*Physical fitness* is a set of attributes that people have or achieve that relate to the ability to perform physical activity." (p. 127)
- *Health* is a dynamic state that ranges from invalidism to optimal levels of functioning in all aspects of life.

This broad concept of health underlies the philosophical approach taken in this chapter, although many of the papers reviewed focus on specific disease endpoints. In research on physical activity or physical fitness on health, health has frequently been defined as avoidance of morbidity or mortality. This is understandable, given the requirements of epidemiological studies to have a specific and measurable endpoint. It has become clear, however, that health is more than the absence of disease.

Physical Activity and Health

It is not surprising that a species with our evolutionary history should require a certain amount of physical activity to maintain good health and a high level of function. Philosophers and physicians from antiquity have recognized the importance of physical activity to health, but only recently have medical scientists conducted controlled studies to document and describe this relationship (Morris & Crawford, 1958; Morris, Heady, Raffle, Roberts, & Parks, 1953; Paffenbarger & Hale, 1975).

Cardiovascular Disease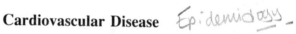

The hypothesis that physical activity is protective against the development of cardiovascular disease arose from the seminal work of Morris and his colleagues in London almost 40 years ago (Morris, Heady, Raffle, Roberts, & Parks, 1953). Those early studies of a population of London Transport workers showed that the drivers of London buses had higher cardiovascular disease rates than the conductors, who were presumably more active as a result of climbing the stairs in the double-decker buses to collect fares. Additional studies in employed populations, perhaps most notably the studies by Paffenbarger et al. of longshoremen, confirm that workers who are physically active on the job are less likely to develop cardiovascular disease than their more sedentary peers (Paffenbarger & Hale, 1975). The active workers had lower rates of cardiovascular disease, coronary heart disease, and sudden death, as well as reduced risk of all-cause mortality.

The protective effects of physical activity do not appear to be limited to occupational activity, but also accrue to individuals who are active in leisure time as well. Morris, Everitt, Pollard, Chave, and Semmence (1980) extended their observations to large groups of executive grade civil servants. In the most recent report, men who reported eight or more bouts of vigorous physical activity per month at baseline were much less likely to develop coronary heart disease than the men who reported no vigorous activity (Morris, Clayton, Everitt, Semmence, & Burgess, 1990). Paffenbarger, Hyde, Wing, and Hsieh (1986) have followed a population of approximately 17,000 Harvard alumni for more than 20 years. Coronary heart disease, cardiovascular disease, and all-cause mortality rates are inversely associated with weekly levels of reported leisure-time physical activity.

Leon, Connett, Jacobs, and Rauramaa (1987) followed a group of men at high risk for developing coronary heart disease who participated in the Multiple Risk Factor Intervention Trial. These men were at risk because of cigarette smoking habits and high blood pressure and cholesterol levels. The 12,138 men were followed for 7 years after an assessment of their leisure-time physical activity. Men in the 2nd and 3rd tertiles of activity had lower coronary heart disease death rates than men in the 1st tertile. There was no advantage for men in the 3rd tertile compared with men in the 2nd tertile of activity.

These three recent studies of physical activity and cardiovascular disease confirm and extend earlier work. The recent studies used relatively detailed physical activity assessment methodology, thorough follow-up with careful documentation of endpoints, and good overall epidemiological methods. A review by Powell, Thompson, Caspersen, and Kendrick (1987) showed that approximately two thirds of the studies on physical activity and coronary heart disease reported an inverse relation between activity and disease. However, in the studies that used good methods, more than 80% of the active individuals showed a reduced risk of coronary heart disease. Thus, it appears that if a study is carefully done, it is virtually certain that a protective effect of physical activity on disease processes will be observed.

Cancer

Studies from as long ago as the 1920s show lower cancer rates in physically active individuals than in sedentary persons (Cherry, 1922; Sivertsen & Dahlstrom, 1922). There have been several recent reports that have reawakened scientists' interest in this topic. Sedentary lifestyle has been evaluated for an association with cancer at several different sites. The type of cancer for which the evidence of an association with inactivity is strongest is colon cancer. Several studies over the past decade show higher colon cancer rates in sedentary individuals than in more active ones (Garabrant, Peters, Mack, & Bernstein, 1984; Gerhardsson, Norell, Kiviranta, Pedersen, & Ahlbom, 1986; Lee, Paffenbarger, & Hsieh, 1991; Whittemore et al., 1990). These studies have been

performed in diverse populations around the world, including the United States, Sweden, and China. There is some evidence of a dose-response gradient across physical activity levels, some of the major potential confounding variables such as cigarette smoking and diet have been adjusted for, and the findings show some consistency across population subgroups.

Exercise may have an impact on sex hormone production and utilization, and thus might be inversely associated with hormonally mediated cancers. There is some tentative evidence that sedentary habits might be related to an increased risk for breast and reproductive cancers in women (Frisch et al., 1985) and to prostate cancer in men (Albanes, Blair, & Taylor, 1989; Lee, Paffenbarger, & Hsieh, 1992). These studies need to be replicated in other populations before conclusions can be drawn.

The mechanisms by which physical activity might affect cancer risk are unclear. The hormone hypothesis may be a factor for some cancers. Other hypotheses that need to be evaluated include the possible role of physical activity in enhancing immune function and contributing to shorter intestinal transit time in active individuals.

Non-Insulin-Dependent Diabetes

Exercise has long been an integral part of blood glucose control management plans, especially in insulin-dependent diabetics. Weight loss and weight control are important cornerstones of patient management in non-insulin-dependent diabetes mellitus (NIDDM), and exercise frequently is included in these plans. There is still considerable disagreement over whether or not exercise is useful in the prevention and treatment of NIDDM. Two recent epidemiological studies provide some important data on this point.

Manson et al. (1991) followed a cohort of 87,253 women for 8 years. The women were initially free of NIDDM, and during follow-up 1,303 women developed the disease. Women who reported performing vigorous exercise at least once per week were 33% less likely to develop NIDDM than their counterparts who were not vigorous exercisers. The inverse association between exercise and development of NIDDM remained after statistical adjustment for body mass index, age, family history of diabetes, and other risk factors.

Helmrich, Ragland, Leung, and Paffenbarger (1991) report on risk of developing NIDDM in a cohort of 5,990 male alumni of the University of Pennsylvania. There were 202 incident cases of NIDDM that developed during follow-up from 1962 to 1976. Risk of developing NIDDM was inversely related to leisure-time physical activity reported at baseline. Age-adjusted risk of developing NIDDM was 6% lower for each 500 kcal increment of physical activity from 500 to 3,500 kcal per week. These findings were unchanged after statistical adjustment for obesity, hypertension, and family history of diabetes.

These two studies provide the first convincing evidence that an active lifestyle may help prevent the development of NIDDM. These results may have considerable public health importance due to the high prevalence of NIDDM, especially in older populations.

Physical Fitness and Health

Studies on physical activity and health have made important contributions to the understanding of the role of sedentary habits in relation to health. One problem with these studies is that it is difficult to measure habitual physical activity. Existing methods typically rely on self-reports of occupational physical activity and participation in sports and other leisure-time activities. Current techniques are crude and imprecise and frequently lead to misclassification of subjects. There are some advantages to using physical fitness as the exposure variable in studies on sedentary lifestyle and health. Although genetic factors make a contribution, the primary determinant of physical fitness is habitual physical activity, thus physical fitness can be viewed as an excellent overall marker for a person's activity level. The advantage of using physical fitness in research studies is that it can be objectively measured, which leads to less misclassification on the exposure variable and presumably gives a more accurate view of the relationship between sedentary habits and health. The obvious disadvantages of adding physical fitness assessments to epidemiological studies are logistical difficulties and expense. Fitness has been added to a few studies in recent years; some of the results are reviewed in this section.

Cardiovascular Disease

Ekelund et al. (1988) followed 4,276 men, aged 30 to 69 years, after a baseline examination that included an assessment of physical fitness by a submaximal exercise test on a treadmill. There were 45 deaths due to cardiovascular disease during 8.5 years of follow-up. There was a strong inverse gradient for all-cause and cardiovascular disease mortality across quartiles of physical fitness. The relative risk for cardiovascular disease mortality was approximately 7.0 when the least physically fit quartile was compared to the most fit quartile.

We have followed a population of 10,224 men and 3,120 women for approximately 8 years after a preventive medical examination at the Cooper Clinic in Dallas (Blair et al., 1989). Physical fitness was assessed by a maximal exercise test on a treadmill. All subjects in this analysis were apparently healthy at baseline, with no history or evidence of myocardial infarction, hypertension, stroke, or diabetes, and all had normal ECGs at rest and during maximal exercise. There were 240 deaths in men and 43 deaths in women during follow-up. We observed a strong inverse relationship between physical fitness and all-cause mortality. Age-adjusted all-cause death rates were 3.44 times higher in the least fit quintile of men when compared to the most fit quintile. The corresponding increased risk in the least fit women was 4.65. Cardiovascular disease mortality was even more strongly associated with physical fitness. Increased relative risks for cardiovascular disease of approximately 8 in men and 7 in women were seen in the low-fit when compared to their high-fit peers.

Cancer

Studies reviewed briefly earlier in this chapter show higher cancer death rates, especially for colon cancer, in sedentary individuals than for physically active individuals. The study of Cooper Clinic patients also evaluated the relationship of physical fitness to cancer mortality (Blair et al., 1989). There were 64 cancer deaths in men and 18 in women. Age-adjusted cancer mortality was much higher in the unfit than in the fit. The low-fit men had a cancer death rate of 20.3 per 10,000 person-years of follow-up and the high-fit men had a cancer death rate of 4.7 per 10,000 person-years of follow-up. The corresponding cancer death rates for women were 16.3 and 1.0 for low-fit and high-fit women, respectively. Questions remain regarding selection versus protection and the elucidation of plausible biological mechanisms, but these preliminary results are striking and more research is urgently needed.

Diabetes

Kohl, Gordon, Villegas, and Blair (1992) followed 8,715 men from the Cooper Clinic for 8.2 years to evaluate the relationship of physical fitness to mortality within glucose tolerance strata. Physically fit men had lower age-adjusted all-cause death rates than unfit men at all levels of glucose tolerance. The age-adjusted death rates for unfit and fit men were 82.5 and 45.9 per 10,000 person-years of follow-up in men with the poorest glucose tolerance (fasting blood glucose of ≥ 7.8 mmol or physician-diagnosed non-insulin-dependent diabetes mellitus). After multivariate analyses that controlled for age, systolic blood pressure, serum cholesterol, body mass index, family history of heart disease, smoking, and length of follow-up interval, the relative risk for all-cause mortality was 1.92 (95% confidence limits = 0.75 and 4.90) in the low-fit compared to the high-fit men.

Descriptive Epidemiology

The objectives of descriptive epidemiology include the evaluation of trends in health; establishment of a basis for the planning, provision, and evaluation of health

Table 4.1 Prevalence of Inactivity in Men and Women in Canada and Australia

Country	Percent of women	Percent of men
Canada[a]		
Persons, age ≥ 10 years, who spend ≤ 1.5 kcal · kg^{-1} per day in leisure-time activity	49%	36%
Persons, age ≥ 15 years, who spend < 3 hours per week in leisure-time activity for fewer than 9 months per year	22%	19%
Australia[b]		
Adults who report no exercise during the previous 2 weeks	19%	21%
Adults classified as sedentary because of low energy expenditure	24%	22%

[a]Stephens and Craig, 1990.

[b]Commonwealth Department of the Arts, Sport, the Environment, Tourism and Territories, 1991.

services; and identification of problems to be studied. Several studies have provided such descriptive data for physical activity. Recent estimates of the prevalence of inactivity in Canadian and Australian men and women are presented in Table 4.1. The prevalence of inactivity in these two populations appears to be at least 20%. The prevalence of inactivity in Canada is higher for the energy expenditure variable (49% for women and 36% for men) than for the other estimates of inactivity. This high prevalence is probably a function of the specific methods used and is likely to be an overestimate of the population at high risk. The epidemiological studies reviewed in this report show that the highest risk group for mortality is the least active 15% to 30% of the population. We conclude that the prevalence of high risk sedentary behavior in Canada and Australia is likely to be in the range of 15% to 25%. In the U.S., 58% of the population 18 years of age and older participates in fewer than three 20-minute sessions of leisure-time physical activity per week, and 29% have no leisure-time activity (Siegel et al., 1991). The three studies reviewed here illustrate the varying definitions of physical activity used by investigators. This variability of methods makes conclusive statements concerning the prevalence of physical activity difficult. However, we estimate, conservatively, that 20% of the adult populations in developed countries are at elevated risk for premature death and disease because of their low level of physical activity.

The potential benefit to the public derived from modification of a risk factor can be calculated as a population attributable risk proportion (PAR). By definition, a PAR is the proportion of an outcome (e.g., death or disease) attributed to an exposure (e.g., physical activity or physical fitness). The PAR reflects both the relative risk and the prevalence of a risk factor in the population. For example, a large proportion of the deaths from lung cancer are due to smoking as represented by the PAR. The high PAR is not only due to the high relative risk for smoking but is also because of the large proportion of smokers in the population. If few people smoked, there would be few lung cancer deaths caused by smoking even if the relative risk due to smoking remained constant. Paffenbarger et al. (1986) calculated a PAR of 16.1% for all-cause mortality due to a sedentary lifestyle. Inactivity was second only to cigarette smoking in its PAR for all-cause mortality. Hahn, Teutsch, Rothenberg, and Marks (1990) investigated the impact of no regular exercise on cause-specific as well as all-cause mortality. The following PARs for lack of exercise were found: 23.3% for all-causes, 34.6% for coronary heart disease, 28.9% for stroke, and 15.0% for colorectal cancer. Blair et al. (1989) found that 9% of the mortality in men and 15% in women in the Aerobics Center Longitudinal Study could be attributed to low physical fitness. Thus, modification of activity patterns could potentially have a major impact on mortality rates in the population. The issue at hand is the challenge of encouraging the least active and fit 20% of the population to become active.

Population Promotion of Physical Activity Via Lifestyle Exercise

The exercise program recommended by the American College of Sports Medicine (3 to 5 times per week, 20 to 40 minutes per time, and at 65% to 90% maximum heart rate) often has been used. With this prescription, cardiovascular benefits as well as physiological changes occur, but the adherence rate in such a program is frequently poor. The drop-out rate for such vigorous exercise programs in both men and women is typically 50% or more after 6 months (Dishman, 1982), but lower drop-out rates, 25% to 35%, are reported for moderate activity. The maintenance of moderate physical activity may be more likely to occur than the maintenance of vigorous physical activity.

It is apparent that new strategies are needed to encourage adults to become more physically active, and to reduce the prevalence of high-risk sedentary behavior in the population. One such approach is a lifestyle exercise concept designed to help individuals integrate physical activity into their daily routines (Blair, 1991; Blair, Kohl, & Gordon, 1992). The lifestyle exercise concept is a new way to help sedentary individuals change their attitude toward physical activity through identification, motivation, verbal persuasion, modeling, support, and feedback. It is the goal of the program to utilize intervention strategies and behavioral psychology principles and techniques to elicit a positive change in behavior in sedentary individuals. This approach can help individuals identify the most appropriate ways to incorporate physical activity into their daily schedules. Physical activity management is addressed to identify the types of activity such as walking, taking the stairs, housework, or recreational activities and how individuals can integrate physical activity into their daily lives.

The psychological, physiological, mental, and social benefits of physical activity are stressed in the lifestyle approach. Long- and short-term realistic goal setting is discussed to help the sedentary individuals regulate their own behavior, monitor their progress toward these goals, and change their environment to be more supportive of these goals. Individual barriers are identified along with possible situations that could contribute to lapse, relapse, and collapse. Individuals are helped to develop a solution that will deal with these issues, to act upon the solution, and to evaluate its effectiveness. The lifestyle exercise approach may not be as intimidating for sedentary persons as the traditional exercise prescription.

Conclusion

The research on health and physical activity or physical fitness reviewed here strongly supports the hypothesis that a sedentary lifestyle is unhealthful. Increased rates of morbidity and mortality are seen in sedentary individuals, when compared with their more active peers.

The prevalence of high-risk sedentary behavior appears to be 20% to 30% in the U.S., Canada, and other industrialized countries. This high prevalence leads to a substantial public health burden for sedentary habits.

Traditional methods of physical activity promotion and intervention are partially effective, but drop-out rates are high and long-term maintenance of exercise behavior is low. New methods to promote increased physical activity in the population, such as the lifestyle exercise or active living programs, need to be developed, implemented, and evaluated.

Acknowledgment

We thank Laura Becker for preparing the manuscript and for proofreading.

References

Albanes, D., Blair, A., & Taylor, P.R. (1989). Physical activity and risk of cancer in the NHANES I population. *American Journal of Public Health*, **79**, 744-750.

Blair, S.N. (1991). *Living with exercise*. Dallas: American Health.

Blair, S.N., Kohl, H.W., III, & Gordon, N.F. (1992). Physical activity and health: A lifestyle approach. *Medicine, Exercise, Nutrition, and Health*, **1**, 54-57.

Blair, S.N., Kohl, H.W., III, Paffenbarger, R.S., Jr., Clark, D.G., Cooper, K.H., & Gibbons, L.W. (1989). Physical fitness and all-cause mortality: A prospective study of healthy men and women. *Journal of the American Medical Association*, **262**, 2395-2401.

Caspersen, C.J., Powell, K.E., & Christenson, G.M. (1985). Physical activity, exercise, and physical fitness: Definitions and distinctions for health-related research. *Public Health Reports*, **100**(2), 126-131.

Cherry, T. (1922). A theory of cancer. *Medical Journal of Australia*, **1**, 425-438.

Commonwealth Department of the Arts, Sport, the Environment, Tourism and Territories. (1991). *Pilot survey of the fitness of Australians*. Adelaide, Australia: University of Adelaide, Department of Community Medicine.

Dishman, R.K. (1982). Compliance/adherence in health-related exercise. *Health Psychology*, **1**, 237-267.

Ekelund, L-G., Haskell, W.L., Johnson, J.L., Whaley, F.S., Criqui, M.H., & Sheps, D.S. (1988). Physical fitness as a predictor of cardiovascular mortality in asymptomatic North American men: The Lipid Research Clinics Mortality Follow-Up Study. *New England Journal of Medicine*, **319**, 1379-1384.

Frisch, R.E., Wyshak, G., Albright, N.L., Albright, T.E., Schiff, I., Jones, K.P., Witschi, J., Shiang, E., Koff, E., & Marguglio, M. (1985). Lower prevalence of breast cancer and cancers of the reproductive system among former college athletes compared to non-athletes. *British Journal of Cancer*, **52**, 885-891.

Garabrant, D.H., Peters, J.M., Mack, T.M., & Bernstein, L. (1984). Job activity and colon cancer risk. *American Journal of Epidemiology*, **119**, 1005-1014.

Gerhardsson, M., Norell, S.E., Kiviranta, H., Pedersen, N.L., & Ahlbom, A. (1986). Sedentary jobs and colon cancer. *American Journal of Epidemiology*, **123**, 775-780.

Hahn, R.A., Teutsch, S.M., Rothenberg, R.B., & Marks, J.S. (1990). Excess deaths from nine chronic diseases in the United States, 1986. *Journal of the American Medical Association*, **264**, 2654-2659.

Helmrich, S.P., Ragland, D.R., Leung, R.W., & Paffenbarger, R.S., Jr. (1991). Physical activity and reduced occurrence of non-insulin-dependent diabetes mellitus. *New England Journal of Medicine*, **325**, 147-152.

Kohl, H.W., Gordon, N.F., Villegas, J.A., & Blair, S.N. (1992). Cardiorespiratory fitness, glycemic status, and mortality risk in men. *Diabetes Care*, **15**, 184-192.

Lee, I.-M., Paffenbarger, R.S., Jr., & Hsieh, C-c. (1991). Physical activity and risk of developing colorectal cancer among college alumni. *Journal of the National Cancer Institute*, **83**, 1324-1329.

Lee, I.-M., Paffenbarger, R.S., Jr., & Hsieh, C-c. (1992). Physical activity and risk of prostatic cancer among college alumni. *American Journal of Epidemiology*, **135**, 169-179.

Leon, A.S., Connett, J., Jacobs, D.R., Jr., & Rauramaa, R. (1987). Leisure-time physical activity levels and risk of coronary heart disease and death: The Multiple Risk Factor Intervention Trial. *Journal of the American Medical Association*, **258**, 2388-2395.

Manson, J.E., Rimm, E.B., Stampfer, M.J., Colditz, G.A., Willett, W.C., Krolewski, A.S., Rosner, B., Hennekens, C.H., & Speizer, F.E. (1991). Physical activity and incidence of non-insulin-dependent diabetes mellitus in women. *Lancet*, **338**, 774-778.

Morris, J.N., Clayton, D.G., Everitt, M.G., Semmence, A.M., & Burgess, E.H. (1990). Exercise in leisure time: Coronary attack and death rates. *British Heart Journal*, **63**, 325-334.

Morris, J.N., & Crawford, M.D. (1958). Coronary heart disease and physical activity of work: Evidence of a National Necropsy Survey. *British Medical Journal*, **ii** (December 20), 1485-1496.

Morris, J.N., Everitt, M.G., Pollard, R., Chave, S.P.W., & Semmence, A.M. (1980). Vigorous exercise in leisure-time: Protection against coronary heart disease. *Lancet*, **ii** (December 6), 1207-1210.

Morris, J.N., Heady, J.A., Raffle, P.A.B., Roberts, C.G., & Parks, J.W. (1953). Coronary heart disease and physical activity of work. *Lancet*, **ii**, 1053-1057, 1111-1120.

Paffenbarger, R.S., Jr., & Hale, W.E. (1975). Work activity and coronary heart mortality. *New England Journal of Medicine*, **292**, 545-550.

Paffenbarger, R.S., Jr., Hyde, R.T., Wing, A.L., & Hsieh, C-c. (1986). Physical activity, all-cause mortality, and longevity of college alumni. *New England Journal of Medicine*, **314**, 605-613.

Powell, K.E., Thompson, P.D., Caspersen, C.J., & Kendrick, J.S. (1987). Physical activity and the incidence of coronary heart disease. *Annual Review of Public Health*, **8**, 253-287.

Siegel, P.Z., Brackbill, R.M., Frazier, E.L., Marious, P., Sanderson, L.M., & Waller, M.N. (1991). Behavioral risk factor surveillance, 1986-1990. *Morbidity and Mortality Weekly Report*, **40**(SS-4), 1-47.

Sivertsen, I., & Dahlstrom, A.N. (1922). The relation of muscular activity to carcinoma. A preliminary report. *Journal of Cancer Research*, **6**, 365-378.

Stephens, T., & Craig, C.L. (1990). *The well-being of Canadians: Highlights of the 1988 Campbell's Survey*. Ottawa: Canadian Fitness and Lifestyle Research Institute.

Whittemore, A.S., Wu-Williams, A.H., Lee, M., Shu, Z., Gallagher, R.P., Deng-ao, J., Lun, Z., Xianghui, W., Kun, C., Jung, D., Teh, C.-Z., Chengde, L., Yao, X.J., Paffenbarger, R.S., Jr., & Henderson, B.E. (1990). Diet, physical activity, and colorectal cancer among Chinese in North America and China. *Journal of the National Cancer Institute*, **82**, 915-926.

5

Physical Activity and Health Outcomes in Women

Barbara L. Drinkwater

All of us would like to believe that "active living" improves the quality of life for women and enhances their well-being. Personal experience, anecdotal evidence, and research have established that the female body responds to increased physical activity with improved performance fitness just as the male body does. However, when it comes to identifying data to support the claim that physical activity will decrease a woman's risk of developing health problems associated with a sedentary lifestyle, there are little research data to draw on.

For example, a long-term study of the relationship of lifestyle factors to cholesterol levels and heart disease, appropriately called MR FIT (Multiple Risk Factor Intervention Trials), included 15,000 men and no women. A 1984 report from the Baltimore Longitudinal Study of Aging on "Normal Human Aging" contained no data on women, ignoring the reality that women live longer than men and comprise a larger proportion of the older population.

It is not surprising then to find that data defining the role of physical activity in improving health-related fitness for women is inadequate, particularly relative to the physiologic changes specific to women, such as pregnancy and menopause, or diseases more common in women, such as eating disorders and osteoporosis. Until definitive data are available, conclusions drawn from studies involving only men or from the few studies including women must be tentative. The following sections briefly outline current knowledge in some of these areas and identify areas where more knowledge is needed in order to plan and conduct activity programs for women that will promote health-related fitness.

Physical Activity and Health Outcomes for Young Women

Pregnancy

Many young women who exercise regularly wish to continue their activity during pregnancy. Other less active women have heard that physical activity has benefits for both the pregnant woman and her fetus and want to start an exercise program. While there are still many unanswered questions about the effect of exercise on pregnancy outcomes, there are sources that can assist health professionals plan a safe exercise program for women during pregnancy. A concise review of research in this area (Wolfe, Ohtake, Mottola, & McGrath, 1989), and a more exhaustive discussion of the physiological changes that accompany pregnancy, how these changes affect the woman's response to exercise, and the practical application of this information (Mittelmark, Wiswell, & Drinkwater, 1991) are valuable sources of information. Although evidence to date does not support the theory that regular exercise will improve pregnancy outcomes, exercise within the constraints recommended by the American College of Obstetricians and Gynecologists (ACOG) guidelines (in press) does seem to improve both the physical and psychological well-being of the mother, preserving muscle tone, strength, and endurance, and enhancing energy level, mood, and self-image.

The cardinal rule, of course, is to do nothing that will harm the mother or the fetus. For that reason, the ACOG guidelines are conservative and designed for the general female population, not the elite athlete. Pushing the boundaries of these guidelines is entering an unexplored area and could expose both the mother and infant to significant risks. Until adequate research is available to document fetal and maternal response to more strenuous exercise, exceeding the ACOG guidelines should only be done with the advice and supervision of a physician. Those tempted to encourage women to go beyond the ACOG guidelines should read Gallup's (1991) chapter, *Legal aspects of exercise prescription and pregnancy.*

Obesity

While obesity is a significant health risk, many women make the mistake of defining obesity by cultural standards rather than health standards. As a result, their forays into dieting are often met with resistance by their own genetic and physiologic makeup leading to a continuous battle against their own biological nature. In all too many cases this battle ends in disappointment and another cycle of weight loss and weight regained. Until our culture accepts the notion that competent and attractive women come in all sizes, fitness and health professionals may have little success in discouraging healthy, nonobese women from joining the thousands of other women in an unrealistic quest for weight loss.

There are, of course, women who should reduce their body fat. Although moderate obesity is defined as 41% to 100% overweight, attendees of a National Institutes of Health consensus conference in 1985 determined that health risks can begin in people who are only 20% overweight (Brownell, 1988). Along with the usual litany of medical conditions associated with obesity are some specific to women, such as menstrual irregularities and cancers of the reproductive tract (Lampman & Schteingart, 1989). Women do have one advantage. Upper body fat, which occurs most often in men, is associated with a higher incidence of cardiovascular morbidity and mortality.

The secret of responsible weight loss is the combination of a sensible diet and a well-designed exercise program. Dieting alone results in a loss of both fat and lean body mass (LBM); adding exercise has been reported to spare LBM (Hagan, Upton, Wong, & Whittam, 1986; Zuti & Golding, 1976). The exercise effect on lean tissue may depend on the training protocol and degree of obesity. One study of an extremely obese group on a 600-kcal diet found no difference in body composition changes between those who did or did not exercise in addition to the diet restriction (Lampman & Schteingart, 1989).

Relatively few of the studies that have examined the interaction between exercise and diet on body composition have included women. Gender differences in metabolism, fat deposition, hormones, or essential fat may influence women's response to the combination of caloric restriction and increased energy expenditure as well as to different exercise regimens. One area which has not been addressed is whether exercise can modulate the changes in body composition that occur following menopause.

There are a number of excellent reviews of this topic that should be consulted by anyone planning or conducting exercise programs for the obese (Brownell, 1988; Lampman & Schteingart, 1989; Pollock, Wilmore, & Fox, 1984; Wells, 1991).

Eating Disorders

Desperate attempts to lose weight can lead to serious dietary disturbances (Wilson & Eldredge, 1992). While the etiology of anorexia nervosa and bulimia is still a matter of conjecture, these authors have suggested that there is a continuum of "disordered eating" among women, clinical eating disorders at one end of the scale and subclinical but abnormal eating patterns at the other. Exercise in this setting is frequently used as another technique to control weight, and rather than enhancing health, it may aggravate the problem. Fitness professionals should be alert to behaviors characteristic of these serious disorders (American Psychiatric Association, 1987). The treatment of anorexia nervosa and bulimia is long and difficult and is best handled by professionals who specialize in these disorders.

Sport for some young women has become a risk factor for osteoporosis, a disease usually associated with the elderly. Pressure to reduce body weight for improved performance in some sporting events has pushed susceptible young athletes into a disordered eating pattern. As the severity of the disorder increases, changes in the reproductive cycle result in lowered estrogen levels and, in turn, decreased bone mass. It now appears that some of this loss is irreversible, placing these women at risk for premature osteoporosis (Drinkwater, Bruemmer, & Chesnut, 1990).

Research is urgently needed to establish the relationship between weight control measures and changes in the reproductive cycle. Women should not have to place their future health at risk in order to succeed in sports. An excellent source of information for those who work with athletes is a recent book edited by Brownell, Rodin, and Wilmore (1992).

Menstrual Cycle

The menstrual cycle has little effect on the activity of women who exercise moderately for fun and fitness, nor is activity likely to affect their cycle (Wells, 1991). Instead, concern today is focused on the elite athlete and other women who exercise vigorously and experience menstrual irregularities ranging from an inadequate luteal phase to primary and secondary amenorrhea. Exercise per se cannot be identified as the single causative factor in these disturbances. Warren (1992) suggests that other factors such as low body weight or fat, diet, psychological stress, sudden weight loss, and prior menstrual history determine which athletes will experience menstrual dysfunction.

Too many athletes simply assume that these conditions are a normal consequence of serious training and do nothing about them. In fact, there are a number of pathological states which cause cessation of menses and which can and should be treated. Even when these conditions are ruled out, bone loss in the untreated hypoestrogenic athlete may place her at risk for premature osteoporosis (Drinkwater et al., 1984). Because the most rapid phase of bone loss occurs in the 3 or 4 years following the decrease in endogenous estrogen, decisions regarding therapeutic interventions must be made soon after the condition becomes evident. The optimal therapy is a slight decrease in activity and a slight increase in caloric intake, which usually results in resumption of normal menses within 2 to 3 months. If menses does not resume or the woman is unwilling or unable to make these adjustments, pharmacological intervention may be necessary to prevent bone loss. Although a number of physicians are prescribing estrogen and progesterone combinations, there are no prospective studies examining the efficacy of the various formulations and dosages.

Prevention of menstrual dysfunction among active women should be a top research priority. Further discussion of this topic can be found in Brownell et al., (1992) and Wells (1991).

Physical Activity as Adjunct Therapy for Health Problems of Older Women

Hypertension

Although hypertension is more common in women than men after age 65, with a concomitant two- to threefold increase in the risk for stroke, women have been underrepresented in studies of the effect of chronic exercise on blood pressure. Only 4 of 32 studies cited by Tipton (1984), in reviews of exercise, training, and hypertension, included women. While the results were generally positive, the studies were far from definitive for women's health. More recently, Blair et al. (1989) provided a link between fitness level, hypertension, and mortalitiy rates. Among women with a systolic pressure above 140 torr, there were 347 deaths in the low fit group, 19 among the moderately fit, and none in the high fitness group.

There have been no studies examining the effect of gender related differences in hypertension on the response to habitual physical activity. Since risk factors for hypertension in women include menopause, use of oral contraceptives, hysterectomy, and nonuse of hormone replacement therapy following menopause, the interaction of these factors with physical activity and hypertension should be investigated.

Coronary Heart Disease

Mortality rates from coronary heart disease (CHD) in men and women begin to converge after age 50. By age 65, deaths from CHD are approximately the same for both sexes. Yet few of the studies relating physical activity to the reduction of risk factors for CHD involve women. On the surface, it would seem that the positive effect of exercise on the primary risk factors for CHD, cholesterol, hypertension, and obesity, would be independent of sex. However, Gibbons, Blair, Cooper, and Smith (1983) found that fitness, as measured by treadmill time, accounted for only a small portion (0.3% to 2.3%) of the variance in risk factors in a group of 1,700 Caucasion women. When age and body mass index (BMI) were added, the percent ranged from 2% to 21%.

Is it possible that other risk factors, independent of activity level, are important in determining women's risk for CHD? For example, no mention was made of estrogen status in the aforementioned study. Yet premenopausal women have a lower incidence of CHD than men of comparable age, and estrogen replacement therapy (ERT) appears to have a strong protective effect against cardiovascular disease in postmenopausal women. Is treadmill time the best indication of "fitness" in women? What is the interactive effect of estrogen and fitness?

Peripheral Vascular Disease

There are several vascular problems, such as Raynaud's disease and migraine headaches, that are more common in women than in men. Both appear to be related to hormonal influence on the sympathetic control of cutaneous blood flow. Women also have a greater susceptibility to inflammatory vascular diseases, such as lupus and other autoimmune disorders, and venous thrombosis. The effect of physical activity in the prevention of these disorders is largely unknown. Walking has been shown to increase exercise tolerance in patients with claudication, independent of gender. Before prescribing exercise, however, it is important to ascertain whether the woman has cardiac insufficiency as well as peripheral vascular problems.

Osteoporosis

Weightbearing physical activity is an essential requirement for bone health. Without the beneficial effect of gravitational or mechanical loading on the axial and appendicular skeleton, there is a rapid and marked loss of bone. Whether the generalized decrease in physical activity as one ages has a cumulative negative impact on bone mass is unknown. However, there is ample evidence that active individuals have a greater skeletal mass than those who are inactive. There are also data to support the concept that those who are sedentary can increase bone mass by becoming more active.

Active postmenopausal women have a higher bone mass than sedentary women (+6.8%) and when sedentary older women participate in long-term activity programs (>8 months) there is usually a slight increase in their lumbar bone mineral density (BMD). The most important question is whether exercise can prevent osteoporosis, which is defined as a disease characterized by low bone mass and microarchitectural deterioration of bone tissue leading to enhanced bone fragility, and a consequent increase in fracture risk.

Three epidemiologic studies (Astrom, Ahnqvist, Beertema, & Jonsson, 1987; Cooper, Barker, & Wickham, 1988; Wickham et al., 1989) have reported fewer hip fractures among women with a history of physical activity than in a less active group. While this is encouraging, the studies were limited in their control of confounding factors. The final assessment of the protective effect of exercise awaits further study.

General principles of physical conditioning, which apply to other physiologic systems, may apply to the skeleton as well and should be considered in planning or evaluating an exercise program to promote bone health. These include the following:

- *The Principle of Specificity*: Exercise provides a local osteogenic effect.
- *The Principle of Overload*: The need for a progressive increase in the intensity of the exercise for continued improvement.
- *The Principle of Reversibility*: The positive effect of exercise on bone will be lost if the exercise program is discontinued.
- *The Principle of Initial Values*: Those who have the lowest bone mass should have the greatest percent improvement.
- *The Principle of Diminishing Returns*: As the biological ceiling is approached, more and more effort will be required to obtain further gain.

In spite of its beneficial effect on bone, there is no evidence that exercise can substitute for hormone replacement therapy (HRT) as a means of preventing bone loss in postmenopausal women. Physical activity can be an important adjunct to HRT by helping older women improve coordination, balance, and muscle strength which may decrease the likelihood of fracture independent of bone mass by preventing falls and/or minimizing the trauma of a fall.

Cancer

Studies of the relationship between physical activity and cancer in women have been retrospective and very limited. Most of the information comes from a single group of college alumnae (Frisch, Wyshak, Albright, Albright, & Schiff, 1989; Frisch et al., 1985). The authors examined the incidence of cancer in women identified as either athletes or non-athletes during their college years. The definition of athlete was very liberal; any woman who was a member of an intramural team in college was considered an athlete. Since these teams seldom practiced or trained, the actual fitness level of these women was unlikely to have been equivalent to that of present day female athletes.

The relative risk for breast cancer and cancers of the reproductive system, thyroid, lung, bladder, and digestive system was significantly higher for nonathletes. Frisch et al. (1985) suggest that early participation in sports establishes a lifestyle that in some way decreases the risk of cancer. For example, 73.5% of former athletes still exercised regularly while only 57% of the nonathletes were currently active. However, there are a number of potential confounding factors as well as the problem of self selection in these studies. While the data are interesting, it is premature to assume physical activity per se is protective against cancer.

Physical Activity and Independence in the "Golden Years"

Exercise and Menopause

One of the more serious concerns many women have about aging revolves around the question of independence. Will they be healthy and vigorous enough to remain independent throughout their postmenopausal years? Fortunately, this is one area where there are data to demonstrate convincingly that older women respond to physical conditioning programs by improving those physiological parameters essential to independence—aerobic capacity, strength, and flexibility. In fact, active older women may be as much as 1 or 2 decades younger physiologically than their inactive peers. While no one can guarantee that exercise will prolong life, it certainly will enhance the quality of life for older women who value their independence.

Maintaining Functional Abilities

As a result of the changes in the oxygen transport system, as well as other changes at the tissue level, aerobic power tends to decrease with age. If a woman remains sedentary throughout her life, the progressive loss in aerobic power may eventually reach a point where she is unable to handle the basic physical demands of daily living. While some of the functional changes that occur with aging are permanent, others can be reversed to some degree through physical training programs. For example, the improvement in aerobic power of older women as a result of physical training is relatively the same as that of younger women, an increase of about 18%.

Changes in lean body mass, including a decrease in muscle mass, declining numbers of Type I, "slow twitch," fibers, and smaller Type II, "fast twitch," fibers may account for part of the decline in strength with aging. However, as recent studies have shown, strength training can result in remarkable gains even in the very old (Fiatarone et al., 1990).

Decreases in flexibility observed with age occur primarily in joints that are seldom used, therefore suggesting that inactivity contributes to the apparent aging effect. As with the other components of fitness, the range of motion about the joints can be improved through a physical training program.

It is heartening to see how many of the decreases in functional capacity in older women can be reversed in well-planned physical activity programs. For older women, performance fitness can be as important as health-related fitness in enabling them to maintain their independence.

Summary and Conclusions

Women of all ages benefit from physical activity. The improvements in performance fitness following a physical conditioning program are well documented. Although the current emphasis appears to focus on health-related fitness, the importance of performance fitness for women should not be overlooked. The demands of everyday living make it imperative that women attain and maintain a satisfactory level of aerobic power, strength, and flexibility.

There are areas of concern specific to women, such as pregnancy, menses, and menopause, where the effect of exercise on both health and performance fitness has not been thoroughly investigated. While it is likely that women as well as men will gain health benefits from a regular program of physical activity, there are not sufficient data to state unequivocally what those benefits may be.

With the exception of osteoporosis and pregnancy, the health-related benefits of physical activity for women have been largely ignored. Data to support a role for active living in preventing diseases more common in or specific to women, such as menstrual dysfunction or arthritis, are either inconclusive or nonexistent. If women are to gain positive health benefits from the active living concept, a greater effort must be made to identify and address the health-related fitness concerns of women.

References

American College of Obstetricians and Gynecologists. (in press). *ACOG guidelines: Exercise during pregnancy and the postnatal period.* Washington, DC: Author.

American Psychiatric Association. (1987). *Diagnostic and statistical manual of mental disorders* (3rd ed., rev. ed.).Washington, DC: Author.

Astrom, J., Ahnqvist, S., Beertema, J., & Jonsson, B. (1987). Physical activity in women sustaining fracture of the neck of the femur. *Journal of Bone and Joint Surgery*, **69-B**, 381-383.

Blair, S.N., Kohl, H.W., Paffenbarger, R.S., Clark, D.G., Cooper, K.H., & Gibbons, L.W. (1989). Physical fitness and all-cause mortality: A prospective study of healthy men and women. *Journal of the American Medical Association,* **262**, 2395-2401.

Brownell, K.D. (1988). Weight management and body composition. In S.N. Blair, P. Painter, R.P. Pate, L.K. Smith, & C.B. Taylor (Eds.), *Resource manual for guidelines for exercise testing and prescription* (pp. 355-361). Philadelphia, PA: Lea & Febiger.

Brownell, K.D., Rodin, J., & Wilmore, J.H. (1992). *Eating, body weight and performance in athletes.* Philadelphia, PA: Lea & Febiger.

Cooper, C., Barker, D.J.P., & Wickham, C. (1988). Physical activity, muscle strength, and calcium intake in fracture of the proximal femur in Britain. *British Medical Journal*, **297**, 1443-1446.

Drinkwater, B.L., Bruemmer, B., & Chesnut, C.H., III. (1990). Menstrual history as a determinant of current bone density in young athletes. *Journal of the American Medical Association*, **263**, 545-548.

Drinkwater, B.L., Nilson, K., Chesnut, C.H., III, Bremner, W.J., Shainholtz, S., & Southworth, M.B. (1984). Bone mineral content of amenorrheic and eumenorrheic athletes. *New England Journal of Medicine*, **311**, 277-281.

Fiatarone, M.A., Marks, E.C., Ryan, N.D., Meredith, C.N., Lipsitz, L.A., & Evans, W.J. (1990). High-intensity strength training in nonagenarians. *Journal of the American Medical Association*, **263**, 3029-3034.

Frisch, R.E., Wyshak, G., Albright, N.L., Albright, T.E., & Schiff, I. (1989). Lower prevalence of non-reproductive system cancers among female former college athletes. *Medicine and Science in Sports and Exercise*, **21**, 250-253.

Frisch, R.E., Wyshak, G., Albright, N.L., Albright, T.E., Schiff, I., Jones, K.P., Witschi, J., Shiang, E., Koff, E., & Marguglio, M. (1985). Lower prevalence of breast cancer and cancers of the reproductive system among former college athletes compared to non-athletes. *British Journal of Cancer*, **52**, 885-891.

Gallup, E. (1991). Legal aspects of exercise prescription and pregnancy. In R. A. Mittelmark, R. A. Wiswell, & B. L. Drinkwater (Eds.), *Exercise in pregnancy* (pp. 293-297). Baltimore, MD: Williams & Wilkins.

Gibbons, L.W., Blair, S.N., Cooper, K.H., & Smith, M. (1983). Association between coronary heart disease risk factors and physical fitness in healthy adult women. *Circulation*, **67**, 977-982.

Hagan, R.D., Upton, S.J., Wong, L., & Whittam, J. (1986). The effects of aerobic conditioning and/or caloric restriction in overweight men and women. *Medicine and Science in Sports and Exercise*, **18**, 87-94.

Lampman, R.M. & Schteingart, D.E. (1989). Moderate and extreme obesity. In B.A. Franklin, S. Gordon, & G.C. Timmis (Eds.), *Exercise in modern medicine* (pp. 156-174). Baltimore, MD: Williams & Wilkins.

Mittelmark, R.A., Wiswell, R.A., & Drinkwater, B.L. (Eds.) (1991). *Exercise in pregnancy*. Baltimore, MD: Williams & Wilkins.

Pollock, M. L., Wilmore, J.H., & Fox, S.M. (1984). *Exercise in health and disease* (pp. 29-46, pp. 97-125). Philadelphia, PA: W.B Saunders Co.

Tipton, C.M. (1984). Exercise, training, and hypertension. In R.L. Terjung (Ed.), *Exercise and sport sciences reviews* (pp. 245-306). Baltimore, MD: Williams & Wilkins.

Warren, M.P. (1992). Eating, body weight, and menstrual function. In K.D. Brownell, J. Rodin, and J.H. Wilmore (Eds.), *Eating, body weight, and performance in athletes* (pp. 222-234). Philadelphia, PA: Lea & Febiger.

Wells, C.L. (1991). *Women, sport, and performance* (pp. 219-235). Champaign, IL: Human Kinetics Books.

Wickham, C.A.C., Walsh, K., Cooper, C., Parker, D.J.P., Margetts, B.M., Morris, J., & Bruce, S. A. (1989). Dietary calcium, physical activity, and risk of hip fracture: A prospective study. *British Medical Journal*, **299**, 889-892.

Wilson, G.T., & Eldredge, K.L. (1992). Pathology and development of eating disorders: Implications for athletes. In K.D. Brownell, J. Rodin, and J.H. Wilmore (Eds.), *Eating, body weight, and performance in athletes* (pp. 115-127). Philadelphia, PA: Lea & Febiger.

Wolfe, L.A., Ohtake, P.J., Mottola, M.F., & McGrath, M.J. (1989). Physiological interactions between pregnancy and aerobic exercise. In K.B. Pandolf (Ed.), *Exercise and sport sciences reviews* (pp. 295-351). Baltimore, MD: Williams & Wilkins.

Zuti, W. B., & Golding, L. (1976). Comparing diet and exercise as weight reduction tools. *Physician and Sportsmedicine*, **4**, 49-53.

6

Potential Health Benefits of Active Living for Persons With Chronic Conditions

Michael T. Sharratt
Jacqueline K. Sharratt

There is mounting evidence that apparently healthy, but otherwise sedentary, men and women can benefit from an increase in physical activity levels. An equally strong case can be made for the potential health benefits of active living for those with chronic conditions. The difficulty is that in the latter case there may be a functional limitation which can complicate the prescription for increased physical activity. The magnitude of this challenge is growing steadily as the population ages. For example, of the 3.3 million Canadians (12% of the population) who have a functional limitation or disability, 40% are 65 years of age or older and not yet institutionalized (Lavigne & Morin, 1991). By the year 2011, it is estimated that 25% of the entire population will exceed 55 years of age. Therefore, the implications for health care expenses and personal well-being in the golden years warrant an approach to life which prolongs independent living. The nature and severity of the functional limitation determine the extent to which this is a realistic goal.

The challenge is to get these people moving, because almost one-half of the Canadian population reporting functional limitations are sedentary. Thus, the functional status and well-being of people with chronic conditions is measurable and capable of substantial improvement in response to active living, if only they can be persuaded to take the first step.

Epidemiology of Functional Limitations

The premise in this paper is that impairment should be related primarily to the functional limitation, rather than the chronic condition, that caused the problem. For example, the extent of the impairment may extend from troublesome (e.g., allergic rhinitis) to crippling but not

life-threatening (e.g., rheumatic arthritis) with inclusion of those chronic conditions which are almost always fatal (e.g., lung cancer) (Powell, Caspersen, Koplan, & Ford, 1989). Consequently, one has to be cautious not to generalize either the extent of impairment or the nature of the intervention based simply on the disease entity.

In the context of this paper, a disability or functional limitation is defined as, "any restriction or lack (resulting from an impairment) of ability to perform an activity in the manner or within the range considered normal for a human being" (World Health Organization, 1980, p. 143). Furthermore, the nature of a disability may be defined or characterized in terms of mobility (i.e., limited ability to walk and/or carry objects), agility (i.e., limited dexterity related to bending, dressing, or grasping), seeing, hearing, speaking, and learning.

As the population ages the older cohort will live longer, and there is an increased likelihood that they will live with more than one disabling condition. For example, there has been a progressive trend toward decreased mortality for coronary heart disease (Canadian Centre for Health Information, 1989) without a concomitant decrease in incidence. Meanwhile, the onslaught of osteoarthritis is virtually inevitable with advancing age. The challenge will be to remain physically active in spite of musculoskeletal and cardiorespiratory limitations. Failure to meet the challenge will result in a lifestyle characterized by immobility, dependency, and compromised well-being.

Common Chronic Conditions Resulting in Functional Limitations

The most prevalent disabling conditions in Canada are associated with diseases of the musculoskeletal system and connective tissue (Department of the Secretary of

State of Canada, 1986). Specifically, arthritis and rheumatism (attributed primarily to aging) and "other musculoskeletal problems" (attributed primarily to accidents) dominate (37%) as causes of disability. Sight and hearing disorders are the second largest cause of disability (21%) with diseases of the circulatory system (e.g., ischemic heart disease and stroke) being third (14%). Diseases of the respiratory system (e.g., emphysema and asthma) and endocrine disorders (e.g., diabetes) are of the same magnitude (5%) but substantially less prevalent than the former disease states.

Impact of Functional Limitations

In the past, investigators have often used inappropriate outcome measures to justify the efficacy of a physical activity intervention. From a patient's point of view, it is more salient to describe the impact of limitations on daily functioning and well-being than to appreciate typical mortality and morbidity statistics.

Stewart et al. (1989) report the first large-scale attempt to describe the profiles of the functioning and well-being of patients with a variety of chronic conditions. She and her colleagues developed a general health survey which is sensitive to those health aspects considered to be most relevant to the patients. The six health concepts are physical, social, and role functioning; mental health; health perception; and bodily pain. When the health survey was administered to over 9,000 patients, half of whom had at least one of nine chronic conditions, those with the chronic conditions reported markedly worse health concepts than patients with acute medical problems. In addition, each condition had a unique profile among the various health components. The significance of this innovative study is that it now provides a potential tool for assessing the efficacy of intervention designed to change quality of life. It may prove to be even more effective than the Nottingham Health Profile which was recently validated by O'Brien, Buxton, and Patterson (1992).

Active Living as a Health Promotion Strategy

There has been a growing awareness by Canadians over the past 25 years that the potential benefits of regular physical activity involve more than the well-documented increases in physical fitness. The adaptations which occur within various body systems in response to systematic and prolonged physical activity are unequivocal. However, it is noteworthy, in the most recent position statement by the American College of Sports Medicine (ACSM, 1990) that the classic recommendations of duration, intensity, and frequency have been modified to accommodate the notion of lower-intensity, long-duration activities yielding similar improvements to higher-intensity, shorter-duration activities *if* the total energy costs of the activities are equal.

Concurrent with the ACSM statement, the American Heart Association (AHA) also issued its *Statement on Exercise* intended for health professionals (McHenry et al., 1990). After summarizing the known benefits of "physical training," the authors provide the following recommendation regarding implementation: "Persons of all ages should be encouraged to develop a physically active lifestyle as part of a comprehensive program for disease prevention and health promotion" (p. 397). A companion document was also published by the American Heart Association (Fletcher, Froelicher, Hartley, Haskell, & Pollock, 1990) in which the standards and guidelines for exercise testing and training were outlined in great detail. These guidelines were designed for persons free of clinical manifestations of cardiovascular disease, and for those with known cardiovascular disease. In either case, the question arises as to how much exercise or physical activity is needed for an "optimum effect." An elegant response to that perennial question is apparent in the AHA report. It suggests that the threshold of intensity to achieve benefit is variable between individuals and may be consistent with walking for many people. The important point is that intensity is less important than the total amount of activity for promoting health.

In summary, the classic physiological benefits of systematic physical activity have been well documented and noted in the position papers. In addition, both expert groups have recognized the health benefits that might be associated with low intensity physical activity. This point of view is totally consistent with the concept of active living and clearly embraces those individuals with one or more chronic conditions. Therefore, the notion of active living as a viable health promotion strategy is intuitively obvious and strongly endorsed by the scientific community.

Empirical Evidence for Tertiary Health Benefits of Active Living

It seems reasonable to assume that the most cost-effective way to attenuate or at least forestall the onset of chronic conditions is through primary prevention. To the extent that lifestyle "diseases of choice" can be influenced by wise behavior decisions, this seems to be a worthy goal. Unfortunately, the prevailing medical model has focused on disease control, cure, and eradication, where possible. In this context, both the mind set and the resources attend to people who are already sick rather than to those who may yet have an alternative.

Once a chronic disease entity is in place, there is no expectation that active living will remove it. Furthermore, those who would promote the longevity benefits of a physical activity intervention are misguided and generally lack support from carefully designed studies. However, the real payoff is too often under-reported or presented in an apologetic tone. For example, in the coronary heart disease literature, it is not uncommon to note the lack of a statistically significant mortality improvement in spite of a systematic exercise intervention over time. Then, almost as an aside, there might be the comment that most of the intervention group felt much better as a result of exercise and had an improved quality of life. Unfortunately, the efficacy of psychosocial studies related to cardiac rehabilitation has been questioned severely for a lack of methodological soundness (Greenland, 1991; Leon et al., 1990).

The rest of this section deals with four chronic conditions as examples of causes of functional limitations which can be influenced positively by physical activity interventions. Arthritis and cardiovascular disease are major afflictions in Canada in terms of functional limitations. In addition, chronic obstructive pulmonary disease and diabetes compromise the quality of life on a daily basis. Active living holds the promise of ameliorating these difficulties for some and enhancing coping strategies for others.

Arthritis

Arthritis is the most prevalent chronic condition in Canada (Statistics Canada, 1990) and is cited most often as the principal cause of role limitations by middle aged and older women. Men of those ages cite it as the second-ranked cause of limitations after diseases of the heart (Laplante, 1988). Arthritis takes many forms with the degree of pain and disablement dependent upon the type of arthritis. Rheumatoid arthritis and osteoarthritis are the two broad categories of the disease. In the former case, the synovial membrane surrounding the joint becomes inflamed while the latter is characterized by degeneration of the articular cartilage (Schumacher, 1988). In both cases, the quality of life may be seriously compromised and patients must deal with a decreased sense of well-being.

Intuitively, one might infer that an increase in physical activity, associated with joint mobility, would be painful for arthritis sufferers and contraindicated by default. Certainly, it does not make sense to challenge rheumatoid arthritis during an acute flare, but in the absence of acute inflammation the avoidance of aerobic activity is probably the worst choice that could be made. Ike, Lampman, and Castor (1989) provide an excellent review of arthritis and exercise in which they cite compelling evidence for judicious physical activity. In addition to the physical gains in aerobic capacity, flexibility, functional status, and muscle strength (Minor, Hewett, Webel, Anderson, & Kay, 1989), they point out the equally important subjective components of quality of life, pain tolerance, mood, and social activity. It is remarkable that, in spite of the pronounced effect of arthritis on physical dysfunctions, these people often make

successful accommodations so their roles and daily activities are not seriously affected by the disease (Verbrugge, Lepkowski, & Konkol, 1991). This is exactly the goal which is promoted by an Atlanta-based program called PACE (People with Arthritis Can Exercise). The eight-week program teaches nearly 70 exercises designed to give a complete body workout and encourage socialization (Samples, 1990). Most of the exercises are targeted to the performance of functional daily tasks such as unscrewing lids, pulling up back zippers, doing up buttons, and general mobility activities.

The incidence of rheumatoid arthritis is three times greater amongst women than men, and the vast majority of patients are between 25 and 55 years of age (Fallowfield, 1990). This means that afflicted women will bear the burden of this disease for many years and should adopt optimal coping strategies early in the disease process. For example, it is known that periods of immobility (especially following a night's sleep) tend to worsen the pain and stiffness (Spector, 1990). For this reason, it is particularly important to resist the temptation to maintain immobility throughout the day. Prolonged bedrest increases the probability of muscle atrophy leading to decreased strength, imbalance between agonist and antagonist muscle groups, and contracture of surrounding soft tissues and tendons (Hicks, 1990). Hicks also points out the insidious trap of putting a pillow behind the knees at night to decrease the pain associated with a full extended knee. This practice may lead to joint contracture, inappropriate use of the quadriceps muscle, and an ultimate restraint on muscle function integral to daily activities. One intervention that has proven successful in terms of reversing muscle weakness and atrophy is the use of exercise therapy in a heated swimming pool (Danneskiold-Samsoe, Lynberg, Risum, & Telling, 1987). However, this must be instituted before major contractures set in. Another attractive exercise alternative is bicycling. Namey (1990) presents a strong case for this weight-supported activity in terms of both physical and psychological benefits. However, one of the strongest arguments in favor of this physical activity modality is the renewed sense of independence which is quickly achieved by overcoming a physical limitation.

Osteoarthritis tends to be the result of degenerative changes in the cartilage with secondary changes around the joints (Fallowfield, 1990). The weight bearing joints such as the hips and knees have been found to be especially affected. Consequently, there is speculation that regular exercise may lead to this degenerative problem. Millions of people have responded to the message that physical inactivity is an independent risk factor for coronary artery disease. However, they require reassurance that they are not trading premature coronary heart disease for long term pain and disability. This question was addressed systematically by Panush and Brown (1987) in their review of exercise and arthritis. Although many studies hypothesize that sports stress and repetitive trauma lead to osteoarthritis, there are serious design flaws and misinterpretations which require better research. Pascale and Grana (1989) suggest that running and other impact-loading sports do not cause arthritis in normal weight-bearing joints but can accelerate the disease in damaged joints. Not enough attention has been paid to the characteristics of the participant and the activity environment. Nevertheless, it seems reasonable that the severe torque which is required of specific joints during football, baseball, or gymnastics, for example, would eventually challenge the integrity of the tissues surrounding the joint. Of equal concern is the potential deterioration which might be associated with more modest activities of mass participation (e.g., brisk walking, swimming, cycling). The interpretation of Panush and Brown (1987) is that modest physical activity carried out over many years need not lead to inevitable joint injury as long as there is no underlying joint abnormality.

Cardiovascular Disease

Cardiovascular Disease (CVD) has been the leading cause of death in Canada since the first national mortality statistics were published in 1921. CVD accounts for almost half of all deaths each year (Canadian Centre for Health Information, 1989) with 46,000 deaths due to ischemic heart disease in 1987, which includes 26,000 deaths due to acute myocardial infarction. The good news is that mortality rates have declined 42% for males and 58% for females between 1951 and 1987. This decline in CVD mortality rates contributes to approximately 20,000 fewer male and 12,000 fewer female deaths in 1987. Not surprisingly, the prevention or at least modification of major independent risk factors has contributed substantially to this decline. For example, encouraging trends have provided optimism for the preventive role of systematic physical activity (Powell et al., 1989; Powell, Thompson, Caspersen, & Kendrick, 1987) especially since sedentary lifestyle is the most prevalent (58%) modifiable risk factor for coronary heart disease (Centres for Disease Control, 1990). Nevertheless, there still remain millions of men and women in Canada and the United States with clinically diagnosed CVD who have eluded or survived premature cardiac events and must cope with the disease on a daily basis. About 25% of all disability pensions paid by the Canada Pension Plan before age 65 are based on a diagnosis of cardiovascular disease (Canadian Centre for Health Information, 1989). Therefore, the search continues for optimal programs of rehabilitation which will enhance the quality of life and perhaps forestall a subsequent fatal cardiac event. In any case, the field has come a long way from the days in 1956 when it was recommended that after myocardial infarction, "patients should be confined to bed at once and remain there 3 to 6 weeks, or longer" (Wood, 1956).

One of the most sophisticated of the major cardiac rehabilitation trials was conducted by Rechnitzer et al. (1983) in the late 1970s. A total of 733 men with carefully documented myocardial infarction were randomly assigned to a vigorous or a light exercise program. It was anticipated that reinfarctions would be decreased by 50% in the high intensity exercise program over the course of 4 years. However, the entry criteria were so rigid that the mortality rate was much less than anticipated. A number of additional factors contributed to the observation that the overall reinfarction rates were not significantly different between groups. Nevertheless, one unintended finding was the beneficial effect of low intensity exercise combined with social support. This combination resulted in an overall reinfarction rate reduction of 13%.

In total, there have been about 14 major studies of tertiary prevention involving over 5,000 patients. In only one of these studies (Kallio, 1981) has a significant reduction in cardiovascular mortality been noted and even this result became nonsignificant when all causes of death were considered. It has become abundantly clear, over a period of 20 years, that no single research study will be able to test the exercise hypothesis effectively. In fact, Shephard (1989) provides an excellent critique of the studies to date including the factors which hamper the demonstration of a decreasing cardiac mortality rate with exercise. Consequently, there has been growing acceptance of a technique which pools information through meta-analysis. For example, May, Eberlein, and Friberg (1984) combined exercise intervention studies for cardiac rehabilitation and reported a significant 19% decrease in cardiovascular mortality associated with an exercise program. Meanwhile, Oldridge, Guyatt, Fischer, and Rimm (1988) pooled 10 randomized clinical trials comprising 4,347 patients while O'Connor et al. (1989) examined 22 randomized trials of rehabilitation with exercise involving 4,554 patients. In both cases, the pooled odds ratios for cardiovascular death were significantly lower in the exercise rehabilitation groups with no significant difference for nonfatal recurrent myocardial infarction. Lipkin (1990) actually questions the appropriateness of pooling these data in view of the differences in patient populations, mortality, and exercise programs between studies. Certainly, the limitations of male subjects and upper age limits of about 70 years reduces generalizability. Nevertheless, the reduction of 25% for Oldridge and 20% for O'Connor in cardiovascular-related mortality associated with exercise rehabilitation programs is impressive.

Finally, there are several recent papers (Fallen et al., 1991; Fletcher et al., 1990; Greenland, 1991; Leon et al., 1990; Myers & Froelicher, 1990) which have attempted to capture the current status of exercise-based cardiac rehabilitation and management. Each paper brings a wealth of wisdom and experience to the critical issues. Without exception, exercise conditioning is embraced as an integral component within a total program designed to enable patients with cardiac disorders to resume active and productive lives within the limitations imposed by their disease process (Fletcher et al., 1990; Greenland, 1991; Leon et al., 1990). This approach does not preclude clinical judgment based on individual patient needs (Fallen et al., 1991). In fact, this becomes exceedingly relevant when the patient's perceptions differ from those of the health professional (Wenger, 1990). For example, a very high priority for a minority of patients might relate to unrelenting psychosocial challenges. However, a critical question has been raised about how well these data can be quantified with the use of questionnaires (Myers & Froelicher, 1990). Anxiety and depression are common sequelae to a sudden unexpected life-threatening illness, but the symptoms are normally transitory and usually disappear within a few months (Fallowfield, 1990). Nevertheless, for those whose symptoms persist, it would appear that systematic physical activity may be beneficial.

It seems clear that the time is ripe to re-examine the "softer" side of cardiac rehabilitation with better tools and tighter methodology. As Mosteller, Gilbert, and McPeek (1980) report,

> Public impression to the contrary, the bulk of medical and surgical treatment is not life-saving, but is aimed at improving the state or quality of life. Most disease is not dramatically fatal, but chips away at comfort and happiness. (cited in Wenger, 1990, p. 91)

The concept of active living has enormous potential within this framework to impact upon quality of life by improving physical function and enhancing well-being.

Chronic Obstructive Pulmonary Disease

Chronic obstructive pulmonary disease (COPD) affects millions of North Americans and clearly limits exercise performance and even activities of daily living (Gallagher, 1990). Patients are acutely aware of every breath they take, so it is easy for them to avoid physical activity and apparently minimize dyspnea. Regrettably, this is not a wise choice, because most patients would then become more sedentary and further erode their limited mobility. It is generally thought that exercise programs are beneficial (Braun, Fregosi, & Reddan, 1982) even though the mechanisms underlying these improvements are debated (Carter, Coast, & Idell, 1992). In any case, it is essential that a carefully monitored evaluation precede the initiation of a physical activity program to determine any limiting factors or contraindications (Cruver & Solliday, 1982).

In spite of the consistent reduction in symptoms and increase in functional ability associated with systematic exercise, the results of pulmonary function tests do not change (Jones, Berman, Bartkiewicz, & Oldridge, 1987) and the progress of the disease is unimpeded. Nevertheless, the gradual increase in exercise tolerance could

have a profound effect on quality of life. People with chronic lung problems do not perceive themselves to be physically compromised as much as someone who has had a myocardial infarction, and yet their mental health and health perceptions are worse (Stewart et al., 1989). Therefore, the careful integration of systematic physical activity into their lifestyle could have an impact on both physical and mental well-being.

Diabetes

Diabetes (and related complications) is the third leading cause of death in North America following heart disease and cancer. It is a chronic metabolic disorder in which the body's ability to manufacture or utilize insulin has been impaired (Vranic & Wasserman, 1990). These authors suggest that exercise programs are beneficial for noninsulin-dependent diabetes mellitus (NIDDM) when combined with weight loss. However, the success rate for reducing body weight in obese NIDDM diabetics is low. It should also be noted that insulin-dependent diabetes mellitus (IDDM) represents only 5% to 10% of diabetics and presents an even greater challenge to physical activity and glycemic control. Berger and Kemmer (1990) were part of the same Toronto Consensus Conference in 1988 but were less than charitable about the role of physical activity for better management of diabetes. Their only note of encouragement for physical activity relates to long-term studies "on the efficacy of exercise training programs in preventing NIDDM diabetes in individuals who are at risk of developing this disease" (p. 494). The protective benefit of physical activity has been reported in two recent studies (Helmrick, Ragland, Leung, & Paffenbarger, 1991; Manson et al., 1991). In addition, Laws and Reaven (1990) present a compelling case for the well-known deterioration of glucose tolerance with aging to be more a consequence of decreased physical fitness and increased adiposity than of aging itself. Certainly, the benefit of long term risk reduction must always be weighed against the short term risk of complications in diabetics who might exercise vigorously (Staten, 1991). Sustained protection is more likely if the activity habit is established in the early years and systematically maintained for life. For those who have NIDDM diabetes, it would appear that risk factor modification may be more easily achieved than glycemic control. Nevertheless, further research is warranted with careful attention to design and physical activity intensity.

Summary and Conclusions

The Health and Activity Limitation Survey (HALS) provides a comprehensive picture of persons with disabilities in Canada. For most of these people a cure is impossible, but death is also not imminent. Therefore, the management of these chronic conditions should be designed to optimize the health-related quality of life. Specifically, this means enhancing daily functioning and well-being. To that end, the concept of active living presents an attractive opportunity to promote daily physical activity within a context and environment which is safe and fulfilling.

However, if the concept of active living is to gain widespread acceptance as an integral component of medical therapy for persons with chronic conditions, it has to provide outcome measures which are reproducible (Deyo, 1991). Fortunately, there is a growing number of state-of-the-art questionnaires which are not only as rigorous as laboratory techniques, but also measure quality of life dimensions that are salient to the patients.

The challenge currently is twofold: First, it is essential to convince physicians and patients alike that active living should be the norm rather than the exception for persons with chronic conditions. Second, the impact of this approach will only gain widespread approval and implementation within the medical community when the positive outcomes are demonstrated in randomized clinical trials.

References

American College of Sports Medicine. (1990). The recommended quantity and quality of exercise for developing and maintaining fitness in healthy adults. *Medicine and Science in Sports and Exercise*, **22**, 265-274.

Berger, M., & Kemmer, F.W. (1990). Discussion: Exercise, fitness and diabetes. In C. Bouchard, R.J. Shephard, T. Stephens, J.R. Sutton, & B.D. McPherson (Eds.), *Exercise, fitness and health: A consensus of current knowledge* (pp. 491-495). Champaign, IL: Human Kinetics.

Braun, S., Fregosi, R., & Reddan, W. (1982). Exercise training in patients with COPD. *Postgraduate Medicine*, **71**(4), 163-173.

Canadian Centre for Health Information. (1989). Cardiovascular disease in Canada. *Health Reports*, **1**(1), 1-22.

Carter, R., Coast, R.J., & Idell, S. (1992). Exercise training in patients with chronic obstructive pulmonary disease. *Medicine and Science in Sports and Exercise*, **24**(3), 281-291.

Centres for Disease Control (1990). Coronary heart disease attributable to sedentary lifestyle-selected states, 1988. *Morbidity and Mortality Weekly Report*, **39**(32), 541-544.

Cruver, N., & Solliday, N. (1982). Fundamentals of exercise stress testing for lung disease. *Respiratory Care*, **27**(9), 1050-1057.

Danneskiold-Samsoe, B., Lyngberg, K., Risum, T., & Telling, M. (1987). The effect of water exercise therapy given to patients with rheumatoid arthritis. *Scandinavian Journal of Rehabilitation Medicine*, **19**, 31-35.

Department of the Secretary of State of Canada. (1986). *Report of the Canadian Health and Disability Survey* (Catalogue 82-555E). Ottawa: Statistics Canada.

Deyo, R.A. (1991). The quality of life, research and care. *Annals of Internal Medicine*, **114**(8), 695-697.

Fallen, E.L., Armstrong, P., Cairns, J., Dafoe, W., Frasure-Smith, N., Langer, A., Massell, D., Oldridge, N., Peretz, D., Tremblay, G., & Williams, W.L. (1991). Report of the Canadian Cardiovascular Society's consensus conference on the management of the postmyocardial infarction patient. *Canadian Medical Association Journal*, **144**(8), 1015-1025.

Fallowfield, L. (1990). *The quality of life: The missing measurement in health care*. London: Souvenir Press.

Fletcher, G.F., Froelicher, V.F., Hartley, L.H., Haskell, W.L., & Pollock, M.L. (1990). Exercise standards. *Circulation*, **82**(6), 2286-2322.

Gallagher, C.G. (1990). Exercise and chronic obstructive pulmonary disease. *Medical Clinics of North America*, **74**(3), 619-641.

Greenland, P. (1991). Efficacy of supervised cardiac rehabilitation programs for coronary patients: Update 1986-1990. *Journal of Cardiopulmonary Rehabilitation*, **11**, 197-203.

Helmrick, S.P., Ragland, D.R., Leung, R.W., & Paffenbarger, R.S. (1991). Physical activity and reduced occurrence of non-insulin-dependent diabetes mellitus. *New England Journal of Medicine*, **325**(3), 147-152.

Hicks, J.E. (1990). Exercise in patients with inflammatory arthritis and connective tissue disease. *Rheumatic Disease Clinics of North America*, **16**(4), 845-868.

Ike, R.W., Lampman, R.M., & Castor, C.W. (1989). Arthritis and aerobic exercise: A review. *Physician and Sports Medicine*, **17**(2), 128-138.

Jones, N., Berman, L., Bartkiewicz, P., & Oldridge, N. (1987). Chronic obstructive respiratory disorders. In J. Skinner (Ed.), *Exercise testing and exercise prescription for special cases*. Philadelphia: Lea and Febiger.

Kallio, V. (1981). Evaluation of earlier studies: Europe. In L.S. Cohen, M.B. Mock, & I. Ringquist (Eds.), *Physical conditioning and cardiovascular rehabilitation* (pp. 257-270). New York: Wiley.

LaPlante, M. (1988). *Data on disability from the National Health Interview Survey, 1983-85*. Report issued by the National Institute on Disability and Rehabilitation Research, U.S. Department of Education. Washington, D.C.: U.S. Government Printing Office.

Lavigne, M., & Morin, J.P. (1991). Leisure and lifestyles of persons with disabilities in Canada. *Special Topic Series from The Health and Activity Limitations Survey* (Catalogue 82-615). Ottawa: Statistics Canada.

Laws, A., & Reaven, G.M. (1990). Effect of physical activity on age-related glucose intolerance. *Clinics in Geriatric Medicine*, **6**(4), 849-863.

Leon, A.S., Certo, C., Comoss, P., Franklin, B., Froelicher, V., Haskell, W.L., Hellerstein, H.K., Marley, W.P., Pollock, M.L., Ries, A., Sivarajan, E.F., & Smith, L.K. (1990). Position paper of the AACVPR—Scientific evidence of the value of cardiac rehabilitation services with emphasis on patients following myocardial infarction—Section 1: Exercise conditioning component. *Journal of Cardiopulmonary Rehabilitation*, **10**, 79-87.

Lipkin, D.P. (1990). Is cardiac rehabilitation necessary? *British Heart Journal*, **65**, 237-238.

Manson, J.E., Rimm, E.B., Stampfer, M.J., Colditz, G.A., Willett, W.C., Krolewski, A.S., Rosner, B., Hennekens, C.H., & Speizer, F.E. (1991). Physical activity and incidence of non-insulin-dependent diabetes mellitus in women. *Lancet*, **338**, 774-778.

May, G.S., Eberlein, K.A., & Friberg, C.D. (1984). Secondary prevention after myocardial infarction: A review of long-term trials. *Progress in Cardiovascular Diseases*, **24**, 331-351.

McHenry, P.L., Ellestad, M.H., Fletcher, G.F., Froelicher, V., Hartley, L.H., Mitchell, J.H., & Froelicher, E.S. (1990). Statement on exercise. *Circulation*, **81**(1), 396-398.

Minor, M.A., Hewett, J.E., Webel, R.R., Anderson, S.K., & Kay, D.R. (1989). Efficacy of physical conditioning exercise in patients with rheumatoid arthritis and osteoarthritis. *Arthritis and Rheumatism*, **32**, 1396.

Myers, J., & Froelicher, V.F. (1990). Predicting outcome in cardiac rehabilitation. *Journal of the American College of Cardiology*, **15**(5), 983-985.

Namey, T.C. (1990). Adaptive bicycling. *Rheumatic Disease Clinics of North America*, **16**(4), 871-885.

O'Brien, B.J., Buxton, M.J., & Patterson, D.L. (1992). *Relationship between functional status and health-related quality of life after myocardial infarction* (pp. 1-15). (Analysis Working Paper #92-1). Hamilton, Ontario: McMaster University Centre for Health Economics and Policy.

O'Connor, G.T., Buring, J.E., Yusuf, S., Goldhaber, S.Z., Olmstead, E.M, Paffenbarger, R., & Hennekens, C.H. (1989). An overview of randomized trials of rehabilitation with exercise after myocardial infarction. *Circulation*, **80**(2), 234-244.

Oldridge, N.B., Guyatt, G.H., Fischer, M.E., & Rimm, A.A. (1988). Cardiac rehabilitation after myocardial infarction. Combined experience of randomized clinical trials. *Journal of the American Medical Association*, **260**, 945-950.

Panush, R.S., & Brown, D.G. (1987). Exercise and arthritis. *Sports Medicine*, **4**, 54-64.

Pascale, M., & Grana, W.A. (1989). Does running cause osteoarthritis? *The Physician and Sports Medicine*, **17**(3):157-166.

Powell, K.E., Caspersen, C.J., Koplan, J.P., & Ford, E.S. (1989). Physical activity and chronic diseases. *American Journal of Clinical Nutrition*, **49**, 999-1006.

Powell, K.E., Thompson, P.S., Caspersen, C.J., & Kendrick, J.S. (1987). Physical activity and the incidence of coronary heart disease. *Annual Review of Public Health*, **8**, 253-287.

Rechnitzer, P.A., Cunningham, D.A., Andrew, G.M., Buck, C.W., Jones, N.L., Kavanagh, T., Oldridge, N.B., Parker, J.O., Shephard, R.J., Sutton, J.R., & Donner, A. (1983). Relation of exercise to the recurrence rate of myocardial infarction in men. Ontario Exercise-Heart Collaborative Study. *American Journal of Cardiology*, **51**, 65-69.

Samples, P. (1990). Exercise encouraged for people with arthritis. *Physician and Sportsmedicine*, **18**(1), 123-127.

Schumacher, H.R. (1988). Osteoarthritis: State of the art. In H.R. Schumacher (Ed.), *Osteoarthritis: Diagnosis and Therapy* (pp. 5-10). Berlin: Springer-Verlag.

Shephard, R.J. (1989). Exercise in the tertiary prevention of ischemic heart disease: Experimental proof. *Canadian Journal of Sport Science*, **14**(2), 74-84.

Spector, T.D. (1990). Rheumatoid arthritis. *Rheumatic Disease Clinics of North America*, **16**(3), 513.

Staten, M.N. (1991). Managing diabetes in older adults—how exercise can help. *Physician and Sportsmedicine*, **19**, 66-77.

Statistics Canada. (1990). *Health and Activity Limitation Survey Highlights: Disabled Persons in Canada* (Category 82-602). Ottawa: Author.

Stewart, A.L., Greenfield, S., Hays, R., Wells, K., Rogers, W., Berry, S., McGlynn, E., & Ware, J. (1989). Functional status and well-being of patients with chronic conditions. *Journal of the American Medical Association*, **262**(7), 907-913.

Verbrugge, L.M., Lepkowski, J.M., & Konkol, L.L. (1991). Levels of disability among U.S. adults with arthritis. *Journal of Gerontology: Social Sciences*, **46**(2), S71-S83.

Vranic, M., & Wasserman, D. (1990). Exercise, fitness and diabetes. In C. Bouchard, R.J. Shephard, T. Stephens, J.R. Sutton, & B.D. McPherson (Eds.), *Exercise, fitness, and health: A consensus of current knowledge* (pp. 467-490). Champaign, IL: Human Kinetics.

Wenger, N.K. (1990). Quality of life in chronic cardiovascular illness. *Journal of Cardiopulmonary Rehabilitation*, **10**, 88-91.

Wood, P. (1956). *Diseases of the heart and circulation* (2nd ed.). London: Eyre and Spottiswoode.

World Health Organization. (1980). *International Classification of Impairments, Disabilities and Handicaps* (p. 143). Geneva: World Health Organization.

7

Benefits of Physical Activity From a Lifetime Perspective

Robert M. Malina

Physical activity is popularly viewed as having a favorable influence on growth, maturation, and development of children and youth. It also has beneficial effects on the individual that persist into adulthood. Several aspects of physical activity during childhood and adolescence, and the transition into adulthood are considered in this chapter.

Growth, Maturation, and Development

The terms growth, maturation, and development often have different meanings to professionals involved with children and youth. *Growth* refers to changes in size, physique, body composition, and in various systems of the body, many of which are related to growth in body size (e.g., the cardiovascular and respiratory systems).

Maturation refers to the tempo and timing of progress towards biological maturity, for example, sexual, skeletal, and somatic maturity. All individuals attain the mature state, but do so at different rates. Indicators of maturity during childhood and adolescence include skeletal age, appearance of secondary sex characteristics, and the timing of maximum growth during adolescence.

Development refers to the acquisition of competence in a variety of behavioral domains—social, cognitive, emotional, moral and motor competence, and perhaps others. Of course, development occurs within the context of traditions and sanctions set by the particular culture in which the individual lives.

Growth and maturation are biological processes, while development is a behavioral process. The three processes are interdependent and interact to mold the individual's self-concept. Thus, the role of physical activity as a factor influencing growth, maturation, and development must be approached bioculturally or biobehaviorally.

Physical Activity and Fitness

Physical activity includes " . . . any body movement produced by the skeletal muscles and resulting in a substantial increase over the resting energy expenditure" (Bouchard & Shephard, in press). It has many forms and contexts including play, free movement, sport, dance, physical education, and exercise. The context of activity probably has more of an influence on development in contrast to the metabolic effects implicit in the definition. The ability to perform physical activities requires some degree of *physical fitness*, which is operationally defined as having morphological (largely body composition), muscular, motor, cardiorespiratory, and metabolic components (Bouchard & Shephard, in press).

Emphasis on the fitness of children and youth has shifted from a primary motor focus to a health-related focus over the past 15 to 20 years. *Motor fitness* is performance oriented and includes components of skilled movements, that is, agility, balance, coordination, power, speed, strength, and muscular endurance, all of which enable the individual to perform a variety of physical activities. *Health-related fitness* is often operationalized in terms of cardiorespiratory endurance, abdominal and low back musculoskeletal function, and body composition, specifically subcutaneous fatness.

Regular participation in physical activity is related to the development and maintenance of fitness. Components of motor and health-related fitness change as a function of growth and maturation, and several components show distinct growth spurts, particularly in males (Beunen & Malina, 1988; Malina & Bouchard, 1991). Hence, it is difficult to partition the influence of physical activity on fitness from that of normal growth and maturation.

Trends in Physical Activity

There is a need for systematic study of factors which influence or determine interest in, motivation for, and habits of physical activity. Daily physical education is not a feature of the lifestyle of the majority of school children (Dishman, 1989). Physical activity outside the school setting has an important role, and it is not surprising that organized sport is a major form of activity among children and youth. By 7 to 8 years of age, over 50% of children have already begun to participate in sport (Seefeldt & Haubenstricker, 1988). The two primary reasons stated by most children for participation in sport are: (a) to have fun, and (b) to learn new skills. These objectives apply to physical activity in general. Among older children and youth (grades 7 to 12), fun is still the primary objective in sport. Boys place more emphasis on improving skills, while girls place more emphasis on "staying in shape" (Athletic Footwear Association, 1992). Social concerns, for example, to be with friends or to make new friends, and physical fitness are also important reasons for many children and youth.

Participation in organized youth sports reaches a peak at about 12 to 13 years of age, and then declines. Two reasons for the decline are the desire to try new things, and changing interests (Athletic Footwear Association, 1992; Gould & Horn, 1984). These, of course, are normal developmental trends. Additional factors are not having fun, time commitment, more rigid selection criteria, and increased specialization associated with some sports. Parallel observations in Finnish youth suggest a change in motivation for physical activity from performance and competition in early adolescence (11 to 13 years of age) to recreational motivation in late adolescence (Telama & Silvennoinen, 1979). The most commonly stated reasons for involvement in physical activity among young adults are (a) to feel better mentally and physically, (b) to control weight and look better, and (c) for pleasure, fun, and excitement (Canada Fitness Survey, 1983; Wellens, 1989). The fun and pleasure aspects of physical activity persist into adulthood.

The trend in youth sports participation is paralleled in the estimated time spent in physical activity, which increases from middle childhood into mid-adolescence in both sexes, and then declines (Malina, 1986, 1990). The decline occurs in activities which are of medium and heavy intensity (Kemper et al., 1983). The decline in adolescent physical activity occurs after the growth spurt and sexual maturation, and is probably related to the social demands of adolescence, changing interests, and perhaps the transition from school to work or college.

Physical Activity, Growth, and Maturation

Although physical activity is viewed as important for children and youth, data about its role as a factor affecting growth and maturation are quite limited. Data are based largely on comparisons of small samples of active and inactive youth, select samples regularly training for specific sports, and short-term experimental studies (Malina, 1990, in press). Physical activity or training for sport has no effect, positive or negative, on statural growth and on indices of biological maturation commonly used in growth studies. In well-nourished children and youth, these variables are primarily regulated by genetic factors. Much discussion of potential negative effects of training focuses on later menarche in female athletes. These data are associational and retrospective, are based on small samples of late adolescent and adult athletes, and do not control for other factors that may influence menarche (e.g., selective criteria and dietary practices). It is difficult to attribute later maturation to training per se. Caution is essential in extending observations on select samples of athletes to the general population.

Regular physical activity, on the other hand, is important in the regulation of body weight. It is associated with a decrease in fatness in both sexes, and occasionally with an increase in fat-free mass at least in boys. Changes in fatness depend on continued activity (or caloric restriction) for their maintenance. With regard to specific tissues, experimental data indicate that regular physical activity has a favorable influence on the metabolic capacity of skeletal muscle tissue and on the mineralization and density of skeletal tissue. Information on the influence of regular physical activity on adipose tissue metabolism and cellularity of children and youth is lacking.

The Relationship Between Physical Activity and Fitness

Studies of the relationship between physical activity and fitness take several forms, including those that compare the fitness characteristics of active and inactive samples, those that assess the relationship between physical activity and fitness, and those that consider the effects of specific training programs on components of fitness (Malina, 1990, in press). Active individuals generally show higher levels of motor, strength, and aerobic fitness. Children respond to instructional programs with improved motor skill, and to strength training programs with improved strength. The latter occurs without hypertrophy in prepubertal children. In contrast, there is apparently relatively little trainability of maximal aerobic power in children under 10 years of age. It is not certain whether this observation is the consequence of low trainability, initially high activity levels, or inadequacies of training programs. During adolescence, the response to aerobic training improves considerably. Changes in response to short-term programs are not permanent, but depend upon continued regular activity for their maintenance.

Physical Activity and Self-Concept

Self-concept refers to perception of self, while self-esteem refers to the value placed on one's self-concept, though the terms are often used interchangably. Many early studies of physical activity focus on self-concept as a global entity, and those with low self-esteem appear to show greater improvement in their sense of self-worth in association with participation in activity and fitness programs (Gruber, 1986; Sonstroem, 1984; Vogel, 1986). Current emphases in self-concept research indicate different domains and changes in specific domains from childhood, through adolescence into adulthood (e.g., Harter, 1983, 1985, 1989; Shavelson, Hubner, & Stanton, 1976). Of specific relevance are domains related to physical ability and physical appearance, which has lead to the development of scales of physical self-perception (Fox, 1990).

Young children 4 to 7 years old identify four domains of self: cognitive competence, physical competence, peer acceptance, and maternal acceptance (Harter, 1983, 1989). Physical competence is described exclusively in the context of motor skills, for example, "good at climbing," "good at running," "good at hopping," etc. These fundamental movement patterns are developing at these ages. Young children do not distinguish between cognitive and physical skills: "One is either competent or incompetent across these activities" (Harter, 1983, p. 331). However, they do recognize practice and learning as important aspects to development of competence.

The structure of self-concept changes at about 8 years of age and has common domains which persist through adolescence into young adulthood (Harter, 1989). Domains are more clearly differentiated and children make judgments about self-worth. Among children 8 to 12 years of age, five domains emerge—scholastic competence, athletic competence, peer social acceptance, behavioral conduct, and physical appearance; while during adolescence three additional domains emerge—close friendship, romantic appeal, and job competence.

Studies of self-concept do not include actual measures of physical or athletic competence (i.e., skill) and do not include measures of size, physique, and maturity status. The relationship between perceived and actual competence thus merits examination. In one of the few studies addressing this issue, Ulrich (1987) considered the relationship between perceived competence and demonstrated competence in basic motor abilities and sports skills in children about 5 to 10 years of age. Children in the lowest tertile of perceived competence, on average, do not perform as well as children in the other tertiles in basic motor ability tasks and more specialized sports skills. The trends in means suggest a dose-response effect. Children with the highest perceived competence tend to show better levels of motor competence, more so in specialized sport skills than in basic motor ability items. The results also suggest that children have a reasonably accurate perception of their motor competence, and emphasize the need for developmentally appropriate programs of physical education at these ages when basic motor skills are developing. Lack of success in motor activities at young ages may in turn have a significant impact on the motivation to participate in physical activities at later ages.

Data for older ages are not as clear. Indicators of motivational orientation and physical self-perception do not discriminate active from less active 11 to 12 year old boys, while specific subscales of motivational orientation (e.g., challenge, curiosity), and physical self-perception (body attractiveness, physical self-worth), discriminate active and less active girls (Biddle & Armstrong, 1992). On the other hand, youth involved in sports demonstrate greater levels of perceived physical competence compared to those who are not involved (Feltz & Petlichkoff, 1983; Roberts, Kleiber, & Duda, 1981). Currently active young athletes and those with more experience in sport have higher levels of perceived physical competence than those who have dropped out and who have less experience.

Though interesting, these results raise several questions.

- What are the determinants of perceived competence?
- Do motor activities and sport attract children with high levels of perceived competence more so than other activities?
- Do children with lower levels of perceived competence shy away from or avoid physical activities?
- Are they the children who drop out of sport?
- Are higher levels of perceived competence a result of participation and/or success in motor activities and sport?

The contributions of specific domains or competencies to self-worth also have implications for health and physical activity. Among elementary and middle school children (8 to 15 years of age), first physical appearance and then social acceptance have the most impact on children's self-worth, while more specific competencies, that is, scholastic and athletic, contribute relatively little to self-worth at these ages (Harter, 1989). Thus, physical appearance and social acceptability have more impact on a child's sense of self-worth than other competencies during middle childhood and early adolescence. This is, on average, a period of dramatic change in size, physique, body composition, and sexual maturity status, so that it would seem logical to include more direct measures of these biological parameters in assessments of self-concept.

Given the concern for physical appearance and social acceptance among children and youth, regular physical activity has the potential to contribute to self-concept or self-worth. However, such self-evaluation also has the potential to induce negative health behaviors such as eating disorders and perhaps drug use. It would be of interest to examine the print and electronic media, in addition to role models in the sport and entertainment industries, as determinants of this concern for physical appearance. Images of extreme slenderness and leanness, and others related to health habits, dress, or hair style, are regularly aimed at children and youth who are among the largest consumers of these media messages.

Physical Activity and Social Competence

Physical activities occur within a social context so that they have potentially significant implications for the development of social competence, that is, the ability to effectively interact with and become adapted to the cultural milieu of which the individual is a member. Physical activities, however, do not socialize per se. They provide the medium in which socialization may occur. Socialization occurs *into* or *via* specific social roles. The individual is socialized into a specific role, for example, a physically active or inactive lifestyle, an athlete or a spectator. The individual is also socialized through specific roles into the learning of more general attitudes, values, and so on.

It is in the context of socialization *via* physical activity that presumed social benefits of participation are discussed. Physical activities provide a variety of social experiences. A question of interest is whether these experiences contribute to the development of socially competent behavior and a physically active lifestyle. Systematic study of the influence of regular participation in physical activities on the development of social competence is limited. The literature tends to focus on specific social behaviors, values, and characteristics of those who are proficient in motor skills, or those who are involved in sport. For example, in one of the earlier studies, third grade children (five boys, five girls) proficient in motor skills, (i.e., physically competent), "... tended to be active, popular, calm, resourceful, attentive, and cooperative ..." (Rarick & McKee, 1949, p. 150) compared to a corresponding sample of children who were not proficient. Other evidence suggests that elementary school children competent in motor skills attain greater social success and status than the less competent, and that leadership and peer acceptance is related to proficiency in motor skills (Evans & Roberts, 1987). Further, 9 to 10 year old boys and girls involved in sport are rated higher in social competence than those not involved in sport (Roberts et al., 1981). In the context of youth sports, the internal structure of the team sport and skill in particular may be important mediating factors in peer relations (Bigelow, Lewko, & Salhani, 1989).

During the transition into adolescence, variation in the timing of the growth spurt and sexual maturation enters the equation and influences the socialization process. Individual differences in biological maturation and associated changes in size and body composition are a major component of the backdrop against which adolescents evaluate and interpret their social status among peers. Physical performance and success in sports is an important aspect of the evaluative process, particularly among males. Biological maturation has significant correlates in physical skills and the value attached to skills by the peer group. Advanced (early) maturation among boys is associated with proficiency in strength and motor performance, as well as with popularity and social status (Jones, 1949). Early maturation in boys is also associated with success in many youth sports (Malina, 1988), often with resulting advantages in social status.

The situation is different for girls. Differences in strength and performance among girls of contrasting maturity status are not as apparent as among boys during the transition into adolescence. It is often the late maturing girl who experiences success in sport and persists in sport through adolescence (Malina, 1988). This raises an important question and undoubtedly others: Are late maturing girls socialized into sport, or are early maturing girls socialized away from sport? Data on the socialization of young girls into sport or a physically active lifestyle and on the social status of physically active and skilled girls are lacking (see Lewko & Greendorfer, 1988).

Data on socialization into physical activities are not extensive. Young children (4 to 9 years of age) with active parents are more likely to be active than those whose parents are not active (Freedson & Evenson, 1991; Moore et al., 1991). This suggests that socialization into a physically active lifestyle begins early in life.

At older ages, the situation is more complex and probably involves an interaction between socialization processes, that is, into and through physical activity. Among junior high school youth (about 13 to 15 years of age), prior experience in physical activity, current activity habits, and attitudes toward physical activity, in addition to parental attitudes towards activity, are significant determinants of the intention to exercise (Godin & Shephard, 1986; Shephard & Godin, 1986). Attitudes toward physical activity are not stable in upper elementary grade children (about 10 to 12 years of age), while the relationship between attitudes and involvement in activity is more stable (Smoll & Schutz, 1980; Smoll, Schutz, & Keeney, 1976). Attitudes toward physical activity are rather stable in high school students (about 16 to 18 years of age), and involvement in activity is more stable than attitude; however, strength of attitude toward physical activity accounts for only about 20% of the variation in degree of involvement (Schutz & Smoll, 1986).

Transition to Adulthood

Current emphasis on physical activity and fitness for children and youth is usually framed in the context of future health status:

- Regular physical activity during childhood and youth may function to prevent or impede the development of several adult diseases that include physical inactivity in a complex, multifactorial etiology—degenerative diseases of the heart and blood vessels, obesity, musculoskeletal disorders (specifically low back pain), and perhaps others.
- Habits of regular physical activity during childhood and youth may directly and favorably influence physical activity habits in adulthood and, in turn, have a beneficial influence on the health-related fitness and thus the health status of adults (Malina, 1991).

It is thus based on assumption that potential benefits of physical activity and habits of activity carry over from childhood and adolescence into adulthood.

Components of fitness track only moderately from adolescence into adulthood. Among 173 males followed from 13 to 18 years of age and then seen at 30 years of age, indicators of physical fitness vary in their stability (Beunen et al., 1992). Flexibility of the lower back tracks reasonably well, while heart rate recovery after a 2-minute step test (cardiovascular fitness) tracks moderately at best. Interage correlations for measures of subcutaneous fatness, muscular strength and endurance, and motor fitness are intermediate, indicating moderate tracking. Stability is better from late adolescence into adulthood (18 to 30 years of age) than from early adolescence into adulthood (13 to 30 years of age).

Some evidence suggests an association between endurance, strength, and motor fitness in childhood and physical activity in young adulthood. Physically active young adult males, 23 to 25 years of age, had better motor fitness scores as children (10 to 11 years of age) and adolescents (15 to 18 years of age) than inactive young adult males (Dennison, Straus, Mellits, & Charney, 1988). The active adults performed, on average, significantly better than inactive adults in the 600-yard run, sit-ups, the 50-yard dash, and the shuttle run during late childhood and adolescence. Further, boys whose performances on the 600-yard run were below the 20th percentile were at a significantly greater risk for adult physical inactivity.

Interage correlations between sport participation during adolescence and at age 30 in males (n=278) are low but increase with age from 13 to 17 years of age so that the correlation between activity at 17 and 30 years of age is 0.39 (Vanreusel et al., in press). There is no association between sport participation at 13 years of age and activity status at 30 years of age (active = >1 hr/week; inactive = <1 hr/week). Proportionally more active 15 year old boys are active at 30, although there is no discrimination between low, medium, and high activity levels during adolescence. At 17 years of age, however, proportionally more boys with medium and high activity levels are active at 30, while proportionally

more inactive boys and boys with low activity levels at 17 years of age are not active at 30 (Vanreusel et al., in press).

As noted earlier, activity levels decline, on average, through adolescence into young adulthood; subsequently, percentages of active individuals tend to be rather stable (Engstrom, 1986). Interestingly, those who have more prior experiences with sport and physical activity at 15 years of age have higher psychological readiness (operationally defined as having a more positive view of their body and capabilities in sport, and a more positive attitude toward fitness activities) for physical activity at 30 years of age, males more so than females. Individuals with higher psychological readiness also tend to be more active at 30 years (Engstrom, 1986, 1991).

Epilogue

Regular physical activity during childhood and youth has benefits that persist into adulthood. Nevertheless, it is important that physical activity programs during childhood and adolescence consider what is best for the overall development of children and youth, and not necessarily what is best for them if they were adults. This perspective is essential as many programs are presently being encouraged to emphasize health-related fitness activities, specifically aerobics, while many programs neglect and may perhaps eliminate instruction and practice of basic motor skills.

Childhood and adolescence are windows of opportunity to sew the seeds of a physically active lifestyle. Basic movement patterns and skills are established during the elementary school years. The middle and high school years may be a significant time for the establishment of positive attitudes and habits of physical activity. This implies a need for quality programs that provide a variety of opportunities and experiences in physical activities.

Limited evidence indicates a link between fitness level and activity habits during adolescence and activity habits in early adulthood. Regular physical activity is necessary to maintain the functional integrity of skeletal muscle and bone tissue; to regulate fatness during adulthood; and to maintain motor, strength, and aerobic fitness. Regular physical activity may reduce the rate of change in these tissues and functions which ordinarily accompany aging. Physical activity also has important social correlates during adulthood, especially with older adults. Activities are not performed in a social vacuum. Improved fitness associated with activity programs may have significance for self-concept in adults. As in childhood and adolescence, adults are also concerned with physical appearance (Harter, 1989). Although this presentation has focused on childhood, youth, and the transition into adulthood, the potential biobehavioral benefits of physical activity extend through the lifespan.

References

Athletic Footwear Association. (1992). *American youth and sports participation*. North Palm Beach, FL: Author.

Beunen, G., Lefevre, J., Claessens, A.L., Lysens, R., Maes, H., Renson, R., Simons, J., Vanden Eynde, B., Vanreusel, B., & Van Den Bossche, C. (1992). Age-specific correlation analysis of longitudinal physical fitness levels in men. *European Journal of Applied Physiology*, **64**, 538-545.

Beunen, G., & Malina, R.M. (1988). Growth and physical performance relative to the timing of the adolescent spurt. *Exercise and Sport Sciences Reviews*, **16**, 503-540.

Biddle, S., & Armstrong, N. (1992). Children's physical activity: An exploratory study of psychological correlates. *Social Science in Medicine*, **34**, 325-331.

Bigelow, B.J., Lewko, J.H., & Salhani, L. (1989). Sport involved children's friendship expectations. *Sport and Exercise Psychology*, **11**, 152-160.

Bouchard, C., & Shephard, R.J. (in press). Physical activity and fitness as determinants of health: The general model and basic concepts. In C. Bouchard, R.J. Shephard & T. Stephens (Eds.), *Physical activity, fitness and health: International proceedings and consensus statement*. Champaign, IL: Human Kinetics.

Canada Fitness Survey. (1983). *Canadian youth and physical activity*. Ottawa: Author.

Dennison, B.A., Straus, J.H., Mellits, E.D., & Charney, E. (1988). Childhood physical fitness tests: Predictor of adult physical activity levels? *Pediatrics*, **82**, 324-330.

Dishman, R.K. (1989). Exercise and sport psychology in youth 6 to 18 years of age. In C.V. Gisolfi & D.R. Lamb (Eds.), *Perspectives in exercise science and sports medicine, volume 2. Youth, exercise, and sport* (pp. 47-95). Indianapolis: Benchmark Press.

Engstrom, L.–M. (1986). The process of socialization into keep-fit activities. *Scandinavian Journal of Sports Science*, **8**, 89-97.

Engstrom, L.–M. (1991). Exercise adherence in sport for all from youth to adulthood. In P. Oja & R. Telama (Eds.), *Sport for All* (pp. 473-483). Amsterdam: Elsevier Science Publishers.

Evans, J., & Roberts, G.C. (1987). Physical competence and the development of children's peer relations. *Quest*, **39**, 23-35.

Feltz, D., & Petlichkoff, L. (1983). Perceived competence among interscholastic sport participants and dropouts. *Canadian Journal of Applied Sport Sciences*, **8**, 231-235.

Fox, K.R. (1990). *The physical self-perception profile manual*. Dekalb, IL: Office of Health Promotion, Northern Illinois University.

Freedson, P.S., & Evenson, S. (1991). Familial aggregation in physical activity. *Research Quarterly for Exercise and Sport*, **62**, 384-389.

Godin, G., & Shephard, R.J. (1986). Psychological factors influencing intentions to exercise of young students from grades 7 to 9. *Research Quarterly for Exercise and Sport*, **57**, 41-52.

Gould, D., & Horn, T. (1984). Participation motivation in young athletes. In J.M. Silva & R.S. Weinberg (Eds.), *Psychological foundations of sport* (pp. 359-370). Champaign, IL: Human Kinetics.

Gruber, J.J. (1986). Physical activity and self-esteem development in children: A meta-analysis. In G.A. Stull & H.M. Eckert (Eds.), *Effects of physical activity on children* [Monograph of the American Academy of Physical Education Papers No. 19] (pp. 40-48). Champaign, IL: Human Kinetics.

Harter, S. (1983). Developmental perspectives on the self-esteem. In E.M. Hetherington (Ed.), *Handbook of child psychology. Volume IV. Socialization, personality, and social development* (pp. 275-385). New York: Wiley.

Harter, S. (1985). Competence as a dimension of self-evaluation: Toward a comprehensive model of self-worth. In R.L. Leahy (Ed.), *The development of the self* (pp. 55-121). New York: Academic Press.

Harter, S. (1989). Causes, correlates, and the functional role of global self-worth: A life-span perspective. In J. Kolligian & R. Sternberg (Eds.), *Perceptions of competence and incompetence across the lifespan* (pp. 67-97). New Haven, CT: Yale University Press.

Jones, H.E. (1949). *Motor performance and growth*. Berkeley, CA: University of California Press.

Kemper, H.C.G., Dekker, H.J.P., Ootjers, M.G., Post, B., Snel, J., Splinter, P.G., Storm-van Essen, L., & Verschuur, R. (1983). Growth and health of teenagers in the Netherlands. *International Journal of Sports Medicine*, **4**, 202-214.

Lewko, J.H., & Greendorfer, S.L. (1988). Family influences in sport socialization of children and adolescents. In F.L. Smoll, R.A. Magill, & M.J. Ash (Eds.), *Children in sport* (3rd ed.) (pp. 287-300). Champaign, IL: Human Kinetics.

Malina, R.M. (1986). Energy expenditure and physical activity during childhood and youth. In A. Demirjian (Ed.), *Human growth: A multidisciplinary review* (pp. 215-225). London: Taylor & Francis.

Malina, R.M. (1988). Growth and maturation of young athletes: Biological and social considerations. In F.L. Smoll, R.A. Magill, & M.J. Ash (Eds.), *Children in sport* (3rd ed.) (pp. 83-101). Champaign, IL: Human Kinetics.

Malina, R.M. (1990). Growth, exercise, fitness, and later health outcomes. In C. Bouchard, R.J. Shephard, T.

Stephens, J.R. Sutton, & B.D. McPherson (Eds.), *Exercise, fitness, and health: A consensus of current knowledge* (pp. 637-665). Champaign, IL.: Human Kinetics.

Malina, R.M. (1991). Fitness and performance: Adult health and the culture of youth. In R.J. Park & H.M. Eckert (Eds.), *New possibilities, new paradigms?* [Monograph of the American Academy of Physical Education Papers No. 24] (pp. 30-38). Champaign, IL: Human Kinetics.

Malina, R.M. (in press). Physical activity: Relationship to growth, maturation, and physical fitness. In C. Bouchard, R.J. Shephard, & T. Stephens (Eds.), *Physical Activity, Fitness and Health: International proceedings and consensus statement.* Champaign, IL: Human Kinetics.

Malina, R.M., & Bouchard, C. (1991). *Growth, maturation, and physical activity.* Champaign, IL: Human Kinetics.

Moore, L.L., Lombardi, D.A., White, M.J., Campbell, J.L., Oliveria, S.A., & Ellison, R.C. (1991). Influence of parents' physical activity levels on activity levels of young children. *Journal of Pediatrics,* **118**, 215-219.

Rarick, G.L., & Mckee, R. (1949). A study of twenty third-grade children exhibiting extreme levels of achievement on tests of motor proficiency. *Research Quarterly,* **20**, 142-152.

Roberts, G.C., Kleiber, D.A., & Duda, J.L. (1981). An analysis of motivation in children's sport: The role of perceived competence in participation. *Journal of Sport Psychology,* **3**, 206-216.

Schutz, R.W., & Smoll, F.L. (1986). The (in)stability of attitudes towards physical activity during childhood and adolescence. In B.D. McPherson (Ed.), *Sport and aging* (pp. 187-197). Champaign, IL: Human Kinetics.

Seefeldt, V., & Haubenstricker, J. (1988). Children and youth in physical activity: A review of accomplishments. In R.M. Malina (Ed.), *Physical activity in early and modern populations* [Monograph of the American Academy of Physical Education Papers No. 21] (pp. 88-103). Champaign, IL: Human Kinetics.

Shavelson, R.J., Hubner, J.J., & Stanton, G.C. (1976). Self-concept: Validation of construct reinterpretation. *Review of Educational Research,* **46**, 407-441.

Shephard, R.J., & Godin, G. (1986). Behavioral intentions and activity of children. In J. Rutenfranz, R. Mocellin, & F. Klimt (Eds.), *Children and exercise XII* (pp. 103-109). Champaign, IL: Human Kinetics.

Smoll, F.L., & Schutz, R.W. (1980). Children's attitudes towards physical activity: A longitudinal analysis. *Journal of Sport Psychology,* **2**, 144-154.

Smoll, F.L., Schutz, R.W., & Keeney, J.K. (1976). Relationships among children's attitudes, involvement, and proficiency in physical activities. *Research Quarterly,* **47**, 797-803.

Sonstroem, R.J. (1984). Exercise and self-esteem. *Exercise and Sport Sciences Reviews,* **12**, 123-155.

Telama, R., & Silvennoinen, M. (1979). Structure and development of 11 to 19 year olds' motivation for physical activity. *Scandinavian Journal of Sport Sciences,* **1**, 23-31.

Ulrich, B.D. (1987). Perceptions of physical competence, motor competence, and participation in organized sport: Their interrelationships in young children. *Research Quarterly for Exercise and Sport,* **58**, 57-67.

Vanreusel, R., Renson, R., Beunen, G., Claessens, A., Lefevre, J., Lysens, R., Maes, H., Simons, J., & Vanden Eynde, B. (in press). Adherence to sport from youth to adulthood: A longitudinal study on socialization. In W. Duquet, P. DeKnop, and L. Bollaert (Eds.), *Youth sport, a social approach.* Brussels: Free University of Brussels Press.

Vogel, P.G. (1986). Effects of physical education programs on children. In V. Seefeldt (Ed.). *Physical activity and well-being* (pp. 455-509). Reston, VA.: American Alliance for Health, Physical Education, Recreation, and Dance.

Wellens, R.E. (1989). *Activity as a temperamental trait: Relationship to physique, energy expenditure and physical activity habits in young adults.* Unpublished doctoral dissertation, University of Texas, Austin.

8

Beneficial and Deleterious Effects of Training on the Health of the Child With a Chronic Disease

Oded Bar-Or

The relevance of physical activity to the health of adults has long been recognized. Much information has been generated, for example, regarding the use of the exercise "stress test" as a diagnostic tool, and the importance of enhanced physical activity during adult years in prevention and rehabilitation of coronary heart disease. Less is known about the relevance of physical activity to pediatric disease. Research on the effects of physical training on children's health has lagged behind that on adults, mostly because of ethical and methodological constraints.

Training programs are often used to nonspecifically improve the patient's fitness, well-being, and general exercise capacity. Some beneficial effects, however, are specific to certain pediatric diseases. Several of these have been proven experimentally, whereas others have been suggested but not yet proven.

Enhanced physical activity is not always beneficial. To the child with a chronic disease, it can sometimes be detrimental. Often, beneficial and deleterious effects occur in the same disease. The benefits usually develop through a training program, whereas the deleterious changes are usually triggered by an acute bout of exercise.

My objective is to outline some of the recent information regarding the health-related effects of training, both beneficial and deleterious, to the child with a chronic disease. Table 8.1 is a summary of such effects. Because of space limitation, I will address only some of the most prevalent pediatric chronic diseases. For earlier reviews and monographs see Arensman, Christiansen, and Strong (1989); Bar-Or (1983, 1985, 1990); Bar-Or and Inbar (in press); Beekman (1986); Despres, Bouchard, and Malina (1990); Neijens (1989); Orenstein (1988); Parker and Bar-Or (1991); Rowland (1990); and Walberg and Ward (1985).

Asthma

In addition to nonspecifically benefiting maximal aerobic power in children with asthma, training can decrease morbidity, increase lung volumes and flows, and reduce the frequency and intensity of exercise-induced bronchoconstriction (EIB). The latter effect is controversial, though, because several intervention studies (King, Noakes, & Weinberg, 1989; Leisti, Finnila, & Kiura, 1979) reported no change in EIB. Among those that did report a reduction in the degree of EIB, four (Henriksen & Nielsen, 1983; Oseid & Haaland, 1978; Svenonius, Kautto, & Arborelius, 1983; Swann & Hanson, 1983) included asthmatic controls that did not train, but in only one of them were the controls randomly selected (Swann & Hanson, 1983). In that study, both the intervention and the placebo treatment given to the controls resulted in a reduced intensity of EIB.

Swimming is the most commonly prescribed activity for asthmatics. A swim training program improves aerobic fitness (Fitch, Morton, & Blanksby, 1976; Schnall, Ford, Gillam, & Landon, 1982; Szentagothal, Gyene, Szocska, & Osvath, 1987; Svenonius et al., 1983) and reduces morbidity, as determined by frequency of asthma attacks, need for medication and hospitalization, or school absenteeism (Fitch et al., 1976; Huang, Veiga, Sila, Reed, & Hines, 1989; Tanizaki, Komagoe, Sudo, & Morinaga, 1984; Szenthagotal et al., 1987). This has been shown in most intervention studies, but only in one of them (Huang et al., 1989) were the controls and experimental group randomly assigned. Table 8.2 is a summary of the changes in morbidity indicators, as monitored in that study for 12 months following the intervention.

EIB is a thoroughly researched deleterious effect of exercise in asthma. Much information has been published regarding the ways EIB can be prevented or

Table 8.1 **Specific Exercise-Related Benefits and Deleterious Effects Reported to Occur in the Child With a Chronic Disease**

Disease	Reported benefits	Reported deleterious effects
Asthma	Reduced morbidity, increased lung volumes and flow, reduced EIB	EIB, enhanced diving reflex
Cerebral palsy	Enhanced ambulation, reduced spasticity, prevention of contractures	
Cystic fibrosis	Increased endurance of respiratory muscles, enhanced clearance of bronchial mucus, increased lung volumes and flows	Oxygen desaturation, dehydration and excessive heat strain, EIB
Diabetes mellitus (insulin-dependent)	Decreased need for insulin, increased diabetic control	Hypoglycemia, hyperglycemia, ketoacidosis
Hypertension	Reduced BP at rest	Exaggerated BP response to acute exercise
Myopathies	Stronger residual muscle, enhanced ambulation, prevention of contractures, controlled weight	Faster muscle deterioration, abnormal serum CK
Obesity	Controlled weight and fatness, improved lipoprotein profile, increased insulin sensitivity, enhanced socialization and self-esteem	Exaggerated BP response to acute exercise

EIB = exercise-induced bronchoconstriction; BP = arterial blood pressure; CK = creatine kinase.

Table 8.2 **Effects of Swim Training on Asthma Morbidity**

Variable	Study group	Controls
Frequency of attacks	↓ 78	↓ 11
Change in PEF at 12 months	↑ 63	↑ 25
Wheezing days	↓ 66	↓ 20
Days requiring medication	↓ 61	↓ 17
Emergency room visits	↓ 89	↓ 13
Rate of hospitalizations	↓ 84	↓ 19
Absent school days	↓ 82	↓ 17

PEF = peak expiratory flow.

Note. Variables were assessed during a 12-month period after a 2-month swim program. Subjects were 90 6- to 12-year-old patients randomly assigned to a training and a control group. Values are percentage change from pretraining period. All between-group differences were statistically significant ($p<0.01$). Adapted by permission from Huang et al. (1989).

ameliorated by the use of medication, modification of the mode of activity, prior warmup, and the warning and humidification of inspired air (for reviews see Anderson, 1985; Katz, 1987; Neijens, 1989). Using these means it is very seldom that an asthmatic child should be exempted from exercise and sports. Two potentially detrimental effects are related to swimming: The diving reflex that occurs with water immersion may induce

bronchoconstriction in asthmatics, secondary to parasympathetic drive (Sturani, Sturani, & Tosi, 1985); and, mostly in indoor pools, chlorine and its derivatives may irritate the airways and trigger bronchoconstriction (for a review, see Bar-Or & Inbar, in press). The clinical relevance of these effects has not been ascertained.

Cystic Fibrosis (CF)

Enhanced physical activity has been recommended for patients with CF to improve their respiratory muscle endurance (Keens et al., 1977; Orenstein et al., 1981), to increase lung volumes and flows (Jankowski, 1987), and to enhance the clearance of mucus from the airways (Orenstein et al., 1981; Zach, Purrer, & Oberwaldner, 1981). The latter effect has been suggested based on larger quantities of sputum collected on days when the child is active than on days when he or she is sedentary. This method is indirect and crude and it depends markedly on compliance.

Arterial O_2 desaturation during maximal or near-maximal effort has been well documented (Cerny & Armitage, 1989; Henke & Orenstein, 1984), mostly among patients with advanced lung disease. It is unclear whether such a response is a contraindication to participation in exercise. Another detrimental effect is the loss of large quantities of the NaCl in the sweat, which suppresses the patient's thirst and induces dehydration during prolonged exercise in hot climates. This may lead to excessive heat strain (Bar-Or et al., 1992). Educating the child and parents about the importance of drinking beyond thirst in hot climates is an effective way of preventing dehydration in these patients.

Hypertension (HT)

In adults with HT, aerobic training has been shown to induce a decrease of 5 to 25 mmHg in the resting systolic blood pressure (BP) and a 3 to 15 mmHg decrease in diastolic BP (for reviews see Seals & Hagberg, 1984; Tipton, 1984). Several recent cross-sectional studies with children and adolescents have shown an inverse relationship between resting BP (mostly systolic) and aerobic fitness or habitual activity (Fraser, Phillips, & Harris, 1983; Harshfield et al., 1990; Hoffman et al., 1987; Panico et al., 1987; Strazullo et al., 1988). This relationship, which is more common in males than in females, has been used to suggest that physical activity and fitness in children and adolescents can help to keep a low BP, possibly through lowering of peripheral vascular resistance. Conformation of this claim through longitudinal studies, however, is inconclusive.

There are very few training intervention studies in adolescents—and none in prepubescents—with HT. A 6-month, 3 sessions-per-week jogging program induced an 8 mmHg reduction in systolic BP and a 5 mmHg reduction in diastolic BP (Hagberg et al., 1983) of 14- to 18-year-old girls and boys whose BP had been above the 95th percentile of the general population. A subgroup of those boys carried on with a 5-month weight training program at the end of the jogging program, which induced a further decrease in BP (Hagberg et al., 1984). This study included controls, but they were not randomly selected. An uncontrolled 2-month weight training program in boys with HT did not induce changes in BP (Laird, Hines, Fixler, & Swanbom, 1979). The BP lowering effect of training seems shortlived. When Hagberg's subjects were retested 9 to 10 months after the programs, their BP had reverted to its preprogram values.

A potential problem for the patient with HT is that an acute bout of high-intensity exercise may induce a major rise in BP. Intraarterial pressure of young adults may exceed 350/250 mmHg during high-resistance weight training (MacDougall et al.,1985). There are no comparable data for children, but during a maximal aerobic test, the systolic pressure of adolescents often reaches 200 mmHg. It is somewhat higher in adolescent athletes (Dlin, 1986) and those with established HT (Nudel et al., 1980).

Should training be recommended for adolescents with HT? The Sixteenth Bethesda Conference on cardiovascular abnormalities in athletes (Frohlich, Lowenthal, Miller, Pickering, & Strong, 1985) endorsed unlimited participation in sports among adolescents whose resting diastolic BP does not exceed 115 mmHg and who have

no target organ damage. In secondary HT, or whenever a target organ has been affected, participation should be limited to low-intensity, noncontact sports. Likewise, the Task Force on Blood Pressure Control in Children (1987) recommends that, in spite of the potentially excessive BP response to exercise, "restriction in sports or other activities should be limited only to those few individuals with severe hypertension who have not yet had adequate response to therapy (p. 15)."

Obesity

Because of its high—and increasing—prevalence, childhood obesity presents a major public health challenge in North America. Although tracking obesity from childhood to adulthood is only fair, an obese child has a higher likelihood of becoming an obese adolescent and adult than does a lean child (Seidman, Laor, Gale, Stevenson, & Danon, 1991).

Enhanced physical activity has been recognized as an important component in the management of childhood obesity; two others are dietary changes and behavior modification. Table 8.3 is a summary of physiologic changes, other than aerobic fitness, that may result from training. Following are some comments regarding these changes.

It has commonly been accepted that aerobic training induces a decrease in percent body fat. Very few data (e.g., Parizkova & Vamberova, 1967; Sasaki, Shindo,

Table 8.3   Training Effects Reported for the Obese Child

Function	Effect of physical training *
Body composition	
Body weight	o/−
% body fat	−
Fat-free mass	o/+
Appetite	o/−
Biochemical changes	
Plasma insulin	−
Sensitivity to insulin	+
Glucose tolerance	+
FFA mobilization	+
Low-density lipoprotein	−
Serum triglycerides	−
Total serum cholesterol	o/−
High-density lipoprotein	+
Blood pressure	−
Energy expenditure	
Resting	Counteracts reduction by diet
Total	+

* − = decrease; o = no change; + = increase. Adapted by permission from Parker & Bar-Or (1991).

Tanaka, Ando, & Arakawa, 1987), however, are available to confirm this effect in obese children. Multimodality interventions, such as by Ylitalo (1981) will not be discussed here. The study by Sasaki et al. (1987) is unique in that the intervention was prolonged (2 years). Their subjects responded with a 30% to 40% decline in "an index of adiposity." This contrasts with an earlier prolonged study (Moody, Wilmore, Girandola, & Royce, 1972), in which 15- and 29-month interventions resulted in a very mild (2.53% and 3.14%) decrease in percent fat of obese female adolescents. These conflicting findings may be explained by the lower training dose in Moody's program.

The inconsistent effect of training raises the possibility that the increase in calorie expenditure, anticipated as a result of training, is different from that actually induced by the intervention. For example, would a prescribed training program induce a compensatory decrease in the spontaneous physical activity of obese children such that their overall additional calorie expenditure would be less than that expected from the program itself? This question was recently addressed by Blaak, Westerterp, Bar-Or, Wouters, and Saris (1992), who found that mildly obese 11- to 12-year-old boys did not change their spontaneous activity while undergoing a laboratory-based 1-month program of daily cycling sessions. Their total energy expenditure (doubly labeled water) increased beyond the values expected from the program itself. It remains to be seen whether the same pattern will hold for children from other societies and with higher adiposity levels.

Very-low-calorie diets may induce a negative nitrogen balance. A question of importance for the growing child is whether the anabolic effect of exercise can prevent such a diet-induced protein loss. Two recent experiments show that this may be the case. In one (Blaak, Bar-Or, Westerterp, & Saris, 1990), a loss of fat-free mass occurred in 11- to 12-year-old boys following a 3-week very-low-calorie diet (750 kcal per 24 h). In contrast, a 4-week aerobic program that raised the daily energy expenditure of such obese boys by 10% to 15%, was accompanied by an increase in fat-free mass (Blaak et al., 1992). No studies are available, however, that directly compare equicalorie exercise and dietary interventions and their effect on protein flux and balance.

Future Directions

Most studies on training-induced specific benefits in children with chronic disease have used subpar experimental design, a small sample size, or an insufficient training dose. Conclusions derived from such research therefore are tentative, at best. More studies are indicated that use randomly controlled interventions of optimal dosage. Even if the available patient pool for any given project is small, the use of such a design will allow for subsequent pooling of the data by metaanalysis to draw definitive conclusions.

Even though single-discipline interventions are needed to understand the mechanisms by which training imparts its benefits, it is likely that maximal and sustained benefits will require multidisciplinary interventions. Examples are the combination of diet, training, and behavior modification in juvenile obesity, and the use of medications, nutritional supplementation, training, and physical therapy in cystic fibrosis. A future challenge therefore is to study the efficacy of such multidisciplinary interventions, using well-defined dosages for each.

Much of the data on the deleterious effects of exertion have been derived from case studies and anecdotal information. Indeed, ethical constraints preclude conducting intervention studies, the end point of which is damage to the child's health. To obtain better insight into such potential damage (e.g., exercise-induced seizures in epilepsy; enhanced damage to muscle cells as a result of intense exertion in muscular dystrophy; excessive heat strain in children with cyanotic heart defects), the onus is on clinicials and scientists to describe cases with sufficient details regarding, for example, the type, intensity, and duration of the exercise provocation; the prevailing climatic conditions; and any objective data documenting damage.

References

Anderson, S.D. (1985). Exercise-induced asthma: The state of the art. *Chest*, **87** (Suppl.), 191S-195S.

Arensman, F.W., Christiansen, J.L., & Strong, W.B. (1989). Juvenile hypertension and exercise. In O. Bar-Or (Ed.), *Advances in pediatric sport sciences* (pp. 203-221). Champaign, IL: Human Kinetics.

Bar-Or, O. (1983). *Pediatric sports medicine for the practitioner: From physiologic principles to clinical applications*. New York: Springer-Verlag.

Bar-Or, O. (1985). Response to physical conditioning in children with cardiopulmonary disease. *Exercise and Sport Sciences Reviews, 13*, 305-334.

Bar-Or, O. (1990). Disease-specific benefits of training in the child with a chronic disease: What is the evidence? *Pediatric Exercise Science, 2*, 299-312.

Bar-Or, O., Blimkie, C.J.R., Hay, J.A., MacDougall, J.D., Ward, D.S., & Wilson, W.M. (1992). Voluntary dehydration and heat intolerance in cystic fibrosis. *Lancet, 339*, 696-699.

Bar-Or, O., & Inbar, O. (in press). Swimming and asthma: Benefits and detrimental effects. *Sports Medicine*.

Beekman, R.H. (1986). Exercise recommendation for adolescents after surgery for congenital heart disease. *Pediatrician, 13*, 210-219.

Blaak, E.E., Bar-Or, O., Westerterp, K.R., & Saris, W.H.M. (1990). Effect of VLCD on daily energy expenditure and body composition in obese boys. *International Journal of Obesity, 14*(Suppl. 2), 86.

Blaak, E.E., Westerterp, K.R., Bar-Or, O., Wouters, L.J.M., & Saris, W.H.M. (1992). Total energy expenditure and spontaneous activity in relation to training in obese boys. *American Journal of Clinical Nutrition, 55*, 777-782.

Cerny, F.J., & Armitage, L.M. (1989). Exercise and cystic fibrosis: A review. *Pediatric Exercise Science, 1*, 116-126.

Despres, J.P., Bouchard, C., & Malina, R.M. (1990). Physical activity and coronary heart disease risk factors during childhood and adolescence. *Exercise and Sport Sciences Review, 18*, 243-261.

Dlin, R. (1986). Blood pressure response to dynamic exercise in healthy and hypertensive youths. *Pediatrician, 13*, 34-43.

Fitch, K.D., Morton, A.R., & Blanksby, B.A. (1976). Effects of swimming training on children with asthma. *Archives of Disease in Childhood, 51*, 190-194.

Fraser, G.E., Phillips, R.L., & Harris, R. (1983). Physical fitness and blood pressure in school children. *Circulation, 67*, 405-412.

Frohlich, E.D., Lowenthal, D.R., Miller, H.S., Pickering, T., & Strong, W.B. (1985). Task Force IV: Systemic arterial hypertension. *Journal of American College Cardiology, 6*, 1218-1221.

Hagberg, J.M., Ehsani, A.A., Goldring, D., Hernandez, A., Sinacore, D.R., & Holloszy, J.O. (1984). Effect of weight training on blood pressure and hemodynamics in hypertensive adolescents. *Pediatrics, 104*, 147-151.

Hagberg, J.M., Goldring, D., Ehsani, A.A., Heath, G.W., Hernandez, A., Schechtman, K., & Holloszy, J.O. (1983). Effect of exercise training on the blood pressure and hemodynamic features of hypertensive adolescents. *American Journal of Cardiology, 52*, 763-768.

Harshfield, G.A., Dupaul, L.M., Alpert, B.S., Christman, J.V., Willey, E.S., Murphy, J.K., & Somes, G.W. (1990). Aerobic fitness and the diurnal rhythm of blood pressure in adolescents. *Hypertension, 15*(6), 810-814.

Henke, K.G., & Orenstein, D.M. (1984). Oxygen saturation during exercise in cystic fibrosis. *American Reviews of Respiratory Disease, 129*, 708-711.

Henriksen, J.M., & Nielsen, T. (1983). Effect of physical training on exercise-induced bronchoconstriction. *Acta Paediatrica Scandinavica, 72*, 31-36.

Hoffman, A., Walter, H.J., Connelly, P.A., & Vaughn, R.D. (1987). Blood pressure and physical fitness in children. *Hypertension, 9*, 188-191.

Huang, S.W., Veiga, R., Sila, U., Reed, E., & Hines, S. (1989). The effect of swimming on asthmatic children—participants in a swimming program in the city of Baltimore. *Journal of Asthma, 26*, 117-121.

Jankowski, L.W. (1987). Exercise testing and exercise prescription for individuals with cystic fibrosis. In J.S. Skinner (Ed.), *Exercise testing and exercise prescription for special cases* (pp. 189-202). Philadelphia: Lea & Febiger.

Katz, R.M. (1987). Coping with exercise-induced asthma. *Physician and Sportsmedicine, 15*, 101-108.

Keens, T.G., Krastins, I.R.B., Wannamaker, E.M., Levison, H., Crozier, O.N., & Bryan, C. (1977). Ventilatory muscle endurance training in normal subjects and patients with cystic fibrosis. *American Reviews of Respiratory Disease, 116*, 853-860.

King, M.J., Noakes, T.D., & Weinberg, E.G. (1989). Physiological effects of a physical activity program in children with exercise-induced asthma. *Pediatric Exercise Science, 1*, 137-144.

Laird, W.P., Hines, H., Fixler, D.E., & Swanbom, C.D. (1979). Effect of chronic weight lifting on the blood pressure in hypertensive adolescents (abstract). *Preventive Medicine, 8*, 184.

Leisti, S., Finnila, M.-J., & Kiura, E. (1979). Effects of physical training on hormonal responses to exercise in asthmatic children. *Archives of Diseases in Childhood, 54*, 524-528.

MacDougall, J.D., Tuxen, D., Sale, D.G., Moroz, J.R., & Sutton, J.R. (1985). Arterial blood pressure response to heavy resistance exercise. *Journal of Applied Physiology, 58*, 785-790.

Moody, D.L., Wilmore, J.H., Girandola, R.N., & Royce, J.P. (1972). The effect of a jogging program on the body composition of normal and obese high school girls. *Medicine and Science in Exercise and Sports, 4*, 210-213.

Neijens, H.J. (1989). Exercise and the child with bronchial asthma. In O. Bar-Or (Ed.), *Advances in pediatric sport sciences* (pp. 191-201). Champaign, IL: Human Kinetics.

Nudel, D.B., Gootman, N., Brunson, C.S., Stengler, A., Shenker, R., & Gauthier, B.G. (1980). Exercise performance of adolescent hypertensives. *Pediatrics, 65*, 1073-1078.

Orenstein, D.M. (1988). Exercise tolerance and exercise conditioning in children with chronic lung disease. *Journal of Pediatrics, 112*, 1043-1047.

Orenstein, D.M., Franklin, B.A., Doershuk, C.F., Hellerstein, H.K., Germann, K.J., Horowitz, J.G., & Stern, R. (1981). Exercise conditioning and cardiopulmonary fitness in cystic fibrosis. The effects of a 3-month running program. *Chest, 80*, 392-398.

Oseid, S., & Haaland, K. (1978). Exercise studies on asthmatic children before and after regular physical training. In B. Eriksson & B. Furberg (Eds.), *Swimming medicine IV* (pp. 32-41). Baltimore: University Park Press.

Panico, S., Celentano, E., Krogh, V., Jossa, F., Farinaro, E., Trevisan, M., & Mancini, M. (1987). Physical activity and its relationship to blood pressure in schoolchildren. *Journal of Chronic Diseases*, **10**, 925-930.

Parizkova, J., & Vamberova, M. (1967). Body composition as a criterion of the suitability of reducing regimens in obese children. *Developmental Medicine and Child Neurology*, **9**, 202-211.

Parker, D.F., & Bar-Or, O. (1991). Juvenile obesity: The importance of exercise—and getting children to do it. *Physician and Sportsmedicine*, **19**, 113-125.

Rowland, T.W. (1990). *Exercise and children's health.* Champaign, IL: Human Kinetics.

Sasaki, J., Shindo, M., Tanaka, H., Ando, M., & Arakawa, K. (1987). A long-term aerobic exercise program decreases the obesity index and increases the high density lipoprotein cholesterol concentration in obese children. *International Journal of Obesity*, **11**, 339-345.

Schnall, R., Ford, P., Gillam, I., & Landau, L. (1982). Swimming and dry land exercises in children with asthma. *Australian Paediatric Journal*, **18**, 23-27.

Seals, D.R., & Hagberg, J.M. (1984). The effect of exercise training on human hypertension. *Medicine and Science of Sports and Exercise*, **16**, 207-215.

Siedman, D.S., Laor, A., Gale, R., Stevenson, D.K., & Danon, Y.L. (1991). A longitudinal study of birth weight and being overweight in late adolescence. *American Journal of Diseases of Children*, **145**, 782-785.

Strazzulo, P., Cappuccio, P., Trevisan, M., De Leo, A., Krogh, V., Giorgione, N., & Mancini, M. (1988). Leisure-time physical activity and blood pressure in schoolchildren. *American Journal of Epidemiology*, **127**, 726-733.

Sturani, C., Sturani, A., & Tosi, I. (1985). Parasympathetic activity assessed by diving reflex and by airway response to metacholine in bronchial asthma and rhinitis. *Respiration*, **48**, 321-328.

Svenonius, E., Kautto, R., & Arborelius, M. (1983). Improvement after training of children with exercise-induced asthma. *Acta Paediatrica Scandinavica*, **72**, 23-30.

Swann, I.L., & Hanson, C.A. (1983). Double-blind prospective study of the effect of physical training on childhood asthma. In S. Oseid & A.M. Edwards (Eds.), *The asthmatic child in play and sport* (pp. 318-322). Bath, England: Putnam Press.

Szentagothal, K., Gyene, I., Szocska, M., & Osvath, P. (1987). Physical exercise program for children with bronchial asthma. *Pediatric Pulmonology*, **3**, 166-172.

Tanizaki, Y., Komagoe, H., Sudo, M., & Morinaga, H. (1984). Swimming training in a hot spring pool as therapy for steroid-dependent asthma. *Arerugi*, **33**, 389-395.

Task Force on Blood Pressure Control in Children. (1987). Report of the Second Task Force on Blood Pressure Control in Children–1987. *Pediatrics*, **79**, 1-25.

Tipton, C.M. (1984). Exercise, training, and hypertension. *Exercise and Sport Science Reviews*, **12**, 245-306.

Walberg, J., & Ward, D. (1985). Role of physical activity in the etiology and treatment of childhood obesity. *Pediatrics*, **12**, 82-88.

Ylitalo, V. (1981). Treatment of obese schoolchildren with special reference to the mode of therapy, cardiorespiratory performance, and the carbohydrate and lipid metabolism. *Acta Paediatrica Scandinavica* (Suppl. 290), 1-108.

Zach, M., Purrer, B., & Oberwaldner, B. (1981). Effect of swimming on forced expiration sputum clearance in cystic fibrosis. *Lancet*, **2**, 1201-1203.

9

An Active and Fit Way-of-Life Influencing Health and Longevity

Ralph S. Paffenbarger, Jr.
Robert T. Hyde
Alvin L. Wing
I-Min Lee
James B. Kampert

The positive benefits of physical activity and physical fitness on health and longevity are best appreciated when contrasted to the sluggishness or negative consequences associated with inactivity or sedentary living. This can be depicted in a pair of schema. The first pattern shows that where exercise is adequate, fitness is likely to be maintained or improved, good health is preserved, quality of life is favorable, chronic disease is avoided or deferred, and length of life is maximal:

Physical Activity → Physical Fitness → High Quality of Life → Low Chronic Disease Risk → Long Life.

The second pattern shows the likely consequences of a downward trend of existence where lack of exercise reduces fitness to unfitness or debilitation, lifestyle and quality of life become unfavorable, health deteriorates toward chronic disease, and risk increases of premature death or shortened life:

Physical Inactivity → Physical Unfitness → Low Quality of Life → High Chronic Disease Risk → Short Life.

The important relation between these two schemata is that avoidance or correction of the problems inherent in the downward path of the second may result in an adherence or return to the beneficial status represented by the first. Inactive individuals may become more physically active, unfit people may regain fitness, their lifestyles may become more favorable to the avoidance of early chronic disease, and they may expect to live longer, healthier, and more satisfying lives than if they had not adjusted their habitual activity patterns.

Current Status of Knowledge

Both physical activity and physiological fitness include optional variables capable of favoring health and longevity, but with fundamentally different implications, because physical activity is a behavior and fitness is a condition. In this sense, physical activity is a dynamic, ongoing concept, and fitness a static or cross-sectional concept. Yet these are intertwined, where fitness establishes bench marks and limitations for physical activity, and activity modifies fitness from one cross-sectional status to another.

Since beneficial physical activity may fend off chronic disease, especially coronary heart disease (CHD) (Berlin & Colditz, 1990; Kendrick, Williamson, & Caspersen, 1991; Paffenbarger, Hyde, Wing, & Hsieh, 1986a; Powell, Thompson, Caspersen, & Kendrick, 1987), and postpone mortality, we now are asking how to promote such exercise and how to anticipate that our longer and more active lives will be blessed with satisfaction and a realization of the higher quality of life that our improved health can make possible. Optimum healthful longevity is the ultimate objective of all preventive medicine, the desired result that makes the entire program cost-effective (Bunker, Gomby, & Kehrer, 1989; Russell, 1986; Shephard, 1990). An ounce of prevention is worth a pound of cure, a stitch in time saves nine, and an apple a day keeps the doctor away if you hike to the orchard and pick the apple yourself.

The achievement of good quality of life is of paramount importance today, but we are only beginning to examine the ways and means by which we can put our constructive efforts to best use.

Physical Activity and Health

A few recent or current studies have been looking at physical activity, fitness, and longevity. Professor J.N. Morris of the London School of Hygiene and Tropical Medicine, who with his colleagues, pioneered studies of vigorous exercise and CHD (Morris, Heady, Raffle, Roberts, & Parks, 1953; Morris, Kagan, Pattison, Gardner, & Raffle, 1966), has extended those analyses to all-cause mortality or longevity among 9,376 British civil servants, aged 45 to 65 years (Morris, Clayton, Everitt, Semmence, & Burgess, 1990; Morris, Everitt, Pollard, Chave, & Semmence, 1980).

For vigorous sportsplay in a 9-year follow-up, they showed that men aged 45 to 54 years required more energy expenditure to achieve beneficial levels of exertion against CHD than their elders, aged 55 to 64 years, who had lower functional capacity with advancing age. Nonvigorous sportsplay showed little benefit in reducing CHD risk over none at all.

With regard to all-cause mortality and longevity in this study population, Morris et al. (1990) reported: "When noncoronary deaths were added to those from CHD, total death rates were lower in men with an exercise related reduction in CHD, and their survival through middle age and into old age greater than in other men."

Socioeconomic and other differences between the British and American study populations were considered among possible explanations for the varying outcomes described. Morris et al. (1990) had characterized their study population as more active than average Britons and perhaps more fit and active than age-comparable Harvard alumni. The alumni might, therefore, show benefit from less exercise than the British to improve their health. Differing methods of activity assessment also might be involved, although the ratio of less active to more active individuals was about 2:1 in both populations.

Patterns of physical activity and mortality among 9,484 elderly Seventh Day Adventist men, during 1960 to 1985, were reported by Linsted, Tonstad, and Kuzma (1991). Men who reported moderate physical activity were older and had lower death rates than those who were deemed highly active or those who reported little or no physical activity.

A multivariate analysis of all-cause mortality showed that interaction between activity level and age was significant for both moderate activity and high activity. At age 50 the respective relative risks were about equal. Moderate activity continued protective beyond age 80, but higher activity lost statistical significance at age 70.

The analysis showed that crossover of risk for moderate activity occurred at 95.4 years of age, and for higher activity at 78.2 years of age. Crossover is the experience point at which the relative risk reaches 1.0; where inactivity and activity no longer influence survival differentially. However, these findings reveal that moderate physical activity continues to be important well into old age, but at each age class all-cause death rates were higher for the highly active than the moderately active.

Kaplan, Seeman, Cohen, Knudsen, and Guralnik (1987) studied physical activity status and mortality data on 4,174 adults aged at least 38 years in 1964, as a cohort of the Alameda County (California) Study. In this age-specific analysis intended to focus on the elderly aged 60 years and older, two younger groups were included for comparison. The findings showed that physical activity benefits continue into the later years of life beyond middle age.

Leisure-time physical activity among male U.S. railroad workers for relation to death from CHD and all causes in a 17- to 20-year follow-up period was studied by Slattery, Jacobs, and Nichaman (1989). Some 3,000 had been queried as to activity patterns and examined for other characteristics between 1957 and 1960. They were reexamined from 1962 to 1964 and followed until 1977. The relative risk of CHD death was 1.28 for men who expended 40 kcal per week as compared with very active men who expended 3,632 kcal per week; the corresponding relative risk for all-cause mortality was 1.21. Leisure-time energy expenditure in light and moderate activities, as well as that of intense effort, showed independent relations to both CHD and all-cause mortality.

Professor A. Gerald Shaper and his colleague, Mr. G. Wannamethee, from the Royal Free Hospital School of Medicine in London have been examining the relation between physical activity and risks of CHD and stroke in middle-aged men, randomly chosen from general medical practices in 24 British towns, which are representative of the socioeconomic distribution of men in that country (Shaper & Wannamethee, 1991; Wannamethee & Shaper, 1992). Research nurses administered a standard questionnaire asking about physical activity, social habits, and a medical history. They made physical measurements, and took electrocardiograms and blood samples, the latter for biochemical and hematological assessments. The questions on leisure-time physical activities led to a complex classification system of six grades of energy expenditure that combine total effort and intensity of effort into six groups from inactive, occasional, light, moderate, moderately vigorous, and vigorous. All men, whether or not they showed evidence of CHD at initial examination, were followed for CHD morbidity and all-cause mortality through established procedures in the British health care system. Men aged 40 to 59 years at entry were followed for CHD events over an 8-year period; men aged 45 to 59 years were followed for stroke events over an 8.5-year period.

With respect to physical activity and CHD, risk decreased with increasing physical activity. The groups reporting moderate or moderately vigorous activity experienced less than half the rate for inactive men. Vigorously active men experienced higher rates, similar to those classified as occasionally or lightly active. Men who entered with symptomatic CHD experienced a lower rate of recurrence at occasional, light, and moderate levels of physical activity, but an increased rate at the moderately vigorous level. Men who entered with asymptomatic CHD experienced a higher rate of recurrence at light and moderate levels, with a decline again at moderately vigorous levels. Overall, men who reported sportsplaying (vigorous) activities weekly had lower CHD rates than men reporting no sportsplaying. After excluding sportsplaying from the analysis, there remained a significant inverse relation between physical activity and CHD incidence in the 8-year follow-up.

Physical activity was inversely related to risk of stroke, both in men free of CHD and stroke at entry and in those with one or the other of these conditions. However, in asymptomatic men at entry, sportsplaying (vigorous) activity now was associated with an increased rate of CHD as compared with that for men engaged in moderate or moderately vigorous activity. And, in men symptomatic from CHD or stroke, those engaged in moderately vigorous or vigorous activity tended to experience a higher risk of CHD than that of inactive men.

These observations by Shaper and Wannamethee (1991, 1992) suggest that moderate physical activity (frequent walking or cycling, very frequent recreational activities, or sportsplaying once a week) is associated with lower rates of CHD and stroke in men both with and without pre-existing CHD. They offer a cautionary note, however, suggesting no further lowering of rates from either disease among men engaging in the most vigorous activities. In fact, frequent sportsplay and recreational (competitive?) activities may be associated with higher rates than those for less vigorous, regular physical activities.

Physiological Fitness and Health

Dr. S.N. Blair (1989) and his colleagues at the Cooper Institute for Aerobics Research in Dallas, Texas, assessed fitness by treadmill performance in 10,244 men and 3,120 women aged 20 to 60+ years and followed them for more than 8 years, for all-cause mortality. Mortality rates were lowest among the most fit and highest among the least fit men and women, parallelling closely the results from studies of physical activity levels and mortality.

Since physical activity habits and fitness often are linked, these findings may imply that the beneficial effects of physical activity on health and survival are mediated via fitness status. Beneficial exercise is known to influence many body systems favorably, while systemic conditions may have roles in determining physiological fitness, for example, cardiovascular-respiratory fitness.

In a 7-year follow-up of a representative sample of the Canadian population, Arraiz, Wigle, and Mao (1992) used a home fitness test to distinguish 807 subjects (37%) with a recommended level of fitness, 375 (17%) with minimally acceptable levels, and 992 (46%) with unacceptable levels. Compared with the most fit, the relative risk of all-cause mortality was 1.6 (95% confidence interval = 0.6-4.2) for subjects with minimally acceptable fitness levels and 2.7 (95% confidence interval = 1.4-5.5) for unacceptable levels. Their findings by fitness levels were similar for cardiovascular disease mortality but unrelated to risks of death from cancer of all sites.

Physical Activity and Mortality

Rates and relative risks of death, from 1977 to 1985, among 11,864 Harvard alumni, by patterns of physical activity assessed in 1977 were studied by Paffenbarger, Hyde, Wing, Lee, and Kampert (in press). These alumni had self-reported the absence of physician-diagnosed CHD on each of two mail questionnaires returned either in 1962 or 1966 and in 1977. Findings agree closely with earlier results among 16,936 alumni (including some of the same men) assessed in 1962 or 1966 and followed for all-cause mortality through 1978 (Paffenbarger et al., 1986a; Paffenbarger, Hyde, Wing, & Hsieh, 1986b). The impact of new, popular interest in physical activity and fitness appears evident among the alumni, whose habitual participation in exercise such as walking and sportsplaying, as measured by prevalence or percentage of man-years, had increased appreciably by 1977 although 11 to 15 years had elapsed.

Table 9.1 contrasts the effects of presence and absence of each of four adverse patterns of sedentary living—low levels of walking, low levels of stair-climbing, lack of moderate sportsplaying, and leisure-time physical activity totaling less than 2,000 kcal per week. Each risk estimate is adjusted for difference in age, other components of physical activity, cigarette smoking, hypertension, overweight-for-height, and parental mortality before age 65. Over the 9-year follow-up period, alumni walking less than 5 km per week, or climbing fewer than 20 floors (about 400 steps), were respectively at 27% or 22% higher risk of death than men who walked or climbed further. Men who did not engage in sportsplay or other recreational activities requiring 4.5 or more METS of intensity, were at 50% higher risk than classmates who did. Thus, paucity of walking and stair-climbing, and absence of moderately vigorous recreational activities made independent contributions to higher risk of premature mortality. Summing walking, stair climbing, and all sportsplaying into kilocalories expended each week, men with an index below 2,000 were at 40% higher risk of death than men physically more active.

As seen in the population attributable risk estimates in the table, if all 11,864 alumni had walked at least 5 km per week, or climbed 20 or more floors, or played moderately intense games or sports, death rates accordingly might have been 7%, 8%, or 15% lower than were actually observed. In terms of physical activity index, the risk of death might have been reduced by 20% if every man had expended 2,000 or more kcal per week in walking, stair-climbing, and recreational activities, and 146 of the 730 deaths during the 9 years of follow-up might have been delayed beyond 1985.

Changes in Physical Activity and Mortality

Age-adjusted rates and relative risks of all-cause mortality are presented in Table 9.2, by continuities and changes in patterns of physical activity of the 11,864 alumni as determined from their questionnaires of 1962 or 1966, and again in 1977. These men had completed both a first and second questionnaire, and were free of self-reported, physician-diagnosed CHD on both occasions. Moderate sportsplay and physical activity index are tabulated as favorable levels associated with reduced risk of death during the follow-up through 1985. Physical activity options (sportsplay and index) are categorized by four combinations of earlier and later participation status, listed in order of presumed increasing benefit, defined as lowered risk of death:

1) High risk status unchanged
2) Low risk status changed to high risk

3) High risk status changed to low risk
4) Low risk status unchanged

The findings for moderate sportsplay resemble those of the activity index pattern, even though one is defined by metabolic equivalents (4.5+ METS) and the other in kilocalories per week. This might be expected since the index includes all sportsplay in hours per week equated to kilocalories. The few men who dropped moderate sportsplay (3% of man-years) were at 23% increased risk (not significant) over men who never reported such recreation. When men with diagnosed cancer were excluded from the starting population, the added risk from discontinuing moderately intense activities was only 12%. Remarkably, even though these alumni had aged 11 to 15 years since answering the first questionnaire, and were indeed in late middle age (58.2 ± 9.1 years of age), 38% of the man-years represented men who had taken up moderate sportsplay, and 41% more were those who had continued it. Three-fourths of the experience identified alumni who participated in leisure-time activities of at least 4.5 METS intensity in 1977.

By "index," 42% of the man-years represented alumni who had never reported enough activity to reach 2,000 or more kcal per week. Another 16% of man-years was contributed by men who by 1977 had dropped below the 2,000 kcal index level and showed a slightly higher (not significant) death rate during the follow-up through 1985 than men persistently sedentary. Quite in contrast, men (prevalence 19% of man-years) who increased their index to favorable levels achieved a relative risk of 0.74, as low as the 0.79 ratio of their classmates who had been active at 2,000 or more kcal per week all along.

Table 9.1   Relative and Attributable Risks of Death[a] Among Harvard Alumni, 1977 to 1985, by Patterns of Sedentary Living

Sedentary living (weekly)	Man-years (%)	Relative risk of death	Population attributable risk (%)	p value
Walking <5 km	26	1.27(1.08-1.50)	7.1(1.9-12.0)	0.004
Stair-climbing <20 floors	37	1.22(1.04-1.42)	8.5(1.5-15.0)	0.013
No moderate sportsplaying[b]	22	1.50(1.27-1.77)	14.6(8.3-20.4)	<0.001
Physical activity index <2,000 kcal[c]	58	1.40(1.19-1.66)	20.4(10.6-29.1)	0.001

[a]Adjusted for differences in age, other components of physical activity, cigarette smoking, hypertension, overweight-for-height, and parental mortality before age 65; 95% confidence intervals in parentheses.

[b]4.5+ METS intensity.

[c]In walking, stair-climbing, and sportsplaying.

Table 9.2 Rates and Relative Risks of Death[a] Among Harvard Alumni, 1977 to 1985, by Continuities and Changes in Patterns of Physical Activity Between 1962 or 1966 and 1977

Physical activity pattern	Status in 1962 or 1966	Status in 1977	Man-years (%)	Number deaths	Deaths per 10,000 man-years	Relative risk of death	p value
Moderate	No	No	18	234	84.1	1.00	
sportsplaying	Yes	No	3	45	103.1	1.23(0.88-1.63)	0.666
(4.5+ METS	No	Yes	38	184	59.6	0.71(0.57-0.86)	0.007
intensity)	Yes	Yes	41	170	58.4	0.69(0.58-0.90)	<0.001
Physical activity	No	No	42	346	72.9	1.00	
index 2,000+ kcal/wk	Yes	No	16	147	87.6	1.20(0.90-1.56)	0.077
(in walking, stair-	No	Yes	19	87	54.3	0.74(0.58-0.95)	0.011
climbing, and	Yes	Yes	23	118	57.2	0.79(0.63-0.98)	0.023
sportsplaying)							

[a]Adjusted for differences in age, other components of physical activity, cigarette smoking, hypertension, overweight-for-height, and parental mortality before age 65; 95% confidence intervals in parentheses.

Age-specific rates and relative risks are displayed in Figure 9.1. They indicate benefits of taking up moderate sports and increasing physical activity in all four 10-year age brackets between 45 and 85 years. The death rate differential for sportsplay increased slightly from 19% to 34%, while that for index declined from 48% to 11% with advancing age.

Physical Activity and Longevity

If physical activity postpones death, one result should be increased longevity. Table 9.3 gives estimated added years of life associated with maintaining or adopting adequate physical activity versus life expectancy with less energy output. These estimates were derived from modified life-table analyses using the observed alumni mortality experience (1977 to 1985). Extrapolations to a younger age group (35 to 44 years of age) are included. The age-specific benefits decrease with advancing age, since the older men are nearer the natural life-span limit and already have passed through longevity brackets yet to be reached by the younger men. In each age group and overall, the time gained by moderate sportsplay is one-quarter to one-third more than by physical activity index of at least 2,000 kcal per week, as might be anticipated from the death rate analyses described earlier. Also, active Harvard alumni were more likely to feel in control of their own well-being and efforts to achieve satisfactory health, and had lower prevalences of cardiovascular disease and diabetes.

Length of life, or added longevity, has meaning not only in calendar years or months but also in the quality of the life preserved or extended. Quality of life may be defined and assessed in various ways related to fitness, fulfillment, and satisfaction. Besides socioeconomic and

health considerations, there are cultural and philosophical or spiritual aspects beyond price. Current reports reveal that much further study on the subject is needed (Driver, Brown, & Peterson, 1990; King, 1991; Stewart & King, 1991).

Discussion

Evidence accumulates that risks of premature death vis-a-vis increased longevity, are related to physical activity expressed by participation or nonparticipation in moderately vigorous sportsplay and by high or low levels of weekly energy expenditure. Moreover, the findings among Harvard alumni from 1977 through 1985 corroborate closely the results obtained from similar investigations in this population between 1962 or 1966 and 1978 (Paffenbarger et al., 1986a, 1986b; Paffenbarger, Hyde, & Wing, 1990; Paffenbarger et al., in press; Paffenbarger, Hyde, Wing, & Steinmetz, 1984; Paffenbarger, Wing, & Hyde, 1978).

Patterns and trends of data in the present study appear to support further consideration of relations of physical activity, physiological fitness, and survival or longevity. As the population of alumni aged, death rates among the less active (and presumably less fit) were consistently greater than among the more active (and more fit) men of the same ages. As time passed, the original high risk group tended to diminish or eventually almost to disappear by such attrition. Meanwhile, the original low risk group was aging and probably tending to become less active and less fit than in their earlier days. Therefore, in the latest decade of survival, the physical activity and physiological fitness differences between the surviving risk groups have tended to diminish, and their death rates to converge,

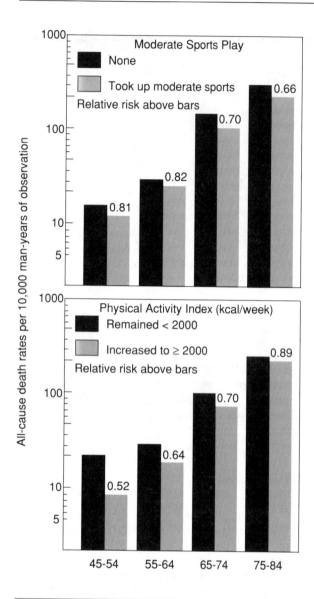

Figure 9.1 Age-specific rates and relative risks of death among Harvard alumni, 1977-1985, by continuities and changes in patterns of physical activity between 1962 or 1966 and 1977. These men had reported themselves free of physician-diagnosed coronary heart disease in 1977.

especially in relation to physical activity index in kilocalories per week. Also, it is likely that the survivors of the original low risk group may have been somewhat more active and fit than their classmates who died sooner. Even in the latest decade, however, the apparent saving influence of moderate sportsplay is still evident from the group differences in death rates and survival. All of these patterns strongly support the hypothesis that adequately vigorous and continuing physical activity is conducive to maximal good health and longevity. Only further follow-up for at least another decade with questionnaires on lifestyles, quality of life, and health status might reveal how long the influences of physical activity on physiological fitness may continue to be important within the normal life span.

The alumni became subject to the influence of national sociomedical and lifeway trends characterized in familiar terms as "the exercise explosion," "fitness-fever," "oil embargo" (eschewing saturated fat), "fiber frenzy" (espousing dietary roughage), "multivitamania," and "weight control," not to mention the "cigarette rebellion," "designated driver," "seatbelt awareness," "drug disdain," and so on. These modern-day trends, each of which may contribute independently and predictably to lowered mortality, are currently fired up by a positive "just-do-it," or a negative "just-say-no" attitude, whichever applies. Changes in ways-of-living and other lifestyle patterns between the 1960s and 1970s, and the ensuing lower all-cause mortality rates through the 1980s among alumni, testify to the favorable impact of at least some of these popular trends. In particular, the hundreds of aging alumni who took up moderately vigorous sportsplay and increased their recreational energy output experienced a substantial reduction in all-cause death rates as contrasted to their less active classmates. And these findings held in all 10-year age classes, 45 to 54 years of age through 75 to 84 years of age, suggesting that it is "never too late to change" and "not too soon to start" (Paffenbarger et al., manuscript submitted for publication).

Thus, we may conclude that the adoption of an active lifestyle may reduce the risk of premature death, and apparently enhance quality of life, or at least satisfaction with life, insofar as that can be measured.

Acknowledgments

This work was supported by U.S. Public Health Service research grants HL 34174 from the National Heart, Lung, and Blood Institute and CA 44854 from the National Cancer Institute.

References

Arraiz, G.A., Wigle, D.T., & Mao, Y. (1992). Risk assessment of physical activity and physical fitness in the Canada Health Survey Mortality Follow-up Study. *Journal of Clinical Epidemiology*, **45**, 419-428.

Berlin, J.A., & Colditz, G.A. (1990). A meta-analysis of physical activity in the prevention of coronary heart disease. *American Journal of Epidemiology*, **132**, 612-628.

Blair, S.N., Kohl, H.W., III, Paffenbarger, R.S., Jr., Clark, D.G., Cooper, K.H., & Gibbons, L.W. (1989). Physical fitness and all-cause mortality: A prospective study of healthy men and women. *Journal of the American Medical Association*, **262**, 2395-2401.

Table 9.3 Added Years of Life[a] to Age 85 From Continuities and Changes[b] in Patterns of Physical Activity as Estimated From the Mortality Experience of Harvard Alumni, 1977 to 1985

Age in 1977	Moderate sportsplay[c] vs. none	Physical activity[d] 2,000+ kcal/wk vs. less	Took up moderate sportsplay[c] vs. none	Physical activity[d] increased to 2,000+ from <2,000 vs. >2,000
[35-44]*	[1.30]	[1.02]	[1.37]	[0.95]
45-54	1.25(0.72-1.79)	0.99(0.53-1.45)	1.31(0.67-1.96)	0.91(0.28-1.54)
55-64	1.07(0.62-1.52)	0.85(0.46-1.25)	1.13(0.58-1.67)	0.79(0.24-1.34)
65-74	0.73(0.42-1.03)	0.58(0.31-0.84)	0.74(0.38-1.09)	0.52(0.16-0.88)
75-84	0.28(0.16-0.39)	0.21(0.11-0.31)	0.26(0.14-0.40)	0.20(0.06-0.33)
45-84	1.06(0.61-1.51)	0.84(0.45-1.23)	1.08(0.55-1.61)	0.77(0.24-1.30)

[a]Adjusted for differences in age, other components of physical activity, cigarette smoking, hypertension, overweight-for-height, and parental mortality before age 65.

[b]Between 1962 or 1966 and 1977.

[c]4.5+ METS intensity.

[d]In walking, stair-climbing, and sportsplaying.

[e]Numbers in brackets are extrapolations.

Bunker, J.B., Gomby, P.S., & Kehrer, B.H. (1989). *Pathways to health; The role of social factors.* Menlo Park, CA: Henry J. Kaiser Foundation.

Driver, B.L., Brown, P.J., & Peterson, G.L. (Eds.) (1990). *Benefits of leisure.* State College, PA: Venture Publishing, Inc.

Kaplan, G.A., Seeman, T.E., Cohen, R.D., Knudsen, L.P., & Guralnik, J. (1987). Mortality among the elderly in the Alameda County Study: Behavioral and demographic risk factors. *American Journal of Public Health*, **77**, 307-312.

Kendrick, J.S., Williamson, D.F., & Caspersen, C.J. (1991). A meta-analysis of physical activity in the prevention of coronary heart disease [Letter to the editor]. *American Journal of Epidemiology*, **134**, 232-234.

King, A.C. (1991). Mini-series: Exercise and aging. *Annals of Behavioral Medicine*, **13**, 87-90.

Linsted, K.D., Tonstad, S., & Kuzma, J.W. (1991). Self-report of physical activity and patterns of mortality in Seventh-Day Adventist men. *Journal of Clinical Epidemiology*, **44**, 355-364.

Morris, J.N., Clayton, D.G., Everitt, M.G., Semmence, A.M., & Burgess, E.H. (1990). Exercise in leisure-time, coronary attack and death rates. *British Heart Journal*, **63**, 325-334.

Morris, J.N., Everitt, M.G., Pollard, R., Chave, S.P.W., & Semmence, A.M. (1980). Vigorous exercise in leisure-time: Protection against coronary heart disease. *Lancet*, **2**, 1207-1210.

Morris, J.N., Heady, J.A., Raffle, P.A.B., Roberts, C.G., & Parks, J.W. (1953). Coronary heart disease and physical activity of work. *Lancet*, **2**, 1053-1057, 1111-1120.

Morris, J.N, Kagan, A., Pattison, D.C., Gardner, M., & Raffle, P.A.B. (1966). Incidence and prediction of ischaemic heart disease in London busmen. *Lancet*, **2**, 552-559.

Paffenbarger, R.S., Jr., Hyde, R.T., & Wing, A.L. (1990). Chronic disease in former college students: XXXVI. Physical activity and physical fitness as determinants of health and longevity. In C. Bouchard, R.J. Shephard, T. Stephens, J.R. Sutton, & B.D. McPherson (Eds.), *Exercise, fitness, and health: A consensus of current knowledge*, (pp. 33-48). Champaign, IL: Human Kinetics.

Paffenbarger, R.S., Jr., Hyde, R.T., Wing, A.L., & Hsieh, C.-c. (1986a). Chronic disease in former college students: XXX. Physical activity, all-cause mortality, and longevity of college alumni. *New England Journal of Medicine*, **314**, 605-613.

Paffenbarger, R.S., Jr., Hyde, R.T., Wing, A.L., & Hsieh, C.-c. (1986b). Physical activity and longevity of college alumni. (Correspondence in reply to four letters.) *New England Journal of Medicine*, **315**, 399-401.

Paffenbarger, R.S., Jr., Hyde, R.T., Wing, A.L., Lee, I.-M., Jung, D.L., & Kampert, J.B. *Changes in physical activity and other lifestyles associated with mortality among college alumni.* (Manuscript submitted for publication.)

Paffenbarger, R.S., Jr., Hyde, R.T., Wing, A.L., Lee, I.-M., & Kampert, J.B. (in press) Chronic disease in former college students: L. Some interrelationships of physical activity, physiological fitness, health, and longevity. In: C. Bouchard, R.J. Shephard, and T. Stephens (Eds.), *Physical activity, fitness, and health: International proceedings and consensus statement*. Champaign, IL, Human Kinetics Books.

Paffenbarger, R.S., Jr., Hyde, R.T., Wing, A.L., & Steinmetz, C.H. (1984). Chronic disease in former college students: XXV. A natural history of athleticism and cardiovascular health. *Journal of the American Medical Association*, **252**, 491-495.

Paffenbarger, R.S., Jr., Wing, A.L., & Hyde, R.T. (1978). Chronic disease in former college students: XVI. Physical activity as an index of heart attack risk in college alumni. *American Journal of Epidemiology*, **108**, 161-175.

Powell, K.E., Thompson, P.D., Caspersen, C.J., & Kendrick, J.S. (1987). Physical activity and the incidence of coronary heart disease. *Annual Reviews of Public Health*, **8**, 253-287.

Russell, L.B. (1986). *Is prevention better than cure?* Washington, DC: Brookings Institute.

Shaper, A.G., & Wannamethee, G. (1991). Physical activity and ischaemic heart disease in middle-aged British men. *British Heart Journal*, **66**, 384-394.

Shephard, R.J. (1990). Costs and benefits of an exercising versus a nonexercising society. In C. Bouchard, R.J. Shephard, T. Stephens, J.R. Sutton, & B.D. McPherson (Eds.), *Exercise, fitness, and health: A consensus of current knowledge* (pp. 49-60). Champaign, IL: Human Kinetics.

Slattery, M.L., Jacobs, D.R., Jr., & Nichaman, M.Z. (1989). Leisure time physical activity and coronary heart disease death: The US Railroad Study. *Circulation*, **79**, 304-311.

Stewart, A.L., & King, A.C. (1991). Evaluating the efficacy of physical activity for influencing quality-of-life outcomes in older adults. *Annals of Behavioral Medicine*, **13**, 108-116.

Wannamethee, G., & Shaper, A.G. (1992). Physical activity and stroke in British middle aged men. *British Medical Journal*, **304**, 597-601.

10

Adjuvants to Physical Activity: Their Proposed Benefits Versus the Research Findings

Jack H. Wilmore
Norman Gledhill
H. Arthur Quinney

The multi-billion dollar business that has sprung from the fitness and slimming industry has resulted in a proliferation of adjuvants to physical activity. Advertising claims continually lure consumers to use a variety of products, while authoritative information concerning their efficacy is scarce. Adjuvants to physical activity are those practices which, because of their potential physiological effects, are used in an attempt to enhance the benefits or reduce the potential detrimental effects of physical activity on fitness and health. In this chapter, the results of the International Conference on Physical Activity, Fitness, and Health (ICPAFH) Consensus Symposium, as it pertains to the intended purpose and scientific evidence regarding electrical stimulation, massage, sauna, sudation garments, questionable exercise devices/spot reduction, and nutritional supplements, will be considered from a practical point of view.

Supplements to Physical Activity

The intended and primary application of *neuromuscular electrical stimulation*, which will be referred to as "electrical stimulation" (ES), is to increase the strength and endurance of patients undergoing rehabilitation. In addition, it has been proposed that ES increases the strength of trained athletes above that which is achieved via normal resistance training. An examination of the scientific literature confirms that ES increases isometric strength (Wigerstad-Lossing et al, 1988). It also increases isokinetic strength at both slow and fast speeds (Snyder-Mackler, Laddin, Schepsis, & Young, 1991; Williams, Morrissey, & Brewster, 1986), with the magnitude of the strength gains inversely proportional to

the initial muscle strength. The latter finding explains why ES works well for patients undergoing rehabilitation, but is of little or no benefit for highly trained athletes. As well, investigators have been unable to substantiate a beneficial effect of ES on muscular endurance beyond the benefits gained from normal resistance training.

It has been proposed that ES accomplishes its rehabilitative effect on strength through augmentation of Type II rather than Type I fibres, which is a reversal of the accepted order of recruitment (Wigerstad-Lossing et al, 1988). For this reason, ES may bring about additional benefits in muscular strength and/or endurance that have not yet been noted. One aspect of ES, which makes it useful in rehabilitation, is its ability to increase the function of injured muscle without the pain that accompanies voluntary contractions. However, this possibility necessitates the warning that patients should be cautious in using ES during rehabilitation, because pain is usually present so that further injury is not incurred.

In summary, the efficacy of ES in the rehabilitation of injured or postsurgical patients has been substantiated scientifically. However, ES has no proven additional benefit in enhancing the development of muscular strength and endurance beyond that gained from resistance training.

The use of *massage* as an adjuvant to physical activity is widespread and long standing. Massage involves manual manipulation of the soft tissue. It has been proposed to enhance neuromuscular relaxation and joint mobility, to prevent and alleviate muscle cramps, soreness, and pain following exercise, and to facilitate the healing of soft tissue. However, these proposed effects are not necessarily supported by the scientific evidence. In fact, there appears to be a significant placebo effect in many of these applications rather than a measurable effect. Nevertheless, the placebo effect in itself may be very important if it enables individuals to perceive that they are recovering faster. An increased alpha motor neuron excitability plus a slight increase in joint range of motion and a slight increase in cutaneous and muscle blood flow has been reported to result from massage. In one study intensive massage caused a decrease in performance (Ahonen, Salorinne, & Weber, 1985). No effect of massage has been documented on muscle strength, circulatory responses to submaximal exercise, or short-term recovery from intense exercise. In addition, to date, researchers have shown no effect of massage on serum beta endorphins.

Sauna involves the use of mild to severe heat in a confined area to bring about an increase in body temperature and sweating. The proposed beneficial effects of sauna are: as a warm-up technique before training or competition, as a mental or physical relaxation technique before and after training or competition, to facilitate mental and physical recovery, to reduce weight, and to prevent or treat musculoskeletal injuries plus respiratory infections. Saunas have also been proposed as a method of training the circulatory system and enhancing the body's acclimatization to heat. Investigators have documented that saunas are effective for achieving acute weight reduction, but the weight loss is simply fluid and not body fat. Saunas have also been reported to have beneficial effects on neuromuscular relaxation and heat acclimation when used in conjunction with exercise, (Hasan, Karvonen, & Piironen, 1966, 1967; Rowell, 1983), but this remains to be proven. In addition, favorable psychosomatic effects have been reported, including the facilitation of recovery from strenuous effort, and decreased post-exercise symptoms of muscular and skeletal soreness.

It is also important to consider the potential risks associated with using saunas. There is definitely potential for cardiovascular complications and thermal injury, and the concern is greater for the elderly as well as for those who are infrequent users, are pregnant, or have cardiovascular disease. There is also concern when saunas are combined with traditional cold exposure such as snow or cold water immersion, particularly with higher risk populations.

Sudation garments are garments such as rubberized suits which induce sweating during exercise and provide a barrier to the evaporation of sweat. They create a microclimate for the individual which could lead to severe thermal stress. The proposed beneficial effects of sudation garments are to enhance exercise heat tolerance and promote weight loss. The limited scientific evidence concerning the effects of sudation garments does not support any beneficial effects. In fact, they are no more effective at enhancing heat tolerance than training at

the same environmental temperature wearing normal exercise clothing (Dawson & Pyke, 1988; Dawson, Pyke, & Morton, 1989). Further, neither normal exercise clothing nor sudation garments are as effective as training in a hot climate. Hence, training in sudation garments is not a substitute for training in the heat. Undoubtedly there is an increased fluid loss with exercise in sudation garments, but the utility of such an acute weight loss appears to be only of value in "making weight" transiently for a sport. Similar to the concern with saunas, when using sudation garments there is also a concern about excessive fluid loss producing potential risks of hyperthermia, dehydration, thermal injury, and reduced exercise capacity.

Questionable Practices and Devices

Exercises designed to bring about *spot reduction* are the most common questionable practices encountered in the slimming and figure control industry. In fact, the practice of spot reduction is the basis of the claimed beneficial effects of most questionable exercise devices. Limited scientific evidence exists concerning the efficacy of spot reduction. In 1965, Mohr observed significant decreases in abdominal skinfold thicknesses following a 4 week program in which 6 isometric abdominal contractions were each held for 6 seconds. However, no control group was employed in this study and only the abdominal skinfolds were measured. Hence, although this study has been cited as providing support for a beneficial effect of spot reduction, the evidence is not conclusive.

In a well-controlled study, Olson and Edelstein (1968) reported a significant decrease in triceps skinfold thickness in the exercised arm but not in the nonexercised arm following a 10 week program of single arm biceps curls and triceps extensions. A similar study was conducted earlier by Roby (1962). Employing the same design as Olson and Edelstein, Roby found a significant decrease in the triceps skinfold thickness, but the decrease was the same for both the trained and untrained arms after the 10 week program of forearm extension weight training exercises. Hence, two studies which were very similar in design arrived at quite different conclusions.

Noland and Kearney (1978) examined the issue of spot reduction in two groups of women who underwent training. One group followed a general conditioning program and the other a spot reduction conditioning program. They found significant changes before and after the program in skinfold thicknesses and girth measurements, but they were essentially identical for both the general and the spot reduction programs. That is, the group that was trying to focus the exercise specifically on one area showed no greater change in that area than the group that was following a general conditioning program.

In a very interesting study, Gwinup, Chelvam, and Steinber (1971) examined a number of professional tennis players and found that the forearm and upper arm girths of their dominant arms were substantially larger, but there were no differences in skinfold thicknesses. Although the dominant arm received considerably more exercise than the control arm (and as a result there was substantial muscle hypertrophy in the dominant arm), there were no differences in the associated skinfold measurements. In a similar study, Taaffe and Lewis (1992) likewise found no differences in forearm skinfold thickness between the dominant and nondominant arms of male and female tennis players in spite of a significant hypertrophy in the dominant arm.

A more sophisticated study on this topic was conducted by Katch, Clarkson, Kroll, McBride, and Wilcox (1984). They examined fat cells taken from the abdominal, subscapular, and gluteal depots. Their subjects performed 5000 sit-ups over a 27 day period and they observed an overall reduction in fat cell diameters but no preferential use of fat from the abdominal depots compared to the subscapular and gluteal regions. That is, there was a generalized utilization of fat rather than a specific utilization in the area being exercised.

Therefore, it can be concluded from the scientific investigations conducted to date that spot reduction does not appear to be effective. This conclusion also casts considerable doubt on many of the questionable exercise devices that are based on the efficacy of spot reduction.

Regular vigorous exercise on a treadmill, cycle ergometer, or resistance training equipment generally leads to changes in body composition. However, there are a number of "exercise devices" that have questionable value, and most of them are marketed on the basis that the consumer will receive significant benefit with minimal effort. They are primarily passive exercise devices which cause no major energy expenditure on the part of the user. Scientific evaluation of these devices is very scarce and generally does not support the advertising claims.

One such questionable exercise device is the *vibrating machine*, which has been available in health clubs for many years and supposedly brings about spot reduction and weight loss. This was the first questionable device that was investigated scientifically and reported in research literature (Hernlund & Steinhaus, 1957). These authors examined the oxygen consumption of subjects during and after 15 minutes of mechanical vibration. They also examined an equivalent period of time on an alternate day when the subjects simply sat and rested, and they found a negligible difference. Hence, they concluded that there is little or no beneficial effect on energy expenditure and body composition from the use of a vibrating machine.

Another example of a questionable exercise device is "*Slim Skins*," which are plastic pants tied at the thighs and above the waist. A length of tubing attaches them to a vacuum device. They are also advertised as "Vacu Pants" in the literature. While wearing the "Slim Skins" with the vacuum operating, the subject does some knee bends and side bends, walks in place for 15 minutes, and then leaves the vacuum running during a 15 minute seated postexercise period. An advertisement illustrated identical twins with one claiming to lose 17 inches in 25 minutes. The advertisement guaranteed that without dieting users would lose 9 to 18 inches from the waist, abdomen, hips, and thighs in just 3 days.

This product was one of three that the U.S. Postal Service contracted Jack Wilmore to investigate in 1983. Previously, the U.S. Postal Service had attempted to stop the Mark Eden Company from distributing a product called the *Bust Developer*, but they lost their case in federal court. The reason cited for the failure of the Post Office in court was that although both sides marshalled a number of experts, only the Mark Eden Company provided "scientific" evidence at the trial concerning the effectiveness of the device. A physiologist from the University of California, San Francisco had reported previously that the bust developer brought about the claimed improvements.

Wilmore's study on the effectiveness of "Slim Skins" was the very first research contract conducted for the U.S. Postal Service, which is responsible for investigating and prosecuting all frauds involving use of mail. Wilmore found no evidence of any fat loss from the abdomen, hips, and thighs following a 3 day program of "Slim Skins" exercises which adhered to the precise instructions of the manufacturer (Wilmore et al., 1985a).

Another device, the "*Astro Trimmer*," was investigated in the same experiment (Wilmore et al., 1985a). The manufacturers claimed that it brought about the loss of over 3 inches from the waistline in just ten minutes, nearly 5 inches off the waistline in less than an hour, and 4-1/2 inches from the waistline on the first day. The Astro Trimmer is a 5-inch-wide belt that circles the waist. It has a black, rubber-like section made of a special composition which supposedly makes the fat around the waist disappear. Presumably it is necessary for the user to move the belt to other locations, because 5 inches in just one area would look rather strange. The device can be attached to a doorknob via a short rubber cord and you simply lean back or if you want to you can walk or jog on the spot. With the Astro Trimmer, Wilmore found no evidence of fat loss at the abdominal girth after the recommended 5 day program. The trial was conducted, exactly as prescribed, and contrary to the claims in the advertisements, there was no evidence of fat loss.

The Mark II *Bust Developer* promised instant development of the bust; 2 inches the first day, 3 inches the first week. The exercise program involved six upper body exercises using the device. The advertisement stated that "In all the world, only the users of Mark II IVR (infinitely variable resistance) are achieving results like this." Since the Mark Eden Company was realizing a very large profit from the sale of these devices, the court case required precise data to gain a guilty verdict. The researchers came up with several ingenious approaches to accurately measure all the dimensions of the breasts, because the claimed benefits of using the bust developer included lifting, separating, shaping, and firming the bust (Wilmore et al., 1985b). For example, water displacement was employed to measure the precise breast volume. The accuracy of the measurements was within 10 milliliters on repeat trials. Some of the techniques that were developed are now being used for such things as reconstructive breast surgery. Two-thirds of the college women who had utilized this device in the original research study indicated that they felt that there were gains. However, following a 21 day program, the researchers could find no evidence to support their benefits or the company's claims and concluded that there was only a perception of positive changes occurring.

The *Continuous and Assistive-Passive Exercise* (CAPE) device was also investigated for faulty advertising and reported in 1990 (Martin & Kauwell, 1990). With this device, the subject is strapped onto a series of six tables which provide a variety of passive or light resistance exercises for the trunk and extremities by bending at various joints and in various directions. A cohort of women experienced a decrease in their maximal oxygen consumption and no change in body weight and skinfolds over a 12 week CAPE program. It was concluded that these devices are not effective. Hence, in line with the findings concerning the ineffectiveness of spot reduction, the scientific evidence concerning questionable exercise devices does not support the advertising claims.

Nutritional Supplements

A variety of nutritional supplements are aggressively promoted in fitness magazines, and the use of supplemental protein, vitamins, and minerals was examined at the ICPAFH Consensus Symposium. It is commonly believed that protein must be supplemented in large quantities in highly active individuals. There are two possible reasons underlying the efficacy of this belief. One possible mechanism of action for a beneficial effect of *supplemental protein* is to provide a more efficient substrate for muscle contraction, especially when glycogen stores are limited. Normally, less than 10% to 15% of the energy for muscle contraction is derived from protein and it has been suggested that protein supplementation might effectively replace more of the energy that is utilized in muscular activity. However, even if a slight increase were accomplished, it would have little or no consequence for health.

A second proposed mechanism of action for supplemental protein is to increase the muscle mass that results from resistance training by enhancing the synthesis of protein. This is the primary reason that body builders, weight trainers, and certain track athletes take protein supplements. However, the rate of protein synthesis decreases in response to an acute bout of exercise. As well, amino acids contribute only 10% to 15% of the total energy expended during exercise and hence the maximum daily protein requirement would be about 2 grams per kilogram of body weight (Brooks, 1987; Viru, 1987). In fact, at the ICPAFH Consensus Symposium, Dr. Gail Butterfield provided a convincing argument that 1.2 to 1.6 grams per kilogram of body weight of protein per day is the maximum that is needed. Hence, there is really no necessity for protein supplementation because almost everyone who exercises on a regular basis would be taking in more than that amount in their normal diet. It has also been suggested that supplementing the diet with branched-chain amino acids may be useful, but there is no evidence to support this proposal. This possibility is purely speculative at this time, but represents an interesting area for further investigation.

Although exercise can increase the need for some vitamins, if an individual's diet is nutritionally well-balanced the scientific evidence does not support the use of *vitamin supplements*. The proposed benefits of vitamin supplementation are mainly with the B complex vitamins plus vitamins C and E. Vitamin B supplementation possibly restores endurance in individuals who are deficient, but it has no effect in those who are not vitamin B deficient. Oxygen free radicals (OFRs) form during normal aerobic metabolism in exercise and, if they accumulate unduly in cells, they can lead to diabetes, cancer, and acceleration of aging. Antioxidants react rapidly with OFRs to protect the body against their harmful effects. Recently, investigators (Alessio, Cao, & Cutler, 1992; Baldi, Sforzo, & Jenkins, 1992) have suggested that vitamin C and E supplements are effective as antioxidants thus reducing tissue damage with exercise and facilitating tissue repair. The reader is referred to the recent review chapter by Clarkson (1991) for more information on both vitamin and other nutritional supplements.

Additional nutritional supplements addressed in the ICPAFH Symposium were: calcium, iron, and electrolyte drinks. Calcium is critical for the formation and maintenance of healthy bones, but the only potential benefit for *calcium supplementation* beyond the recommended daily intake is for amenorrheic or postmenopausal women who have low estrogen levels. Iron is required for the production of hemoglobin and hence it is important for oxygen transport. However, *iron supplementation* is not usually necessary except when iron deficiency is present, and this condition is very rare in normal individuals. On the other hand, the incidence of sports anemia is quite high among endurance-trained athletes, and although the etiology of the problem is unclear (diet or loss), iron supplementation for endurance athletes may be advisable (Gledhill, 1992). Caution must be taken when using iron supplements, as free iron enhances the generation of OFRs, and mega-doses of iron could be problematic. Compared with plain water, commercial *electrolyte solutions* are of small additional benefit in replacing fluid and electrolyte loss due to sweating. The mechanism that accounts for the minor beneficial effect of these solutions is the facilitation of fluid uptake in the small intestine.

In a recent comprehensive, double blind, placebo-controlled investigation of nutritional supplements, 90 days of multivitamin-mineral supplementation had no effect on the aerobic power, endurance run time, or isokinetic strength of healthy physically active males (Singh, Moses, & Deuster, 1992). Hence, to summarize the information regarding nutritional supplements, providing that you are not reducing your total caloric intake, a balanced diet will provide all of the vitamins and minerals that you require. Therefore, there is generally no reason to take nutritional supplements for normal health purposes.

Acknowledgment

The authors would like to acknowledge the contributions of Dr. Ilkka Vuori in the preparation of the initial section on "Supplements to Physical Activity."

References

Ahonen J., Salorinne Y., & Weber T. (1985). Effect of various types of massage on muscular performance and release of muscle enzymes in athletes. *Valmennus ja kuntoilu*, **1**, 60-61.

Alessio, H.M., Cao, G., & Cutler, R.G. (1992). Total antioxidant protection following vitamin E and C supplementation and sub-maximal exercise. *Medicine and Science in Sports and Exercise*, **24**(5), S16.

Baldi, C., Sforzo, C., & Jenkins, R. (1992). The effect of vitamin E and iron supplementation on free radical production in response to exercise. *Medicine and Science in Sports and Exercise*, **24**(5), S16.

Brooks, G.A. (1987). Amino acid and protein metabolism during exercise and recovery. *Medicine and Science in Sports and Exercise*, **19**: S150-S156.

Clarkson, P.M. (1991). Vitamins and trace minerals. In D.R. Lamb & M.H. Williams (Eds.), *Ergogenics: Enhancement of performance in exercise and sport* (pp. 123-176). Dubuque, IA: Brown and Benchmark.

Dawson, B., & Pyke, F.S. (1988). Artificially induced heat acclimation of team game players with sweat clothing: I. Responses to wearing sweat clothing during exercise in cool conditions. *Journal of Human Movement Studies*, **15**, 171-183.

Dawson, B., Pyke, F.S., & Morton, A.R. (1989). Improvement in heat tolerance induced by interval running training in the heat and in sweat clothing in cool conditions. *Journal of Sports Science*, **7**, 189-203.

Gledhill, N. (1992). Hemoglobin, blood volume and endurance. In R.J. Shephard & P.O. Åstrand (Eds.), *Endurance in Sport* (pp. 208-214). Oxford, England: Blackwell Scientific Publications.

Gwinup, G., Chelvam, R., & Steinberg, T. (1971). Thickness of subcutaneous fat and activity of underlying muscles. *Annals of Internal Medicine*, **74**, 408-411.

Hasan, J., Karvonen, M.J., & Piironen, P. (1966). Physiological effects of extreme heat as studied in the Finnish "sauna" bath. Part I. *American Journal of Physical Medicine*, **45**, 296-314.

Hasan, J., Karvonen, M.J., & Piironen, P. (1967). Physiological effects of extreme heat as studied in the Finnish "sauna" bath. Part II. *American Journal of Physical Medicine*, **46**, 1226-1246.

Hernlund, V., & Steinhaus, J. (1957). Do mechanical vibrators take off or redistribute fat? *Journal of the Association of Physical and Mental Rehabilitation*, **11**, 95.

Katch, F.I., Clarkson, P.M., Kroll, W., McBride, T., & Wilcox, A. (1984). Effects of sit-up exercise training on adipose cell size and adiposity. *Research Quarterly Exercise, Sport*, **55**, 242-247.

Martin, D., & Kauwell, G.P.A. (1990). Continuous assistive-passive exercise and cycle ergometer training in sedentary women. *Medicine and Science in Sports and Exercise*, **22**, 523-527.

Mohr, D.R. (1965). Changes in waistline and abdominal girth and subcutaneous fat following isometric exercises. *Research Quarterly*, **36**, 168-173.

Noland, M., & Kearney, J.T. (1978). Anthropometric and densitometric responses of women to specific and general exercise. *Research Quarterly*, **49**, 322-328.

Olson, A.L., & Edelstein, E. (1968). Spot reduction of subcutaneous adipose tissue. *Research Quarterly*, **39**, 647-652.

Roby, F.B. (1962). Effect of exercise on regional subcutaneous fat accumulations. *Research Quarterly*, **33**, 273-278.

Rowell, L.B. (1983). Cardiovascular adjustments to thermal stress. In J.T. Shephard & F.M. Abbound (Eds.), *Handbook of physiology: Section 2. The cardiovascular system Vol. III, Part 2. Peripheral circulation and organ blood flow* (pp. 967-1023). Bethesda, MD: American Physiological Society.

Singh, A., Moses, F.M., & Deuster, P.A. (1992). Chronic multivitamin-mineral supplementation does not enhance physical performance. *Medicine and Science in Sports and Exercise*, **24**(6), 726-732.

Snyder-Mackler, L., Laddin, Z., Schepsis, A.A., Young, J.C., & Massachusestts, B. (1991). Electrical stimulation of the thigh muscles after reconstruction of the anterior cruciate ligament. *Journal of Bone and Joint Surgery*, **73-A**, 1025-1036.

Taaffe, D.R. & Lewis, B. (1992). Hand dominance effects limb tissue composition. *Medicine and Science in Sports and Exercise*, **24**(5), S8.

Viru, A. (1987). Mobilisation of structural proteins during exercise. *Sports Medicine*, **4**, 95-128.

Wigerstad-Lossing, I., Grimby, G., Jonsson, T., Morelli, B., Peterson, L., & Renström, P. (1988). Effects of electrical muscle stimulation combined with voluntary contractions after knee ligament surgery. *Medicine and Science in Sports and Exercise*, **20**, 93-98.

Williams, R.A., Morrissey, M.C., & Brewster, C.E. (1986). The effect of electrical stimulation on quadriceps strength and thigh circumference in meniscectomy patients. *Journal of Orthopaedic and Sports Physical Therapy*, **8**, 143-146.

Wilmore, J.H., Atwater, A.E., Maxwell, B.D., Wilmore, D.L., Constable, S.H., & Buono, M.J. (1985a). Alterations in body size and composition consequent to Astro-Trimmer and Slim-Skins training programs. *Research Quarterly*, **56**, 90-92.

Wilmore, J.H., Atwater, A.E., Maxwell, B.D., Wilmore, D.L., Constable, S.H., & Buono, M.J. (1985b). Alterations in breast morphology consequent to a 21-day bust developer program. *Medicine and Science in Sports and Exercise*, **17**, 106-112.

Part II

Psychological and Sociological Aspects of Physical Activity, Fitness, and Health

There exists an overriding belief that exercise is good, not only for the body but also for the mind. The popularly reported benefits include reduced stress, enhanced well-being, and an exercise "high." Concurrently, although most people recognize that there are physical and psychological benefits of an active lifestyle, only between 10% and 25% of the population exercise at a frequency and intensity sufficient to cause significant positive outcomes. The image of the "couch potato" is more appealing in some circles than the picture of the fit and healthy person. Part II therefore examines scientific data available on the psychological outcomes and determinants of participation in a physically active lifestyle.

Landers and Petruzzello examine the scientific literature that deals with how physical activity and fitness can have a desirable impact on some negative psychological parameters including anxiety and stress reactivity. Landers and Petruzzello conclude that although effects do exist, their underlying mechanisms are poorly if at all understood, and that much more research is required for future interventions. McAuley reverses the tables and addresses whether physical activity and fitness can have an impact on positive psychological parameters such as self-esteem, perceptions of capacity to perform, and global well-being. Following an examination of relevant literature, McAuley concludes that exercise can enhance positive psychological parameters and suggests how exercise environments can be modified to maximize the likelihood of these outcomes.

Gauvin examines the literature dealing with the effects of exercise withdrawal and exercise addiction on psychological functioning and highlights some of the practical applications of the literature on psychological outcomes of physical activity. Gauvin concludes that information about the psychological outcomes of exercise could, if properly disseminated and applied, promote physical activity and fitness in the population. Dishman focuses on the different means that can be used to increase exercise behavior, clearly identifying what is practical and what is effective. Following a review of relevant literature, Dishman identifies those models and concepts most likely to result in changes in exercise behavior. Rejeski and Hobson also examine the issue of motivation for exercise but tailor their practical applications to those practitioners involved in rehabilitative medicine. Rejeski and Hobson suggest that exercise motivation should be approached in a proactive manner through consideration of the psychosocial as well as physiological factors in exercise prescription and application of multiple strategies.

Wankel and Hills also examine the question of exercise motivation, but do so using a social marketing approach. Wankel and Hills suggest that the adoption of active lifestyles be considered as an ongoing process and that interventions address both the product and the stage of involvement of the exerciser. Finally, recognizing that sport participation during childhood and adolescence is crucial in determining participation in adulthood, Duda examines what can be done to maximize the quality of the youth sport experience. Drawing on existing literature, Duda provides a series of principles for developing and applying youth sport programs.

11

The Effectiveness of Exercise and Physical Activity in Reducing Anxiety and Reactivity to Psychosocial Stressors

Daniel M. Landers
Steven J. Petruzzello

Anxiety has become a pervasive social problem. Estimates from earlier reports (Dishman, 1982) suggest that 30 million of the 250 million U.S. citizens have their "normal" lifestyles disrupted due to anxiety or anxiety-related problems and that from 30% to 70% of the patients seen by general practitioners and internists have problems with managing stress.

There is growing interest on the part of many health care professionals in the role that physical activity plays in preventing the onset of emotional problems and in serving as a treatment modality once such problems have developed (Morgan & Goldston, 1987). For example, among 1,756 primary care physicians, 60% of those surveyed indicated that they routinely prescribed exercise for patients with anxiety disorders (Ryan, 1983). Of course, psychotropic drugs are also prescribed, but their administration can produce adverse effects (e.g., withdrawal following treatment termination, potential for negative side effects). Scientific evidence for the anxiolytic (i.e., anxiety-reducing) effect of exercise would help to further promote the use of exercise in preventing the onset of anxiety-related problems or its use as an intervention once these problems have developed. The heightened clinical awareness of the anxiolytic role of exercise has prompted the National Institutes of Mental Health to identify this topic of "immediate concern" (Morgan & Goldston, 1987).

The purposes of the present review are to discuss the general conclusions derived from these research reviews and discuss some of the implications of these conclusions for professional practice.

Definition of Terms and Scope of the Present Review

The conclusions regarding physical activity/fitness and anxiety reduction are based on 27 narrative and 2 meta-analytic published reviews of this literature as well as articles reviewed by Landers and Petruzzello (in press) for the International Consensus Symposium on Physical Activity, Fitness and Health (total of 159 empirical studies). The conclusion regarding exercise and stress reactivity was primarily derived from 34 studies in Crews and Landers' (1987) meta-analytic review. Readers who are unfamiliar with meta-analysis are referred to Petruzzello, Landers, Hatfield, Kubitz, and Salazar (1991).

Before discussing the main conclusions of these reviews, it is first necessary to define what is meant by "anxiety," "stress reactivity," and "physical activity/fitness" which in turn will determine the scope of the present review.

Anxiety and Its Measurement

Coincident with moderate to high arousal levels where the individual's behavior begins to become disrupted (i.e., performance drops, and perception, retention, and decision-making are degraded) is the emergence of a negative form of cognitive appraisal typified by worry, self-doubt, and apprehension. This negative cognitive appraisal is what is termed "anxiety." It arises because the individual perceives a high degree of uncertainty or lack of control over task demands, available resources, behavioral consequences and their meaning, and bodily reactions (Landers & Boutcher, 1986). A more succinct definition (Lazarus & Cohen, 1977) holds that anxiety arises "... in the face of <u>demands that tax or exceed the resources of the system</u> or ... demands to which there are no readily available or automatic adaptive responses" (p. 109).

Because anxiety is fundamentally a cognitive phenomenon, it is measured by a number of questionnaire instruments. By contrast, arousal is usually indexed by physiological measures (Petruzzello et al., 1991). A common distinction in this literature is between trait and state measures of anxiety. *Trait* anxiety is the general predisposition to respond across many situations with high levels of anxiety. *State* anxiety, on the other hand, is much more specific and refers to the subject's anxiety at a particular moment. The instructions for responding to the measures convey the "set" in which subjects should respond to the question, for example, "how I feel in general" (trait) versus "how I feel at this moment" (state). Although the "trait" and "state" aspects of anxiety are conceptually distinct, the available operational measures for state-trait anxiety and other partitions of anxiety (i.e., "cognitive-somatic" anxiety) show a considerable amount of overlap among these subcomponents of anxiety (Smith, 1989).

Stress Reactivity

Studies investigating stress reactivity present subjects with a situational stressor (e.g., electric shock, loud noise, cognitive tasks performed under time pressure) to determine whether being physically fit or having undergone acute or chronic exercise will help to shield the person from the effects of these stressors (i.e., reactivity), and if it will help them return to baseline more quickly (i.e., recovery) than unfit or nonexercising subjects. The effects of stress are inferred from measures of arousal and anxiety which in turn are derived from physiological and questionnaire measures, respectively. Whereas the anxiety-reduction research is analogous to viewing exercise as a "tranquilizer," investigators examining the stress reactivity issues would consider exercise to be more like a "beta blocker."

Physical Activity/Fitness

Cardiovascular efficiency will be emphasized here since it is generally agreed to be the best indicator of fitness and health. Thus, this review will include studies which examine prolonged engagement in physical activities at an intensity which has the potential for improving aerobic (i.e., continuous, rhythmical activities) or anaerobic (i.e., intermittent, strength/power activities) capacity. This review is based on studies of

- trait anxiety of fit and unfit individuals,
- state anxiety response before and after a single bout of exercise (termed acute exercise),

- state and trait anxiety before and after a longitudinal exercise training program (termed chronic exercise), and
- stress reactivity following a single bout of exercise or after a longitudinal training program.

Excluded from this review are studies (a) of swimming skill instruction to reduce fear of the water; (b) of dealing with the trait anxiety of athletes and nonathletes; (c) which are not data-based, or do not show if another treatment modality was combined with exercise; (d) that used exercise for experimental purposes other than to create anxiety reduction following exercise; and (e) dealing with athletes in an overtrained state where anxiety is often increased rather than reduced. Given these definitions of anxiety and physical activity/fitness, the following set of conclusions seemed warranted.

Conclusions and Implications

Anxiety Reduction

Although most of the conclusions which follow are based on questionnaire measures of anxiety, reductions in anxiety following exercise have been observed irrespective of whether self-report, behavioral, or physiological measures are employed. Across all 159 studies there are also consistent findings that are of methodological significance. For instance, studies that had strong research designs (i.e., within-subjects designs or optimal sample sizes) and equality among groups (i.e., random assignment of subjects to groups) were associated with larger anxiety differences between exercise and a no treatment control group.

Conclusion 1: A Small to Moderate Relationship Shows Physically Fit People to Have Less Trait Anxiety Than Unfit People

In previous reviews (Franks & Jetté, 1970), this literature has been summarized as showing:

> ... an inverse relationship between manifest anxiety and physical fitness measures. The correlations have been low to moderate, seldom higher than 0.35 (thus accounting for no more than 10-15% common variance). ... In addition, the correlations between physiological measures that have been used to measure anxiety such as heart rate and blood pressure range from 0.15 to 0.45. (p. 49)

When cardiovascular measures of fitness are emphasized, the studies are supportive of the low correlations noted previously (r values ranging from -0.22 to -0.50). In a large scale multivariate study of 4,351 patients from a preventive medicine clinic, Collingwood, Bernstein, Hubbard, and Blair (1983) examined 23 clinical risk factors of coronary heart disease along with 29 psychological characteristics. In their study, cardiorespiratory fitness was measured from a maximal treadmill test and anxiety was measured by the Clinical Anxiety Questionnaire. The canonical correlations revealed that people who were fit and who exercised were less likely to have somatic complaints or nervous tension.

Despite that these studies are cross-sectional and correlational in nature, they are strikingly consistent in showing that physically fit people have less anxiety than unfit people. Although these findings are meaningful, they do not suggest that exercise or fitness per se is the cause of these anxiety differences. It may be that fit people live more healthy lifestyles (better nutrition, education, and occupation) and thus they tend to be less anxious. In order to better determine if exercise is responsible for changes in anxiety, it is necessary to examine studies that have compared changes in anxiety either before and after an acute bout of exercise or before and after a longitudinal exercise training program.

Conclusion 2: Compared to No Treatment Control Groups, State Anxiety Is Reduced Following an Aerobic Exercise Training Program or Following an Acute Bout of Aerobic Exercise

Regardless of the kind of anxiety measure employed (state or trait) and the exercise paradigm employed (acute versus chronic), the results are consistent in showing that exercise is associated with a reduction in anxiety. These results are not surprising since this was the typical conclusion in the 29 reviews on this topic. These results do not support hypotheses (e.g., Pitts & McClure, 1967) which would predict the opposite result. Although these results are clear, the moderating variables which relate to the physical activity and anxiety reduction relationship are not as readily recognized. In other words, which variables make this relationship stronger and which make it weaker? Answering this question may help to further clarify the finding, which in turn, may have important practical implications and be a first step in the eventual explanation of its occurrence.

Conclusion 3: Reductions in State and Trait Anxiety Are Associated With Activities Involving Continuous, Rhythmical Exercise (i.e., More Aerobic) Rather Than Resistive, Intermittent Exercise (i.e., Less Aerobic)

Very few studies have examined activities that involve resistive or strength training activities. Petruzzello et al. (1991) only located 15 comparisons where exercise was not of a continuous, rhythmical nature. The results for these less aerobic activities were not statistically meaningful and were in the opposite direction of the predicted

anxiolytic effect. For example, activities like handball and strength/flexibility training produced results on the state and trait anxiety questionnaires that were associated with increases in anxiety. There may be something associated with the nature of aerobic activities that is conducive to producing anxiolytic effects. Until future research can determine what this might be, people interested in using exercise to reduce anxiety levels should use continuous, rhythmical forms of exercise that typically produce more aerobic benefit.

Conclusion 4: Anxiolytic Effects of Exercise on State Anxiety Begin Within 5 Minutes After Acute Exercise and Continue for at Least 2 Hours

Several reviewers have indicated that anxiety is reduced for up to 4 to 6 hours following exercise. Unfortunately, these estimates were based on only one study, an unpublished master's thesis by Seemann (1978). In this study, anxiety was only measured a few times following exercise. Thus, all that can be concluded is that somewhere between 4 to 6 hours after exercise, anxiety returned to pre-exercise levels.

Only nine other comparisons of state anxiety before and after exercise have been made beyond 20 minutes following exercise (see Petruzzello et al., 1991). These studies basically confirm Seemann's (1978) finding in showing that the anxiolytic effects of exercise begin within 5 to 6 minutes after exercise and continue for at least 2 hours. The fact that anxiety is reduced for a time after a bout of exercise has led to the suggestion that "the benefits of regular exercise may reside in its ability to reduce anxiety on a daily basis and, hence, prevent the development of chronic anxiety" (Morgan, 1981, p. 306).

Conclusion 5: Trait Anxiety Is Reduced More if the Length of the Training Program Is Beyond 15 Weeks

In examining the results of several studies, Petruzzello et al. (1991) found training programs that ranged from 4 weeks to more than 15 weeks. The average length of most of the programs was between 7 and 12 weeks. Compared to exercise training of less than 9 weeks, anxiety reduction in these studies was much greater if the training program was longer than 15 weeks. Therefore, based on the results of Petruzzello et al. (1991), training programs that are in excess of 15 weeks are recommended to produce more substantial anxiolytic effects.

Conclusion 6: Regardless of Exercise Intensity or Duration, Anxiety Reduction Occurs Following Acute and Chronic Exercise

This is perhaps the most controversial area among the previous reviews of this area. With older subjects, deVries (1981) found that low to moderate exercise was sufficient to reduce tension levels. Franks and Jetté (1970) concluded that moderate exercise reduced trait anxiety better than vigorous exercise. However, the majority of the reviewers adopted the position that exercise needed to be at 70% to 80% of VO_2max to elicit anxiolytic effects. This conclusion was based at the time on walking exercise at between 55% to 72% HRmax and treadmill exercise (HR=100-110 bpm). Although exercise intensity was attributed to the failure to find anxiety reductions in these studies, there were factors other than exercise intensity that could explain these findings (Petruzzello et al., 1991).

Examination of the exercise intensity (percent HRmax or percent VO_2max) across several studies (Petruzzello et al., 1991) showed no significant differences in state and trait anxiety for exercise intensities ranging from 40% to 80%. There are numerous examples in the literature of low intensity exercises like walking and jogging being related to meaningful reductions in post-exercise anxiety. For example, Moses, Steptoe, Mathews, and Edwards (1989) showed that anxiety was reduced with moderate exercise (60% of HRmax), but not with more vigorous exercise (70% to 75% HRmax). Similar results were reported by Franks and Jetté (1970) which led them to conclude that training should be at an intensity that subjects can adjust to. From an examination of these 159 studies in their entirety, it appears that any level of exercise above 40% of maximum intensity is sufficient to lower anxiety.

For both state and trait anxiety, the studies reported in Petruzzello et al. (1991) would at first glance suggest that exercise durations of less than 20 minutes do not yield anxiolytic effects. Upon closer inspection of these studies, however, Petruzzello et al. found other design or methodological characteristics in these studies masked the anxiolytic benefits of exercise. When these problems were corrected, anxiolytic effects were observed even for exercise durations ranging from 5 to 20 minutes. Thus, it is unnecessary to insist that people exercise longer than 20 minutes to achieve anxiety-reducing effects.

Conclusion 7: Individuals Who Are Initially Low Fit or High Anxious Achieve the Greatest Reductions in Anxiety From an Exercise Training Program

Although Petruzzello et al. (1991) did not address this issue, other reviewers have suggested that less fit individuals, who are prone to be more anxious, should benefit the most from a training program (Simono, 1991). The law of initial values would suggest that this is true. If physical activity/fitness and anxiety are related as the aforementioned evidence suggests, then subjects initially scoring low on fitness should be able to make rapid fitness gains and thus lower their anxiety levels.

Likewise, highly anxious subjects, who are typically less fit, can conceivably make more rapid fitness gains than highly fit subjects, and this change should produce greater reductions in anxiety.

In examining the reviews, there is very meager evidence that less fit people experience greater anxiety reductions. Folkins, Lynch, and Gardner (1972) found that although men and women college students improved in fitness, only the women showed significant anxiety reductions after a 12-week jogging program. The authors subsequently discovered that prior to beginning the exercise program the women were less fit and more anxious than the men. By subdividing their sample, Wilfley and Kunce (1986) found similar results in that improvements in anxiety occurred only for those below the sample mean on fitness and anxiety before the start of the exercise program.

There is much more evidence regarding initial levels of anxiety than initial levels of fitness, particularly for measures of trait anxiety. Comparisons within and across trait anxiety studies reveal that compared to normal (nonclinical) subjects there is a tendency for greater anxiety reduction among cardiac rehabilitation patients, psychiatric patients, and highly anxious subjects (Petruzzello et al., 1991). For instance, Jetté (1967) found larger mean differences for highly anxious subjects than subjects with low anxiety. Likewise, other investigators (Sexton, Maere, & Dahl, 1989; Steptoe, Edwards, Moses, & Mathews, 1989) showed very meaningful differences for walking/jogging in before and after anxiety scores of symptomatic neurotics and previously inactive, anxious adults. Of course, with clinical patients, exercise is more often recommended as an adjunct to the primary treatment (e.g., hypertensive, mood altering, or muscle relaxing drugs). However, whether exercise is used as an adjunct or as a primary treatment, the results to date suggest that initially highly anxious individuals with low fitness levels have the most to gain psychologically from an exercise training program.

Conclusion 8: In Most of the State Anxiety Studies, Exercise Has Not Been Shown to Reduce Anxiety Any More or Less Than Other Known Anxiety-Reducing Treatments

With the exception of deVries (1981), most of the reviewers have concluded that exercise is no better than traditional interventions used to alleviate stress and anxiety (e.g., meditation, relaxation, quiet rest/reading). deVries (1981) was not referring to psychological interventions, but instead compared exercise to the tranquilizer drug meprobamate. He concluded that "exercise of an appropriate type and intensity had a significantly greater effect on resting musculature than did meprobamate" (p. 49). There is some support for deVries' conclusion in the trait anxiety literature where there is a meaningful difference between exercise and some other anxiety-reducing treatment (Petruzzello et al., 1991).

Although exercise may differ from tranquilizer drugs, exercise has not been shown to be any different from other psychological interventions for reducing state anxiety (Petruzzello et al., 1991). For example, Bahrke and Morgan (1978) found that regardless of whether subjects exercised, meditated, or rested quietly while reading an article, anxiety was significantly reduced. The point which must be emphasized is that exercise was no worse in reducing anxiety than the other psychological interventions. Obviously, exercise has other *physiological* benefits that are important for health promotion which may not exist for meditation, relaxation, and quiet rest.

Morgan (1981) suggested a "time-out" explanation for these results. This is similar to Gal and Lazarus' (1975) explanation that activities (e.g., exercise, meditation, and quiet reading) unrelated to the cause of the stress, diverts or distracts the person's attention away from the stress cues. Whether exercise produces a "time out" by providing rest breaks from daily activities, remains to be seen. Distraction, however, is not the only psychological explanation. For example, expectations regarding the benefits of exercise and the other anxiety-reducing interventions could also affect anxiety reports during the posttest.

Stress Reactivity

Conclusion 9: Acute or Chronic Aerobic Exercise Reduces Stress Reactivity and Hastens Recovery From the Stressor

Crews and Landers (1987) reviewed 34 studies in which subjects were exposed to one or more stressors either following an exercise training program or following an acute bout of exercise. The acute, short-term psychosocial stressors included:

- cognitive performance tasks such as solving timed arithmetic problems,
- passive response tasks such as viewing films of industrial accidents or medical operations,
- active physical performance tasks such as exercise, and
- passive physical performance tasks such as holding an immersed limb in ice water.

Although studies were coded for eight different moderator variables, none of them were shown to change the basic relationship. Regardless of study and subject characteristics, methodological characteristics, and stressor characteristics, the results demonstrated that aerobically fit subjects had a reduced psychosocial stress response. According to Crews and Landers (1987),

"The underlying assumption for reducing stress response lies in the belief that reduced physiological response to stress or faster physiological recovery results in overall less time spent in stress at perhaps a lower level of stress" (p. S118). Thus, exercise can either act as a coping strategy by reducing autonomic recovery time, or as an "inoculator" by providing repeated, intermittent stress on the sympathetic nervous system through exercise training bouts. Bouts of exercise may be analogous to repeated psychosocial stress in that it produces adaptations in the sympathetic nervous system (Dienstbier, 1988) and leads to cognitions (e.g., increased confidence) that are conducive to handling stress.

Summary

The literature reviews on reduced anxiety and stress reactivity as a function of exercise or fitness show that normal amounts of exercise (i.e., when subjects are not overtrained) can have anxiolytic effects. It is uncertain at this time what causes these effects. There are many psychological and physiological explanations that are currently being investigated (Hatfield, 1991). It is not even known if fitness gains brought about by exercise training programs are implicated in anxiety reduction and stress reactivity. Thus far, studies relating fitness gains to changes in anxiety have found mixed results (Landers & Petruzzello, in press). Considering that aerobic fitness may be independent of emotional state, it can be said that something associated with exercise or the exercise training program produces self-report, behavioral, and physiological changes that have been interpreted as reduced anxiety or stress reactivity.

Although the causal nature of this relationship is still unanswered, the fact remains that a solid relationship does exist, and this relationship has important practical implications. Within a wide range of exercise intensities and durations, aerobic exercise can produce therapeutic effects for up to 2 hours following exercise. Exercise training over a period of 15 weeks or more can produce very large effects, particularly for subjects who initially had low fitness levels or were highly anxious. For short-term stress management, exercise may be no better or worse than other anxiety-reducing psychological interventions. However, for long-term therapeutic intervention, little is known about the additive effects of multicomponent interventions (e.g., exercise combined with relaxation), or the comparative effects of exercise and other anxiety-reducing treatments, even though Dienstbier (1988) has theorized that exercise would be better.

References

Bahrke, M.S., & Morgan, W.P. (1978). Anxiety reduction following exercise and meditation. *Cognitive Therapy and Research*, **2**, 323-333.

Collingwood, T.R., Bernstein, I.H., Hubbard, D., & Blair, S.N. (1983). Canonical correlation analysis of clinical and psychologic data in 4,351 men and women. *Journal of Cardiac Rehabilitation*, **3**, 706-711.

Crews, D.J., & Landers, D.M. (1987). A meta-analytic review of aerobic fitness and reactivity to psychosocial stressors. *Medicine and Science in Sports and Exercise*, **19**, S114-S120.

deVries, H.A. (1981). Tranquilizer effect of exercise: A critical review. *Physician and Sportsmedicine*, **9**(11), 47-55.

Dienstbier, R.A. (1988). Arousal and physiological toughness: Implications for mental and physical health. *Psychological Review*, **96**, 84-100.

Dishman, R.K. (1982). Contemporary sport psychology. *Exercise and Sport Science Reviews*, **10**, 120-159.

Folkins, C.H., Lynch, C., & Gardner, E. (1972). Psychological fitness as a function of physical fitness. *Archives of Physical Medicine and Rehabilitation*, **53**, 503-508.

Franks, B.D., & Jetté, M. (1970). Manifest anxiety and physical fitness. *National College Physical Education Association for Men Annual Proceedings*, **73**, December, Chicago.

Gal, R., & Lazarus, R.S. (1975, December). The role of activity in anticipating and confronting stressful situations. *Journal of Human Stress*, pp. 4-20.

Hatfield, B.D. (1991). Exercise and mental health: The mechanisms of exercise-induced psychological states. In L. Diamant (Ed.), *Psychology of sports, exercise, and fitness: Social and personal issues* (pp. 17-49). Bristol, PA: Hemisphere.

Jetté, M. (1967). *Progressive physical training on anxiety in middle-age men*. Doctoral dissertation, University of Illinois, Champaign-Urbana.

Landers, D.M., & Boutcher, S.H. (1986). Arousal-performance relationships. In J.M. Williams (Ed.), *Applied sport psychology: Personal growth to peak performance*. Palo Alto, CA: Mayfield.

Landers, D.M., & Petruzzello, S. (in press). Physical activity, fitness, and anxiety. In C. Bouchard, R.J. Shephard, and T. Stephens (Eds.), *Physical activity, fitness and health: International proceedings and consensus statement*. Champaign, IL: Human Kinetics.

Lazarus, R.S., & Cohen, J.P. (1977). Environmental stress. In I. Altman & J.F. Wohlwill (Eds.), *Human behavior and the environment: Current theory and research*. New York: Plenum.

Morgan, W.P. (1981). Psychological benefits of physical activity. In F.J. Nagel & H.J. Montoye (Eds.), *Exercise in health and disease*. Springfield, IL: Charles C Thomas.

Morgan, W.P., & Goldston, S.N. (Eds.) (1987). *Exercise and mental health*. Bristol, PA: Hemisphere.

Moses, J., Steptoe, A., Mathews, A., & Edwards, S. (1989). The effects of exercise training on mental well-being in the normal population: A controlled study. *Journal of Psychosomatic Research*, **33**, 47-61.

Petruzzello, S.J., Landers, D.M., Hatfield, B.D., Kubitz, K.A., & Salazar, W. (1991). A meta-analysis on the anxiety-reducing effects of acute and chronic exercise. *Sports Medicine*, **11**, 143-182.

Pitts, F.N., & McClure, J.N., Jr. (1967). Lactate metabolism in anxiety neurosis. *New England Journal of Medicine*, **277**, 1329-1336.

Ryan, A.J. (1983). Exercise is medicine. *Physician and Sportsmedicine*, **11**, 10.

Seemann, J.C. (1978). *Changes in state anxiety following vigorous exercise*. Unpublished master's thesis, University of Arizona, Tucson, AZ.

Sexton, H., Maere, A., & Dahl, N.H. (1989). Exercise intensity and reduction in neurotic symptoms. *Acta Psychiatrica Scandanavia*, **80**, 231-235.

Simono, R.B. (1991). Exercise and mental health: The mechanisms of exercise-induced psychological states. In L. Diamant (Ed.), *Psychology of sports, exercise, and fitness: Social and personal issues* (pp. 51-66). Bristol, PA: Hemisphere.

Smith, R.E. (1989). Conceptual and statistical issues in research involving multidimensional anxiety scales. *Journal of Sport and Exercise Psychology*, **11**, 452-457.

Steptoe, A., Edwards, S., Moses, J., & Mathews, A. (1989). The effects of exercise training on mood and perceived coping ability in anxious adults from the general population. *Journal of Psychosomatic Research*, **33**, 537-547.

Wilfley, D., & Kunce, J. (1986). Differential physical and psychological effects of exercise. *Journal of Counseling Psychology*, **33**, 337-342.

12

Enhancing Psychological Health Through Physical Activity

Edward McAuley

Exercise and physical activity have been consistently and reliably implicated in the reduction of all-cause mortality (Blair et al., 1989), cardiovascular disease, and a host of other debilitating conditions (Bouchard, Shephard, Stephens, Sutton, & McPherson, 1990), however, the robustness of exercise effects on psychological health and well-being is less clear (Hughes, 1984; Plante & Rodin, 1990). Although the scientific and lay press often extol the almost intuitive psychological benefits of physical activity, the nature of these benefits and the mechanisms that drive such effects have yet to be firmly established. The controversies in the literature have in large part been attributed to methodological and conceptual problems and a lack of agreement in definitions of physical activity and psychological health. The extant literature in this area has typically focused on the anxiety-reducing, stress-dampening, and antidepressant effects of exercise and physical activity (e.g., North, McCullaugh, & Tran, 1990; Petruzzello, Landers, Hatfield, Kubitz, & Salazar, 1991). However, the psychological aspect of health has been defined as varying along a positive and negative continuum (Bouchard & Shephard, 1991), suggesting that solely focusing on the amelioration of negative symptomology is a rather restrictive perspective.

Physical Activity and Psychological Health: An Overview

In this chapter, the role of exercise and physical activity in the enhancement of psychological health is reviewed with respect to *positive* psychological effects. That is, exercise appears to have a positive relationship with self-perceptions (e.g., esteem, mastery, efficacy), mood, and affect (McAuley, 1993). It is these positive psychosocial benefits, specifically self-esteem, psychological well-being, and self-efficacy, that will be examined. *Self-esteem*, although often used interchangeably with

the term self-concept, encompasses the favorable views one holds regarding oneself and is considered a focal aspect of psychological health and well-being (Rosenberg, 1985). Several authors have suggested that physical activity may have its greatest potential benefit on psychological health by enhancing self-esteem (Folkins & Sime, 1981; Hughes, 1984).

Psychological or *emotional well-being* for the purpose of this chapter is defined as a psychological state represented by a preponderance of positive over negative affect. In this regard, it is an obvious parallel to what other authors have termed subjective well-being if general satisfaction with life is also included in the definition (see Diener, 1984, for a review). This definition of psychological well-being is in marked contrast to that used by many authors who associate psychological well-being with a reduction in psychological distress (e.g., anxiety, depression, stress-related emotions).

Self-efficacy expectations are concerned with people's beliefs in their capabilities to execute necessary courses of action to satisfy situational demands (Bandura, 1982, 1986) and have been shown to be important determinants of people's choices of activities, the amount of effort expended on such activities, and the degree of persistence demonstrated in the face of failure or aversive stimuli. As a psychological variable, self-efficacy cognitions have, by and large, been studied either as determinants of exercise behavior or as potential mediating mechanisms that might explain the effects of exercise on various aspects of psychological functioning (e.g., Petruzzello et al., 1991). A number of researchers (McAuley, 1991; McAuley & Courneya, 1992b; Sonstroem & Morgan, 1989) have contended that efficacy cognitions are influenced by physical activity participation and in turn influence other psychosocial outcomes. Let us now consider the general effects of exercise and activity on self-esteem, psychological well-being, and self-efficacy.

Self-Esteem

Self-esteem development has long been associated with active engagement in physical activity and a large body of research exists in this area. Several substantive reviews have been published (Doan & Scherman, 1987; Gruber, 1986; Sonstroem, 1984). There is agreement in these reviews and the consensus statements that physical activity can positively influence self-esteem and that the relationship is apparently stronger in people with initially debilitated levels of self-esteem. It should be further noted, however, that the vast majority of this research has focused on self-esteem from a global or general perspective, as opposed to more contemporary views that operationally and conceptually define self-esteem as multidimensional (e.g., Shavelson, Hubner, & Stanton, 1976). Indeed, the relationship between physical self-esteem and physical activity involvement appears to be quite consistent (e.g., Fox & Corbin, 1989; Marsh & Jackson, 1986; Marsh & Peart, 1988), indicating that physical activity participation can enhance one's sense of physical worth but does not necessarily influence other aspects of self-esteem.

What is not clear in this literature is exactly how physical activity participation might influence self-esteem. From a social psychological perspective, sense of mastery or efficacy has been identified by several researchers as an alternative mechanism (Petruzzello et al., 1991; Plante & Rodin, 1990; Sonstroem & Morgan, 1989). As I shall demonstrate, efficacy cognitions appear to be significantly influenced by both acute and long-term exercise participation. Sonstroem and Morgan (1989) have recently adopted this hypothesis in presenting a model of exercise and self-esteem that proposes physical activity information (through physical testing) to influence perceived physical efficacy which, in turn, influences perceptions of physical competence. They propose that physical competence has a direct effect on global self-worth and an indirect effect through perceptions of physical acceptance. They also underscore the necessity of examining perceived importance of physical activity when testing the proposed relationships. The model has, as yet, not been fully tested in the literature but certainly holds some promise for understanding the nature of this relationship.

Psychological Well-Being

The findings in this literature are generally quite positive, supporting the notion that physical activity participation enhances a variety of indexes of psychological well-being. Of particular interest in this group of studies was the obvious attempt to examine the hypothesized relationships in the ''normal'' population. Therefore, positive associations reported may be more generalizable than associations reported in previous reviews.

Evidence from large population-based studies suggests that leisure-time physical activity is positively related to a variety of indexes of well-being and that the relationship is stronger for females and older age groups than males and younger age groups (Stephens, 1988). Whereas many of the studies in this area are correlational, survey-type designs, many involve exercise interventions and report positive effects of physical activity on psychological well-being (King, Taylor, Haskell, & DeBusk, 1989; Moses, Steptoe, Mathews, & Edwards, 1989). However, as in the self-esteem literature, it is not clear whether fitness change plays a role in this association or whether vigorous activity is necessary for affective change to take place. Because many of the interventions employed moderate intensity activity programs and were able to demonstrate positive psychological gains, it does not appear at this point that vigorous bouts of activity are necessary for these gains (Moses et al., 1989). Therefore, activities such as brisk walking, jogging, and cycling may well provide the necessary stimulus for positive psychological benefits.

Although often an ignored fact in the exercise literature, it has been fairly well-established that affect is composed of at least two consistently identified dimensions, positive (PA) and negative (NA) affect. However, few efforts have been directed at determination of whether other affect dimensions exist that are specific to exercise and physical activity. McAuley and Courneya (1982a) have recently reported the development of a three dimension, exercise-induced affect measure assessing NA, PA, and physiological distress affect (PDA). Initial psychometric properties are promising, and the fact that the measure is brief and specific to physical activity may ensure sufficient sensitivity to detect meaningful exercise-induced change in psychological well-being in future endeavors.

In many respects, the data concerning exercise effects on positive psychological well-being are generally quite consistent and represent one of the more exciting and relatively untraveled research avenues in exercise psychology. As methods and measures improve and develop, our knowledge of this area will undoubtedly improve and so to will the contribution exercise and physical activity make to the psychological aspects of active and healthy living.

Self-Efficacy

The consensus statements generally agree that both long-term and acute exercise interventions have a consistent and relatively robust effect on self-efficacy across study design and populations. That is, exercise participation positively influences perceptions of physical capabilities and both acute bouts of activity and longer-term participation appear to have positive effects (Ewart, Stewart, Gillian, & Kelemen, 1986; Ewart, Taylor, Reese, & DeBusk, 1983; McAuley, Courneya, & Lettunich, 1991; Toshima, Kaplan, & Ries, 1990). This effect of exercise on efficacy occurs in both normal asymptomatic and clinical populations. However, it is pivotal to remember that exercise effects on efficacy are specific to the domain of functioning or mode of activity. That is, one would not necessarily expect significant changes in beliefs about one's cardiovascular capabilities following completion of a weight training program because no new information has been presented with respect to aerobic functioning (Ewart et al., 1986). Nevertheless, it is possible that information gained from participation in one type of aerobic activity, such as stationary bicycling, might have the carryover effect of generalizing to one's perceptions of capabilities in other aerobic domains, such as walking and jogging (McAuley et al., 1991).

Unlike the self-esteem and psychological well-being literature in this area, there does seem to be a relationship with perceived self-efficacy and degree of physical capacity or fitness. In those studies assessing fitness levels (Ewart et al., 1983; McAuley & Courneya, 1992b; McAuley et al., 1991; Taylor, Bandura, Ewart, Miller, & DeBusk, 1985) using standard graded-exercise testing, fitter individuals perceived themselves to have a greater exercise self-efficacy. Interestingly, however, even for the extremely unfit, a single bout of exercise provides sufficient mastery information to enhance perceptions of physical capabilities (McAuley et al., 1991; Taylor et al., 1985).

A further note of interest is pertinent to the fact that there appears to be a significant increase in the number of females and older individuals becoming physically active in their leisure time (Stephens, 1988). One recent report (McAuley et al., 1991) examined the effects of acute and long-term exercise participation on exercise efficacy in middle-aged males and females. Prior to the onset of a walking program, males had higher self-efficacy than did females, and both groups demonstrated proportionately equal increases in efficacy as a result of acute activity bouts. However, over the course of the 5-month exercise program females dramatically increased their perceptions of their physical capabilities to the point that they were as efficacious as males with respect to some activities and more so in other activities. The need to be increasingly vigilant in our offerings with respect to physical activity for older, impaired, and sedentary populations is clear. Also clear is the fact that females have been traditionally limited or restricted in the types, quality, and quantity of activities available to them. This in turn may have helped impair efficacy cognitions.

There is considerable evidence to identify self-efficacy as not only a determinant of future behavior and psychosocial outcomes, but also as a psychosocial outcome itself. The exercise and physical activity domain, if structured correctly, can offer myriad opportunities for the growth and development of a strong sense of personal efficacy. Such perceptions subsequently influence choice of future behavior, effort and persistence in that behavior, and affective and self-evaluative responses.

Overview Conclusions

The conclusions regarding the effects of exercise and physical activity on psychological health, as defined here, are as follows:

- Some evidence suggests that exercise and physical activity is positively associated with self-esteem, but recent endeavors indicate this relationship may be best evidenced by examining physical self-esteem, rather than global perceptions of esteem.
- Psychological well-being, defined here as enhancement of positive affect, appears to be consistently influenced by physical activity participation.
- Research suggests that beliefs in personal capabilities or self-efficacy perceptions are enhanced by both acute and longer term physical activity participation.
- Some evidence suggests that self-efficacy mediates other psychosocial outcomes such as affective responses (Ewart, 1989; McAuley, 1991; McAuley et al., 1991) and self-esteem (Sonstroem & Morgan, 1989).

Psychological Health and Active Living

The concept of active living incorporates the philosophy that "physical activity is valued and integrated into daily life" (Fitness Canada, 1991, p. 4). A healthy, happy, and satisfied life is a human objective or aspiration that has as its base psychological health, as typified by the preponderance of positive over negative affect, satisfaction with life, and the relative lack of anxiety, depression, and stress. Therefore, in the remainder of this chapter I will focus on methods and strategies for maximizing the likelihood that physical activity and exercise participation will cultivate positive psychological health.

A model of how physical activity influences positive affect, self-esteem, and self-efficacy is shown in Figure 12.1. In this model, the position is taken that physical activity participation affects self-esteem development and positive affective responsivity through the mediation of self-efficacy percepts. That is, engaging successfully in exercise and physical activity enhances people's beliefs about what they are capable of, and this enhanced sense of mastery in the physical domain leads to increases in evaluation of their physical self-worth (e.g., Sonstroem & Morgan, 1989) and improved positive affect.

Clearly, this model views self-efficacy cognitions not only as an outcome of physical activity participation

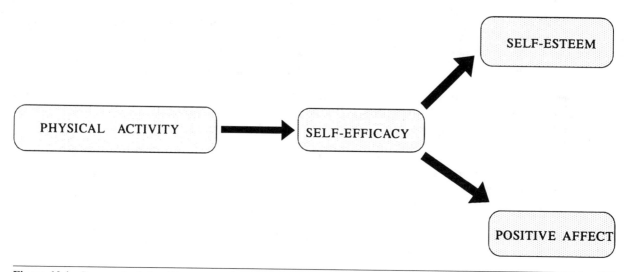

Figure 12.1 Proposed relationships among physical activity participation, self-efficacy, self-esteem, and positive affect.

but also as an important factor in the mediation of such participation on other aspects of psychological health. Because of the pivotal role played by this variable, most of the recommendations for practitioners focus on enhancing self-efficacy.

Structuring the Exercise Environment to Enhance Psychological Health

I now present some general guidelines that might be implemented at multiple levels—practitioner, program, and policy making—of the active living delivery system. These guidelines incorporate determining the nature of participation objectives, maximizing sources of mastery information, determining affective responses that commonly result from activity participation, and structuring the environment to best facilitate these responses.

Determining Participation Objectives

Many program leaders and exercise scientists presume that participants' priority in engaging in exercise programs is the enhancement of cardiovascular fitness and health. While this is undoubtedly true for many, it is equally likely that many others enroll in physical activity programs for nonfitness related reasons (e.g., social interaction, social support for others, stress relief, peer pressure, psychological benefits). Given these differing objectives, how programs are structured to satisfy the needs of the participants will vary. For example, an individual who enters a program for a combination of social (e.g., meeting new people) and health (e.g., wants to lose weight) reasons, and finds the program primarily geared toward high intensity, low interaction aerobic activity, will be unlikely to have his or her needs met

and subsequently be dissatisfied by the program. Alternatively, a program that incorporates varied, interactive activity of a moderate intensity is likely to foster continued, enjoyable involvement and satisfy the needs of the participants. Granted, it is not always possible to please everyone, but offering sufficient variety, having flexible and individually tailored exercise prescriptions, and attempting to incorporate participant interaction may well encourage prospective disengagers to stay with the program and, as they progress, to seek a more demanding type of program.

Influencing Self-Esteem and Positive Affect

Influencing self-esteem and positive affect, it is argued, is most potently achieved by directing efforts at bolstering perceptions of personal efficacy with respect to physical activity and exercise. A subsequent section deals with the sources of efficacy within the physical activity environment. Recent activity-related research in self-esteem has underscored the need to assess the degree of importance that participants place in the various domains of self-esteem (e.g., Fox & Corbin, 1989; Marsh & Peart, 1988; Zaharopoulus & Hodge, 1991), suggesting that it is only when physical activity is seen to be important by the participant that it influences self-esteem, and then only domain-specific self-esteem. This becomes particularly significant in physical activity environments that have the potential but fail to offer a choice of variety of activities. For example, one may wish to enhance one's muscular strength or tone while also improving aerobic conditioning. Therefore, activities that include both of those components will be deemed more important and are likely to encourage continued participation, development of competency (efficacy), and ultimately physical self-esteem. Furthermore, many participants in physical activity and exercise programs engage in many different forms of activity without really knowing why they are doing so. In these instances, the activity leader may, by simply providing information as to why engaging in a specific activity is important and necessary, foster a sense of exercise importance in the participant.

It would seem that promoting a variety of activities, particularly in school-based physical education programs, would increase the number of individuals finding some aspect of physical activity that was important and of interest to them. This might not only influence esteem development, but also encourage lifelong participation. Moreover, a recent study of adolescents reported that engagement in cooperative aerobic activity resulted in increased physical self-esteem, whereas competitive aerobic activity served to decrease self-esteem (Marsh & Peart, 1988). Therefore, cooperative activities can serve a dual purpose. They may lead to self-esteem enhancement and encourage social interaction, another common objective of physical activity involvement.

Apart from the provision of self-efficacy information (to be discussed later) to influence self-esteem, it appears necessary to take into consideration the degree of importance placed on physical activity and the factors that may further underlie esteem development. Variation, choices, and interest appear to be key components to be incorporated.

Although I previously identified some general dimensions of affective responses to exercise involvement (positive, negative, and physiological distress affect), a host of individual affects arise as a function of physical activity involvement, any one of which may take on more or less importance to the participant. Whereas aerobic dance and jogging may result in exhilaration, feelings of competence, and energy for the instructor, it is unlikely that beginning, older, or sedentary participants are likely to experience similar responses. Similarly, a "hard" workout for well-conditioned individuals may give rise to the same affective responses as a "light to moderate" activity session in less fit individuals. Knowledgeable exercise leaders and fitness consultants are acutely aware of the need to bring participants along gradually and safely. However, it is important to realize that the affective response to be obtained from physical activity may be independent of remarkable fitness gains. This is clearly demonstrated in methodologically sound empirical studies in which perceived fitness gains and increases in positive affect are shown to result from moderate intensity home-based exercise programs in the absence of any statistically significant increments in aerobic conditioning (King et al., 1989).

Maximizing Sources of Exercise-Induced Efficacy Information

Because the adoption and maintenance of physical activity is a health behavior that can be controlled and regulated by the individual, it is vitally important for practitioners and programs to provide experiences that maximize individuals' beliefs in their sense of personal capabilities with respect to exercise and physical activity. If practitioners fail to organize, present, and develop their programs in such a way as to cultivate efficacy beliefs, participants are likely to perceive the activity negatively, become disenchanted and discouraged, and discontinue. On the other hand, adequately organizing exercise and physical activity sessions in a manner such that a strong sense of personal efficacy is promoted will result in individuals displaying more positive affect, evaluating their physical self-worth more positively, embracing more challenging activities, putting forth more effort, and persisting longer. In short, they will be in a position to successfully self-regulate their behavior.

Four primary sources of efficacy information can be easily tapped by exercise and fitness leaders. Information regarding personal efficacy is culled from

(1) performance accomplishments or mastery experiences,
(2) social modeling,
(3) social persuasion, and
(4) physiological or emotional states (Bandura, 1986).

Table 12.1 details some examples of how each might be implemented to strengthen efficacy in the physical activity domain.

Mastery Experiences

Mastery experiences or performance accomplishments are considered to be the most effective and influential sources of efficacy information. Whereas successful exercise attainments are likely to enhance perceptions of physical efficacy, failures debilitate perceived capabilities. Encouraging participants to chart their progress with respect to duration of activity, heart rate, perceived exertion, number of days exercised, and distance covered each session is a simple way to provide efficacy information. Such accomplishments also serve as standards by which to gauge future progress and to set subsequent participation goals, thereby further enhancing motivation.

Social Modeling

Social modeling provides a second source of information from which efficacy can be enhanced. Such a source may be particularly salient when participants are sedentary, older, or have little experience in the activity. In such cases it is common to look to other people, especially those that bear similar physical characteristics to ourselves, for motivation and information regarding our own prospects of success. Our research group has employed short videotapes of middle-aged, sedentary adults beginning an exercise program, demonstrating

Table 12.1   Strategies for Strengthening Self-Efficacy Expectations

Mastery experiences
   Treadmills: Gradual increasing of speed, grade, or duration
   Stationary Bicycles: Gradual increase of resistance or duration
   Weights: Gradual increase of load, repetitions, sets
   Daily activities: Walking or biking to work, school, or errands instead of using motor transportation. Using stairs instead of elevators or escalators
   Leisure activity: Walking around golf course instead of riding

Social modeling
   Showing videotape of successful models similar in age, physical characteristics, and capabilities
   Providing frequent leader or expert demonstrations
   Attending orientation sessions at health and exercise facilities to observe others
   Using peer demonstrations frequently
   Employing participant modeling in which gradually diminished aid is provided to participant for more difficult exercises
   Cooperative exercise activities in groups or with partners

Social persuasion
   Providing information and orientation seminars for participants
   Providing videotape and multimedia health promotion information
   Providing articles, magazines, or information pamphlets and booklets for participants
   Developing social support system through "buddy systems" and group social activities
   Providing a telephone hot line or telephone reminders for frequent absentees
   Providing an exercise and health bulletin board and newsletter

Physiological states
   Instruct participants in how to accurately and positively interpret the following:
   Perspiration, heart rate, muscle soreness, weight changes, and general fatigue

effort, persistence, and enjoyment as they progress through the various stages of exercise adoption and maintenance. These videotapes are used as social modeling modalities to provide successful efficacy information in similarly aged and conditioned individuals.

Social Persuasion

Social persuasion is a commonly employed technique for convincing people to do what they initially believe they are incapable of doing. An astute exercise leader will draw upon important aspects of information that when conveyed to a self-doubting participant are capable of bolstering that person's belief in his or her own capabilities. However, it often requires more than a simple positive statement or encouragement for social persuasion to effectively facilitate efficacy. The exercise leader, as well as proffering encouragement and support, must also provide graded-exercise situations that offer opportunities for successful self-attained accomplishments on the part of the participant to accompany the positive feedback. This encourages the maintenance of self-perceptions regarding not only the realistic possibility of success, but also promotion of continued coping in the face of subsequent difficulties. In a combination of social modeling and persuasion, one can implement a *buddy exercise system* in which two or three individuals exercise together, serve as models and social supports, and take on a sense of responsibility for each other.

Physiological States

Teaching participants to modify or reinterpret their impressions of their physiological states during exercise serves as a final source for efficacy information. Obviously when exercising, and especially when beginning an exercise program, the body undergoes considerable physiological stress and strain resulting in fatigue, muscular tension, aches and pains, and increases in cardiorespiratory responses. Having a racing heart, dry throat, and shortness of breath are all natural physical responses to the exercise stimulus, and participants should be taught to interpret gradual change in the degree of those symptoms as markers of improved conditioning and thereby increased physical capabilities. We have participants in our programs frequently complete a 1-mile timed walk and we provide them with feedback regarding improvements in time and heart rate, emphasizing that they are continuing to work at the same intensity but are making marked improvements in performance times.

Focusing on such methods for boosting self-efficacy, being imaginative in identifying mastery experiences and social models, incorporating new methods of social persuasion, and reinterpreting physiological responses will lead to a robust sense of personal efficacy. In turn, this sense of efficacy will safeguard against discouragement, feelings of displeasure and incompetence, a dislike for activity, and a proclivity to give up in the face of any real or perceived adversity and challenge of physical activity. Exercise and program leaders can play a pivotal role in the development and continued fostering of a healthy sense of personal efficacy.

Conclusion

The scientific and lay community are becoming increasingly aware of the multiple positive health benefits to be derived from physical activity participation. From a psychological perspective, some evidence suggests that exercise participation can contribute to an enhanced sense of physical self-esteem, increased perceptions of personal capabilities with respect to physical performance, and elevated psychological well-being. Future endeavors must attempt, through carefully controlled longitudinal studies, to determine what might mediate such relationships and design appropriate interventions to maximize these effects. As has been pointed out by Quinney, Wall, and Gauvin (chapter 1), scientific research is but one of the sources upon which physical activity practice and policy are based. Scientific study and advancement are often driven by practical problems and questions. Indeed, although exercise and physical activity practitioners often have unique solutions that appear to work, it is not always clear *why* they work. Some might say that this is irrelevant, as long as they do work. However, it is only by scientific testing and determination of mechanisms that influence behavior that we can effectively guide policy makers and practitioners to design and offer programs that will effectively promote and maintain active and healthy living in North America. The interaction between scientist and practitioner is vital to the achievement of this objective.

Acknowledgment

Completion of this paper was partially supported by a grant from the National Institute on Aging (#AG07907).

References

Bandura, A. (1982). Self-efficacy mechanism in human agency. *American Psychologist, 37*, 122-147.

Bandura, A. (1986). *Social foundations of thought and action.* Englewood Cliffs, NJ: Prentice Hall.

Blair, S.N., Kohl, H.W., III, Paffenbarger, R.S., Clark, D.G., Cooper, K.H., & Gibbons, L.W. (1989). Physical fitness and all-cause mortality: A prospective study of healthy men and women. *Journal of the American Medical Association, 262*, 2395-2401.

Bouchard, C., & Shephard, R.J. (1991). *Physical activity, fitness, and health: A model and key concepts.* Consensus Doc-017.

Bouchard, C., Shephard, R.J., Stephens, T., Sutton, J.R., & McPherson, B.D. (Eds.) (1990). *Exercise, fitness, and health: A consensus of current knowledge.* Champaign, IL: Human Kinetics.

Diener, E. (1984). Subjective well-being. *Psychological Bulletin, 95*, 542-575.

Doan, R.E., & Scherman, A. (1987). The therapeutic effect of physical fitness on measures of personality: A literature review. *Journal of Counseling and Development, 11*, 28-36.

Ewart, C.K. (1989). Psychological effects of resistive weight training: Implications for cardiac patients. *Medicine and Science in Sports and Exercise, 21*, 683-688.

Ewart, C.K.., Stewart, K.J., Gillian, R.E., & Kelemen, M.H. (1986). Self-efficacy mediates strength gains during circuit weight training in men with coronary artery disease. *Medicine and Science in Sports and Exercise, 18*, 531-540.

Ewart, C.K., Taylor, C.B., Reese, L.B., & DeBusk, R.F. (1983). Effects of early post myocardial infarction exercise testing on self-perception and subsequent physical activity. *American Journal of Cardiology, 51*, 1076-1080.

Fitness Canada. (1991). *Active living: A conceptual overview.* Ottawa: Government of Canada.

Folkins, C.H., & Sime, W.E. (1981). Physical fitness training and mental health. *American Psychologist, 36*, 373-389.

Fox, K.R., & Corbin, C.B. (1989). The physical self-perception profile: Developmental and preliminary validation. *Journal of Sport and Exercise Psychology, 11*, 408-430.

Gruber, J.J. (1986). Physical activity and self-esteem development in children: A meta-analysis. *American Academy of Physical Education Papers, 19*, 30-48. Champaign, IL: Human Kinetics.

Hughes, J.R. (1984). Psychological effects of habitual aerobic exercise: A critical review. *Preventive Medicine, 13*, 66-78.

King, A.C., Taylor, C.B., Haskell, W.L., & DeBusk, R.F. (1989). Influence of regular aerobic exercise on psychological health: A randomized, controlled trial of healthy middle-aged adults. *Health Psychology, 8*. 305-324.

Marsh, A.W., & Jackson, S.A. (1986). Multidimensional self-concepts, masculinity, and femininity as a function of women's involvement in athletics. *Sex Roles, 15*, 391-415.

Marsh, H.W., & Peart, M.D. (1988). Competitive and cooperative physical fitness training programs for girls: Effects on physical fitness and multidimensional self-concepts. *Journal of Sport and Exercise Psychology, 10*, 390-407.

McAuley, E. (1991). Efficacy, attributional, and affective responses to exercise participation. *Journal of Sport and Exercise Psychology, 13*, 382-393.

McAuley, E. (in press). Physical activity and psychosocial outcomes. In C. Bouchard, R.J. Shephard, & T. Stephens (Eds.), *Physical activity, fitness, and health: International proceedings and consensus statement.* Champaign, IL: Human Kinetics.

McAuley, E., & Courneya, K.S. (1992a, March). *The exercise-induced affect scale: Preliminary development and validation.* Paper presented at the annual meeting of the Society of Behavioral Medicine, New York.

McAuley, E., & Courneya, K.S. (1992b). Self-efficacy relationships with affective and exertion responses to exercise. *Journal of Applied Social Psychology,* **22**, 312-326.

McAuley, E., Courneya, K.S., & Lettunich, J. (1991). Effects of acute and long-term exercise on self-efficacy in sedentary middle-aged males and females. *The Gerontologist,* **31**, 534-542.

Moses, J., Steptoe, A., Mathews, A., & Edwards, S. (1989). The effects of exercise training on mental well-being in the normal population: A controlled trial. *Journal of Psychosomatic Research,* **33**, 47-61.

North, T.C., McCullagh, P., & Tran, Z.V. (1990). Effect of exercise on depression. *Exercise and Sport Science Reviews*, **18**, 379-415.

Petruzzello, S.J., Landers, D.M., Hatfield, B.D., Kubitz, K.A., & Salazar, W. (1991). A meta-analysis on the anxiety-reducing effects of acute and chronic exercise. *Sports Medicine,* **11**, 143-182.

Plante, T.G., & Rodin, J. (1990). Physical fitness and enhanced psychological health. *Current Psychology: Research and Reviws,* **9**, 3-24.

Rosenberg, M. (1985). Self-concept and psychological well-being in adolescence. In R.H. Leahy (Ed.), *The development of the self* (pp. 205-246). Orlando, FL: Academic Press.

Shavelson, R.J., Hubner, J.J., & Stanton, G.C. (1976). Self-concept: Validation of construct interpretations. *Review of Educational Research,* **46**, 407-441.

Sonstroem, R.J. (1984). Exercise and self-esteem. In R.L. Terjung (Ed.), *Exercise and sport sciences reviews* (Vol. 12, pp. 123-155). Lexington, MA: Collomore.

Sonstroem, R.J., & Morgan, W.P. (1989). Exercise and self-esteem: Rationale and model. *Medicine and Science in Sports and Exercise,* **21**, 329-337.

Stephens, T. (1988). Physical activity and mental health in the United States and Canada: Evidence from four population surveys. *Preventive Medicine,* **17**, 35-47.

Taylor, C.B., Bandura, A., Ewart, C.K., Miller, N.H., & DeBusk, R.F. (1985). Exercise testing to enhance wives' confidence in their husbands' cardiac capability soon after clinically uncomplicated acute myocardial infarction. *American Journal of Cardiology,* **55**, 635-638.

Toshima, M.T., Kaplan, R.M., & Ries, A.L. (1990). Experimental evaluation of rehabilitation in chronic obstructive pulmonary disease: Short-term effects on exercise endurance and health status. *Health Psychology,* **9**, 237-252.

Zaharopoulus, E., & Hodge, K.P. (1991). Self-concept and sport participation. *New Zealand Journal of Psychology,* **20**, 12-16.

13

Application and Program Implications of the Psychological Outcomes of Exercise and Physical Activity

Lise Gauvin

Other authors (Landers, chapter 11 this volume; McAuley, chapter 12 this volume) have associated increased exercise participation with the alleviation of negative psychological states and the enhancement of psychological well-being. In this chapter, I will examine the effects of exercise withdrawal on psychological parameters and underscore some of the practical applications and program implications of the knowledge on psychological outcomes of exercise and physical activity.

Psychological Outcomes of Exercise Withdrawal

Previous reviews of the literature have dealt with the effects of increasing exercise and physical activity on psychological outcome (North, McCullagh, & Tran, 1990; Petruzello, Landers, Hatfield, Kubitz, & Salazar, 1991). The bulk of the research has focused on the presentation of an exercise stimulus to inactive subjects. This is probably a reasonable strategy because population surveys indicate that 75% to 90% of the North American population do not engage in exercise frequently enough or at a sufficiently high intensity to result in optimal benefits for cardiovascular health.

However, an equally important question pertains to the psychological effects of stopping exercise among the 10% to 25% of the population who regularly participate in vigorous exercise. Understanding the psychological effects of involuntary stoppage of exercise is important for several reasons. First, most people must deal with responsibilities, illness, or travel commitments that sometimes infringe upon their regular exercise schedules. It is important to know how even minor disturbances in exercise regimens might affect the individual because some people have suggested that the

effects can be very detrimental. Also, some authors have suggested that people can become addicted to exercise and demonstrate behaviors and symptoms that are typically observed in substance abuse. If we are to promote active living, we must be aware of the excesses that might occur and what factors seem to promote their occurrence.

Effects of Exercise Withdrawal

When asked how they feel when missing a workout, physically active people overwhelmingly report experiencing guilt (Gauvin, 1989). We must, however, be cautious in interpreting this type of interview data because they may be nothing more than a reflection of what people think they *should* feel like as opposed to what they *actually* feel like.

Nevertheless, a study of female runners (Harris, 1981) documented that a majority of women felt more depressed and tense, less energetic, and fatter when forced to stop running. A study of male and female runners (Robbins & Joseph, 1980) found that people who ran to cope with problems experienced a greater number of withdrawal symptoms (e.g., irritability, nervousness) than people who ran for enjoyment. Yet another study of runners (Carmack & Martens, 1979) found that those people who ran more also reported more discomfort when missing a run compared with those people who ran less. In another survey-type study, Anshel (1991) found that people who reported more addiction to exercise also reported more discomfort when missing a workout. In sum, most active participants report a wide range of negative mood disturbances as a result of their exercise withdrawal. For the reason mentioned previously, however, we must be wary of survey-type data.

More dependable experimental research reveals a similar pattern. In an experimental study (Thaxton,

1982) in which regular runners were asked to stop exercising for 24 hours, it was found that running deprivation resulted in increased depression and anxiety as reflected by selected physiological indexes. Other researchers have found that one week of withdrawal by men who ran regularly resulted in increased reports of physical symptoms, anxiety, insomnia, and strain. Two weeks of withdrawal resulted in more reported depression (Morris, Steinberg, Sykes, & Salmon, 1990). A study of male and female exercisers of all types (Gauvin & Szabo, 1992) found that 1 week of exercise stoppage resulted in reports of more physical symptoms but not of psychological mood changes.

Very few studies (Crossman, Jamieson, & Henderson, 1987) have found that exercise deprivation results in no effects whatsoever. Because the study of the effects of exercise deprivation is so new, researchers have not been able to confirm or disconfirm any theories as to why these effects do or do not occur.

So what does all this mean? What do we know about exercise deprivation? When surveyed about the consequences of exercise deprivation, most people say that their moods are quite negatively affected and that they experience physical discomfort. However, when we experimentally manipulate exercise withdrawal, we observe only some of these negative mood changes and not consistently across studies. We must therefore conclude that while exercise stoppage is related to disturbances, they may not be of the magnitude that are typically reported through surveys.

Similarly, while these effects seem to occur, it is not known why they occur. Presumably they could be due to changes of a physiological nature or to how people interpret the meaning of the exercise withdrawal.

Exercise Dependence: Fact or Fallacy

In discussing the topic of exercise dependence, the first question that must be addressed is whether this condition exists at all. Can people really become addicted to exercise in the traditional sense of the term? Or is some people's high commitment to exercise just a convenient conversation piece or media attention-grabber?

Researchers in this area are split in their opinions and not a great deal of work has been done (deCoverley-Veale, 1987; Polivy, 1992). First, the term exercise *addiction* may not be adequate at all; in discussing dependence, most health professionals consider that addiction to some substance is required before this term can correctly be used. In regard to exercise and physical activity, research has yet to demonstrate that people become physically addicted to some substance that is exercise-related or to exercise per se.

Certain clinical reports and case studies suggest that some people demonstrate behaviors that are reminiscent of substance dependence (Sacks & Sachs, 1984). For example, some reports indicate that persons can become obsessed with the idea of exercising; neglect social, work, or family responsibilities in order to engage in exercise; or become despondent when deprived of exercise. However, statistics on the prevalence of such severe and clearly pathological symptoms are not available. The estimated incidence of such extreme occurrences are fortunately quite minimal. Furthermore, other researchers (cf. Polivy, 1992) have suggested that exercise dependence might be a symptom of another mental health problem, namely eating disorders. As in the area of exercise addiction, little work has been done on this issue but it is frequently observed that persons with eating disorders exercise as a method of burning calories. However, firm conclusions about the nature of the relationship between eating disorders and exercise cannot be drawn at this time.

In sum, the words *exercise dependence* may not adequately describe the phenomenon that can sometimes be observed when a person becomes obsessed with the thought and desire to engage in physical exercise. This obsessiveness does not seem to occur in many exercise enthusiasts, and it is not understood why these thoughts and behaviors occur.

Strategies for Application of Knowledge

In attempting to underscore the practical applications and program implications of the knowledge available on the psychological outcomes of exercise, I was faced with an interesting dilemma. What does one do with information that essentially tells us about the consequences of a given behavior or lifestyle pattern? There are two general strategies for applying this knowledge, namely disseminating the information on psychological outcomes and maximizing the likelihood that positive psychological outcomes will occur.

Disseminating Information About Psychological Outcomes

People may object on several grounds to the suggestion that practitioners should actively disseminate information about psychological outcomes. Research shows that simple awareness of the health and psychological benefits of exercise and physical activity is not sufficient to insure compliance to exercise regimens or to promote adherence to active living (see Dishman, chapter 14 this volume). One response to this objection is that disentangling popular beliefs from accurate scientific information is a prerequisite to continued and sustained participation in an active lifestyle. Accurate information can place exercise at an appropriate level in the person's hierarchy of priorities.

Some people also may object because the public is reasonably aware of the health benefits of exercise and physical activity and generally has a positive view of the role of exercise and physical activity in mental well-being. Thus, disseminating information about the psychological outcomes of exercise serves no useful purpose. The response to this objection is that the public may know a lot less than we imagine about the benefits of physical activity, particularly in regard to psychological outcomes. We must therefore strive to educate the public about the psychological outcomes of exercise.

A survey commissioned by the Canadian Council on Smoking and conducted on a representative sample of more than 1,000 Ontario residents supports this point (Environics, 1991). The purpose of this survey was to assess respondents' awareness of the health hazards of smoking. In general, the survey indicated that despite the numerous and longstanding public awareness campaigns about the ill effects of smoking, the majority of respondents were not aware of the health hazards of smoking. Specifically, in naming the health hazards related to smoking, only 44% of respondents mentioned lung cancer, only 34% mentioned cancer in general, only 20% mentioned heart disease, and only 20% mentioned emphysema. In responding to the question of what percentage of lung cancer cases result in death, 32% had no opinion, and among those who volunteered an answer, the average estimated mortality rate was 64.7%. In reality, about 85% of lung cancer cases result in death. Thus, awareness of the outcomes of smoking is dismally low despite widespread campaigns to enhance public awareness. We might hypothesize that because the psychological benefits of exercise have been studied only recently, people may know even less about their nature and existence than they know about the outcomes of smoking on health.

Misinformation may also be a problem. I'm sure that many practitioners have encountered participants who firmly believe that exercise makes people feel better, look better, deal better with stress, and generally be happier. This message was in fact conveyed in a promotional advertising campaign by a chain of fitness clubs in Montreal in the winter of 1989. Their marketing campaign was based on the idea that members of the club would get rid of a newly coined psychological disorder (essentially the midwinter blues) by joining the club and exercising. While most people recognize this as marketing hype, misinformation about the psychological outcomes of exercise may create false expectations in potential participants. Once people's unrealistic expectations are not met, the chances of continued participation are small. Thus there is ample reason to disseminate scientifically supported information about the psychological outcomes of exercise.

With this in mind, I would like to briefly underscore some of the points raised by other authors in this volume (Landers & Petruzzello, chapter 11; McAuley, chapter 12) and the researchers in the consensus symposium concerning what is known about the psychological outcomes of exercise.

As indicated by McAuley, physical activity seems to enhance self-esteem or feelings of self-worth, particularly in people who have low self-esteem to begin with. Both acute and chronic exercise increases self-efficacy or perceptions of one's capacity to perform a given task. This is particularly noteworthy because some research suggests that higher self-efficacy is also related to higher persistence in an exercise regimen. Physical activity is associated with positive moods, particularly in women and older subjects.

As mentioned by one of the consensus speakers (Thomas, 1992), exercise and physical activity are positively associated with intellectual function, memory, and reaction time.

Furthermore, as discussed by Landers, physical activity results in significant decreases in subjectively and physiologically assessed symptoms of anxiety. Higher levels of fitness are related to lower reactivity to stressors. Another of the consensus speakers (Morgan, 1992) has documented that physical activity and depression are negatively related, indicating that higher physical activity accompanies lower levels of depression.

Finally, as discussed previously, exercise withdrawal in regularly active subjects results in some increases in perception of physical symptoms and perhaps some small mood disturbances. Whether more extreme occurrences of these effects constitute exercise addiction or some other process remains to be demonstrated. The factors that seem to promote obsessive exercise behavior are not well understood nor are their determinants well known.

Maximizing the Psychological Outcomes of Exercise

The second general strategy to the application of the psychological outcomes of exercise consists of maximizing the positive psychological outcomes. To achieve this end, practitioners should bear in mind four general principles.

(1) Type, Frequency, and Intensity of Exercise Required to Accrue Benefits

This is known in the literature as the dose–response issue. In the consensus conference, Rejeski (1992) concluded that there is limited knowledge about the dose of exercise that results in a variety of psychosocial outcomes. This lack of information obviously creates a dilemma for the practitioner. What do you encourage participants to do?

However, as indicated by Rejeski, we do know that moderate exercise results in vigor and exhilaration, but high-intensity exercise tends to result in tension or anxiety. Higher intensity exercise does seem to yield increases in positive moods and decreases in negative moods following exercise. Finally, overtraining may result in decreases in positive moods.

In regard to chronic exercise, the data suggest that lower intensity exercise is better than high-intensity or discontinued exercise in decreasing tension or anxiety and increasing coping skills (Rejeski, 1992). Increases in aerobic fitness levels are not critical in inducing positive psychological outcomes. Finally, it may take 4 to 6 months to optimize the effects of exercise training on the psychological factors of anxiety and depression.

Thus, in prescribing exercise, we must recognize that high-intensity exercise may be psychologically suitable for only certain subsets of the population. We must also be aware that lower intensity exercise may produce better psychosocial outcomes in the long term than high-intensity exercise. Finally, awareness of the 4- to 6-month delay in producing substantive psychological benefits is also important given that the typical exercise prescription spans only a 12-week period.

(2) Participant's Characteristics

As mentioned by McAuley and Rejeski in the consensus symposium, not all people get the same benefits out of exercise. For example, those people who seem to be the worst off in terms of self-esteem are also those who accrue the largest gains in self-esteem. Similarly, the subjective meaning that people ascribe to exercise participation probably influences how they perceive and internalize the experience of physical activity. Thus, in prescribing exercise we must also be aware that the psychological outcomes will differ a great deal among individuals.

(3) Leader's Characteristics

As mentioned by McAuley, many behaviors of the leader can increase self-efficacy, or a person's perception of his or her capacity to perform a given task. For example, providing verbal encouragement along with the exercise and demonstrating the success of others in performing a given task can be helpful in increasing a person's self-efficacy. This suggests that exercise instructors must also develop the social skills of effective teaching and coaching. Therefore, we should demonstrate behaviors that are designed not only to guide exercise behavior as it unfolds but also to increase the perceptions of competence of participants. Such a strategy should not only maximize the likelihood of sustained participation but also maximize the self-efficacy benefits of exercise and physical activity.

(4) Situation Where the Activity Unfolds

As indicated by one study (Pennebaker & Lightner, 1980), subjects who ran a given distance outdoors alternatively on a track and on a cross-country trail, reported identical amounts of fatigue and physical symptoms even though they ran the 1,800m distance significantly faster on the cross-country trail. One would expect performance on the cross-country trail to be slower because running on a cross-country trail is objectively more difficult, especially for the beginning joggers who composed the sample of this study. The finding suggests that the environment in which the exercise unfolds can significantly affect the positive or negative perception that subjects have of the experience of exercise and presumably of the psychological outcomes that might ensue. It is unrealistic to suggest modifying existing facilities that are less than ideal, but changes designed to make the environment more appealing could have a positive effect. Many of the suggestions offered by McAuley are important in this regard.

As a final comment on this matter, an interview study conducted several years ago (Gauvin, 1989) found that the main complaints of regular exercisers had to do with poor air quality and poor shower facilities. Thus program planners and facility managers should attempt to create exercise environments that have high quality air and feature pleasant surroundings.

Conclusion

In closing, I would like to reiterate some of the practical applications and program implications of research on the psychological outcomes of exercise. First, we should make a great effort to accurately inform participants about the psychological outcomes of exercise and physical activity. We must ensure that the information conveyed is accurate and scientifically supported. Second, we should recognize that different types and amounts of exercise may result in different psychological outcomes. The prescription of high-intensity exercise should be approached with caution from a psychological standpoint, and participants should be made aware of the potential delay (4 to 6 months) in gaining psychological benefits. Third, awareness that the greatest positive outcomes are achieved by those who have less favorable psychological profiles calls for targeting exercise programs to these populations if psychological outcomes are actively being pursued. Fourth, the behavior of the exercise leader is instrumental in maximizing any psychological benefits. Exercise leaders and people who interact directly with exercise participants should emulate the social behavior of effective teachers and coaches. Finally, we should strive to create exercise environments that are attractive for the participants.

If some of these guidelines are followed, there is a greater likelihood that desirable psychological outcomes will be achieved through exercise and physical activity participation.

References

Anshel, M.H. (1991). A psycho-behavioral analysis of addicted versus non-addicted male and female exercisers. *Journal of Sport Behavior, 14*, 145-154.

Carmack, M.A., & Martens, R. (1979). Measuring commitment to running: A survey of runners' attitudes and mental states. *Journal of Sport Psychology, 1*, 25-42.

Crossman, J., Jamieson, J., & Henderson, L. (1987). Responses of competitive athletes to lay-offs in training: Exercise addiction or psychological relief? *Journal of Sport Behavior, 10*, 28-38.

deCoverley-Veale, D.M.W. (1987). Exercise dependence. *British Journal of Addiction, 82*, 735-740.

Environics. (1991). *Awareness of health hazards due to smoking*. Ottawa: Canadian Council on Smoking.

Gauvin, L. (1989). An experiential approach to the motivational features of exercise and lifestyle. *Canadian Journal of Sport Sciences, 15*, 51-61.

Gauvin, L., & Szabo, A. (1992). Application of the Experience Sampling Method to the study of the effects of exercise withdrawal on well-being. *Journal of Sport and Exercise Psychology, 14*, 361-374.

Harris, M.B. (1981). Women runners' views of running. *Perceptual and Motor Skills, 53*, 395-402.

Morgan, W.P. (1992, May). *Physical activity, fitness and depression*. Paper presented at the International Consensus Symposium, Toronto.

Morris, M., Steinberg, H., Sykes, E.A., & Salmon, P. (1990). Effects of temporary withdrawal from regular running. *Journal of Psychosomatic Research, 34*, 493-500.

North, T.C., McCullagh, P., & Tran, W. (1990). Effect of exercise on depression. *Exercise and Sport Science Reviews, 19*, 379-415.

Pennebaker, J.W., & Lightner, J.M. (1980). Competition in internal and external information in an exercise setting. *Journal of Personality and Social Psychology, 39*, 165-174.

Petruzello, S.J., Landers, D.M., Hatfield, B.D., Kubitz, K.A., & Salazar, W. (1991). Effects of exercise on anxiety and mood: A meta-analysis. *Sports Medicine, 11*, 143-182.

Polivy, J. (1992, May). *Physical activity, fitness and compulsive behaviors*. Paper presented at the International Consensus Symposium, Toronto.

Rejeski, W.J. (1992, May). *Dose–response issues from a psychosocial perspective*. Paper presented at the International Consensus Symposium, Toronto.

Robbins, J.M., & Joseph, P. (1980). Commitment to running: Implications for the family and work. *Sociological Symposium, 30*, 87-108.

Sacks, M.L., & Sachs, M.L. (1984). *Psychology of running*. Champaign, IL: Human Kinetics.

Thaxton, L. (1982). Physiological and psychological effects of short-term exercise addiction on habitual runners. *Journal of Sport Psychology, 4*, 73-80.

Thomas, J.R. (1992, May). *Physical activity and intellectual performance*. Paper presented at the International Consensus Symposium, Toronto.

14

Predicting and Changing Exercise and Physical Activity: What's Practical and What's Not

Rod K. Dishman

To my knowledge, there are no standardized professional guidelines for practice designed to increase and maintain exercise and physical activity. The influential *Guidelines for Exercise Testing and Prescription* (American College of Sports Medicine, 1991), and its resource manual, published by the American College of Sports Medicine (ACSM), contain practically oriented chapters on behavior change. The American Council on Exercise, a leading industry organization, has included a practical chapter on exercise adherence in its *Personal Trainer Manual* (American Council on Exercise, 1991). Each of these sources is contemporary and offers potentially practical advice, but neither represents a formal consensus by experts or a set of sanctioned and validated professional guidelines. The active living campaign in Canada provides an initiative to examine the current knowledge base that might underlie professional guidelines for promoting exercise adherence.

In this chapter, I discuss my view of the practical aspects of the scientific consensus (Dishman & Sallis, in press) in the area of exercise adherence. The chapter is organized around four questions that characterize the scientific and professional literature compiled during about the past 15 years. These questions are

1. Can exercise and physical activity be predicted with the precision that is adequate for practical purposes?
2. Are behavior-change interventions implementable and effective for increasing physical activity, exercise, and physical fitness?
3. Can existing theories direct effective interventions for increasing and maintaining physical activity, exercise, and physical fitness?
4. Are there valid technologies that are standardized and can be implemented in evaluating the effectiveness of existing theories and interventions currently applied in exercise and physical activity settings?

These questions offer a structure for a constructive criticism of the "state of the art" in exercise adherence. I believe that nothing is as practical as a good theory. A good theory, however, evolves from empirical evaluation and revision by both deductive (tests of exceptions to the rules) and inductive (common observations leading to testable rules) approaches. I hope to show that if the past segregation of methods and levels of scientific inference across the practical questions I have asked is perpetuated, practical gains in our understanding of exercise behavior will not advance.

My perspective presumes that for knowledge to be practical, it must emerge from some method of scientific inquiry. Observations made by clinicians in practical settings can lead to useful principles and practices, but their validity and generalizability require verification by others. Likewise, theoretical models may offer directions for successful programming decisions and interventions in practical settings, but their propositions require testing by reliable observations. Rational, natural-science traditions based on quantitative assessment have been the approach of nearly all exercise adherence studies. Only a handful of studies have used the methods of qualitative assessment (e.g., Gauvin, 1989) based in ethological traditions more common in anthropology and the social sciences.

Past Approaches

Adherence studies generally have employed either a screening or correlational approach to predicting exercise and physical activity or an intervention approach designed to increase participation. Methods using a screening or correlational approach have in most cases been limited to a descriptive level of analysis in which eventual adherents and dropouts are contrasted on personal characteristics such as demographic, biological, and psychological variables that exist at the outset of involvement. These approaches can provide preliminary evidence for the validity of theories that could prove to be practical, and studies using these approaches have shown that several personal attributes are reliably associated with adherence behavior. However, the focus on differences between people on static attributes has not allowed behavioral prediction for individuals, thus limiting the direct clinical significance of the differences observed. There has been no way to quantitatively apply the screening information in a meaningful or practical way to determine if, or for how long, an individual will stay with a given program.

Prediction?

One of the earliest and most systematic adherence studies employing a predictive screening model was initiated by Oldridge (1979) and his associates with a prospective study of male postmyocardial infarction (MI) patients enrolled in the Ontario Exercise-Heart Collaborative Study sponsored by the Ontario Ministry of Health and by Health and Welfare Canada. Ninety-six percent of the patients characterized by four factors: smoked, were inactive in their leisure time, and held blue-collar jobs with low energy expenditure, subsequently dropped out. However, only 22 individuals, 3% of the 751 men screened, fit this characterization. Because 335 patients dropped out, had this diagnostic profile been 100% accurate it still could have accounted for only about 7% (22 of 335 dropouts) of dropout behavior in this setting. Thus, a nominal approach that dichotomizes screening characteristics is limited in the practical advantage it can provide due to its selective elimination of subjects to which it does not apply. Multivariate prediction models assessing psychological variables based on interval (at the least ordinal) data, on the other hand, allow a prediction of variation in behavior among participants that is usually 5% to 30% above a chance prediction. However, studies using this approach have not yielded practically useful prediction accuracy either (Dishman, 1981; Dishman, Ickes, & Morgan, 1980, Sallis, Hovell, & Hofstetter, 1992).

Past prediction studies indicate that even the most precise screening data are associated with substantial prediction error for a given individual. The practical advantage of these approaches remains unclear until better estimates of the specificity (i.e. few false positives) and sensitivity (i.e., few false negatives) are available. Recently, attempts to develop equations to predict adoption or dropout from exercise programs seem to have been abandoned in favor of population studies of theory and interventions. The abandonment of prediction studies may be premature. When exercise settings

and populations are stable, it should be possible to develop predictive equations combining demographic, psychometric, biometric, and historic data that have sufficient accuracy to aid decision making by exercise program staff. Predictions cannot occur, however, without interdisciplinary collaboration, standardization of measures, replication, and cross-validation. It takes time, effort, and a willingness to eschew criticism by deductive theorists to reach these goals.

Interventions?

Facility accessibility and spouse support have been replicated as weak but reliable determinants of supervised and free-living physical activity. These findings suggest that exercise adherence might be facilitated by management of the exercise setting. Early (Sanne, 1973) and recent (King, Taylor, Haskell, & DeBusk, 1988) clinical trials have shown that home-based programs can be associated with enhanced adherence. The principal focus of studies that have intervened in the adherence process, however, has been participant-oriented rather than setting-oriented. Future applications must balance the emphasis to determine which, or in what combination, personal and setting interventions will be most practical.

Behavior modification interventions are directed at the person without an attempt to teach the person skills or to change beliefs, attitudes, or self-perceptions. They generally follow one or both approaches called stimulus control or reinforcement control. Stimulus control manipulates antecedent conditions that can prompt a behavior. Simple examples include the use of posters, written slogans, written agreements to be active, placement of exercise equipment in conspicuous places, travel routes past an exercise facility, and so forth. Reinforcement control manipulates consequent conditions associated with increasing activity. Examples include behavior contracts that specify the conditions of activity and consequences for breaking the contract, token economies whereby rewards are contingent on behavior, and group lotteries where a chance drawing determines the allocation of a reward pool to which each member of the group has contributed. Behavior modification techniques are typically under the supervision of a care provider and are referred to as therapist-centered. Conversely, *cognitive-behavior modification* interventions can employ basic stimulus control and reinforcement control principles, but they are directed at changing psychological variables assumed to be mediators of behavior. The goal of the intervention is to teach skills the person can use to control the antecedent and consequent conditions that prompt and reinforce behavior. They are referred to as client-centered approaches. Simple examples include goal setting, self-monitoring, feedback, and a decision-balance worksheet whereby expected benefits and costs of a new behavior are contrasted and weighted and strategies for overcoming barriers are planned. Most studies done in the past 10 years to increase physical activity or exercise behavior have combined varying features of all these techniques into comprehensive intervention packages.

Until the past 3 or 4 years, most intervention studies have used single dimensional approaches with small numbers of people who were homogeneous in terms of gender, race, ethnicity, health status, and economic and educational status. Recently, community-based interventions have applied psychological and behavioral theories for behavior change (King et al., 1992). These approaches go beyond the traditional practice of individual counseling to include organizational (e.g., community recreation centers, churches, diffusion strategies through schools), environmental (e.g., facility planning), and social (e.g., family interventions) macrochanges, or they use cost-effective or pragmatically convenient avenues (e.g., mailings, telephone) for reaching large numbers of individuals who might not be accessible or amenable to traditional clinically based interventions.

For this conference, I conducted a quantitative meta-analysis of 20 studies conducted during the past 5 years of interventions to increase physical activity or exercise (Dishman & Sallis, in press). Results from the studies were transformed to a correlation coefficient (r) according to procedures outlined by Friedman (1968) and Rosenthal (1984). Consistent with Cohen (1977), population values of r approximating .01, .30, and .40 can be regarded as small, moderate, and large, respectively. Because it is useful to view the results of interventions in terms of success rates, r effects can be presented as binomial effect sizes (BES) according to Rosenthal and Rubin (1982). The BES can be interpreted as a measure of the success of an intervention (i.e., the change in the proportion of exercise adherents in the experimental group compared to a control group). A zero binomial effect reflects a 50-50 chance for success. This approximates the median success rate for supervised exercise programs involving both healthy adults and coronary heart disease (CHD) patients.

The behavior change interventions analysis summarized in Table 14.1 suggests the following conclusions about recent interventions:

- Studies typically support that health education and behavior modification or cognitive-behavior modification principles can be implemented with exercise programs and are accompanied by increased frequency of activity or time spent in activity for limited periods of time.
- With the exception of studies closely linked with on-site programs or periodic supervision (e.g., work sites, clinics, or schools), the studies do not demonstrate that exercise intensity or total activity has been increased enough to reliably increase

physical fitness or to reduce risk for future morbidity or mortality.

- The quasiexperimental or uncontrolled designs used in about half of the literature limit confident conclusions about the cause-and-effect nature of the increased physical activity that has accompanied the interventions.
- Most studies have used indirect measures of physical activity (e.g., self-report) or indirect estimates of physical fitness based on heart rate or treadmill time; thus, their validity is uncertain. Only a few studies have attempted to verify self-reports of activity with expected increases in fitness.
- The effect size for increased fitness when $\dot{V}O_2$ peak was measured is typically small, even when the effects for self-reported activity were large.
- A contributor to the uncompelling nature of the existing evidence has been the failure of most exercise studies to base interventions on broader theoretical models of behavior change such as stage theories (Dishman, 1982; Prochaska & Marcus, in press) and to consider the companion literature on the determinants of physical activity.

Educational counseling (which includes instruction about benefits of physical activity and guidelines for safely increasing fitness), health-risk appraisal and fitness testing, as well as behavior modification and cognitive-behavior modification interventions, have shown potential *efficacy* (they can work) for increasing exercise and physical activity, but their *effectiveness* (do they work?) for increasing exercise, physical activity, fitness, or health in the population remains unclear. Interventions, regardless of tradition or content, usually are associated with moderate binomial effect sizes for frequency of physical activity, suggesting that exercise programs that experience success rates of about 40% (when adherence is defined as attendance) might have increased success to about 60% with a behavioral intervention. The impact on changes in intensity and duration of physical activity is less clear. The effect sizes for educational counseling, behavior modification, and cognitive-behavior modification are comparable to those found for lowered intensity, duration, and frequency of exercise prescriptions in fitness-training studies for white males (Pollock, 1988). Thus, the superiority of behavior change interventions over modifications in traditional fitness programming merits direct testing. Uncontrolled case studies and quasi-experimental, multiple-baseline studies published prior to 1988 have commonly reported increases in the frequency of physical activity of 50% to 200% (Dishman, 1991). However, the absolute levels of the increased activity typically fall below the frequency, duration, and intensity required to increase physical fitness (American College of Sports Medicine, 1990) and may not reach the level required to optimally decrease risk for disease morbidity or all-cause mortality (Blair et al., 1989).

Table 14.1   Behavior Change Interventions, 1988-1992 [20 studies: 61 effects]

Type	Activity measure	Study design
Educational counseling 0.18±0.25	Self-report 0.14±0.18	Randomized 0.17±0.20
BM 0.23±0.21	Heart rate 0.19±0.20	Nonequivalent control 0.17±0.28
BM/CBM 0.19±0.28	Treadmill time 0.29±0.20	Uncontrolled cohort 0.41±0.16
Exercise dose 0.14±0.05	V0$_2$ peak 0.02±0.11	0.195l±0.24

Summary of a meta-analysis of behavior change interventions for exercise and physical activity from 1988 to February, 1992. Effect sizes are presented as mean correlation coefficients ± standard deviations for different types of interventions, activity measures, and study designs. The value in the lower right hand corner represents the mean correlation for all 20 studies. BM is behavior modification. CBM is cognitive-behavior modification.

Only about one half of the studies reported a follow-up to the intervention, and they typically showed that as follow-up time elapsed, increases in physical activity or fitness associated with the interventions diminished. Minimally effective intervention conditions for control comparisons have been rare. Therefore, generalizations are not possible about specific components of the interventions that are effective for specific populations. Many types of interventions have been associated with increased physical activity, but the superiority of these interventions has not been directly established. It can be concluded that using any of the interventions appears better than doing nothing. However, it is not clear that the components of the interventions employed exert a practical, meaningful influence on physical activity beyond that exerted by social support and reinforcement. The superiority of behavior change interventions over increased attention from professionals still has not been convincingly shown.

Effects of self-reported physical activity (0.14 ± 0.18) appear larger than effects for changes in V̇O$_2$max (0.02 ± 0.11). In general, the size of effects is inversely associated with the scientific quality of the study. The effect size for uncontrolled studies (0.41 ± 0.16) is twice that of randomized or quasi-experimental studies. The effect of the several interventions based on health education and fitness testing is comparable to behavior modification (BM) and cognitive-behavior modification (CBM). However, the scientific quality is poor for most studies that have reported an effect of health education and fitness testing on exercise behavior.

Until the methodological and design limitations of the intervention literature are resolved, it will not be possible to evaluate the true practical impact of behavior change strategies for increasing physical activity. Many interventions can be implemented, but their success has not been scientifically validated. However, until the science matures, practitioners can still do something! Based on my limited meta-analysis, I believe the first step is to modify traditional exercise programming guidelines to deliver moderate-intensity activities of a broader variety of types than traditionally employed, and to tailor to individual or population-segmented preferences determined from more formalized activity histories and goals assessments. This face-to-face approach can easily be implemented within the professional competencies of traditionally trained exercise specialists with modest additional training (e.g., a course and practicum in exercise psychology at the master's level). Population-based media campaigns in Australia (Donovan & Owen, in press) and Canada (e.g., the Particip-ACTION program) and community-based clinical programs delivered by Stanford University in the U.S. (e.g., King et al., 1988) present good models for extending traditional fitness programming to a mediated counseling approach. In these programs, telephone prompts and mailouts for education, monitoring, support, and problem-solving self-help kits appear as effective as traditional full-fledged behavior modification and are much more practical for fitness and health education personnel. These interventions can also be modeled after existing theories of behavior change from the fields of social psychology and marketing, with the addition of a qualified behavioral scientist to the traditional fitness programming staff. All of the contemporary intervention packages I am aware of that have been tested for effectiveness have been centered around

- setting goals based on initial fitness and desired outcomes;
- identifying personal costs and expected barriers to adoption and maintenance of an activity routine;
- developing strategies for preventing or minimizing the impact of barriers to participation and for increasing support and reinforcement from friends, family, or house members;
- planning a gradual progression of difficulty to optimize success and facilitate self-efficacy so the client has growing confidence in both the ability to be active and the ability to maintain the new pattern of activity;

- receiving feedback from fitness testing and self-monitoring of activity and progress by the client; and

- developing personal strategies for returning to activity after a period of relapse to inactivity due to flagging motivation, injury, vacation, and so forth.

Using Theory to Guide Interventions?

In early studies from supervised exercise programs (Andrew et al., 1981; Danielson & Wanzel, 1977) dropouts were simply asked why they stopped. Self-reports implicated lack of goal attainment, inconvenient program accessibility, and schedule incompatibility with other commitments such as work. Lack of spouse support for involvement was associated with a threefold increase in the dropout rate in the Ontario Exercise-Heart Collaborative Study (Andrew et al., 1981). Although these factors were examined using traditions of social psychology, the findings lacked a theoretical context that could guide interventions designed to decrease dropout.

There is recent, replicated evidence that theoretically derived psychological variables such as attitudes (including outcome-expectancy values and perceived barriers of time and effort), self-efficacy (confidence in being active), and intentions are prospectively associated with physical activity in both supervised and free-living settings (Dishman & Sallis, in press; Godin, in press; King et al., 1992). However, the lack of studies that control for past physical activity habits limits our confidence about how much of the observed relationship between cognitive determinants and activity is causal and how much reflects a selection effect; that is, active individuals report strong attitudes, self-efficacy, and intentions due to past success, but the past success was caused by factors other than attitudes, self-efficacy, or intentions. Education and persuasion campaigns can improve knowledge and attitudes about physical activity and show models that build self-efficacy in the inactive, but the effectiveness of interventions to accomplish this has not been widely quantified (Ewart, Taylor, Reese, & DeBusk, 1983).

It is unlikely that population interventions will be perfectly effective in increasing cognitive variables, so effect sizes estimated from correlational data will overestimate actual causal effects. As shown in Figure 14.1, it is more likely that the behavioral impact of interventions designed to influence knowledge and attitudes will be diminished markedly from initial public awareness, to changes in intention, to volitional attempts to be active, to successful maintenance.

Correlations between self-reports of physical activity and social-cognitive variables like self-efficacy, attitudes, and intentions commonly approximate .50 (Dzewaltowski, Noble, & Shaw, 1990; Godin & Shephard, 1990). Expressed as a binomial "effect size," a correlation of .50 suggests that a success rate in adopting

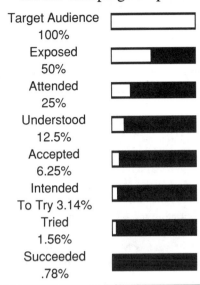

Media Campaign Impact

Target Audience
100%

Exposed
50%

Attended
25%

Understood
12.5%

Accepted
6.25%

Intended
To Try 3.14%

Tried
1.56%

Succeeded
.78%

Figure 14.1 Illustration of the decline in the diffusion impact of a media campaign with no additional intervention. This example assumes a 50-50 chance effect or a zero binomial effect[1] (adapted from Donovan & Owen, in press).

or maintaining exercise of 25% under control conditions would increase to 75% following an intervention whereby attitudes, self-efficacy, or intentions were increased. But, Figure 14.1 illustrates that the use of a media campaign to accomplish an increase in intentions will typically produce a much smaller behavioral effect. If, as shown, only 3% of a sedentary audience intended to become active as the result of a media campaign, the effect would still be practically important for the 3 in 100 people helped by the intervention. But this example illustrates that "effect sizes" estimated from correlational studies will far overestimate the real causal effect implied by the predictive relationship.

Alternatively, direct behavioral change may not be a reasonable standard for evaluating the practical effectiveness of population interventions. Reasonable outcomes of education campaigns and advice to begin a safe and effective exercising program, when they are applied in a community or a population base, are probably limited to changing awareness or consciousness about the importance of physical activity, rather than the measurable change in exercise behavior.

The purpose of the following sections is to overview two prominent theoretical models of behavior change, the relapse prevention model (Marlatt & Gordon, 1985) and the transtheoretical model (Prochaska & DiClemente, 1985), that show promise for guiding screening and intervention approaches in both population-based and clinically-based settings. A case example of a practical intervention, the PACE (physician-based assessment and counseling for exercise) project (Pender, Sallis, Long, & Calfas, in press), will illustrate the application of these models to changing exercise behavior.

The Relapse Prevention Model

Even among the habitually active, unexpected disruptions in activity routines or settings can interrupt or end a previously continuous exercise program. Relocation, medical events, and travel can impede the continuity of activity reinforcement and create new activity barriers. It is believed, however, that interruptions and life events have less impact as the activity habit becomes more established (Dishman, 1982); their impact may also be diminished if the individual anticipates and plans for their occurrence, recognizes them as only temporary impediments, and develops self-regulatory skills for preventing relapses to inactivity.

A popular example of relapse prevention was developed by Marlatt and Gordon (1985), of which the application to exercise has been described by Knapp (1988). The main components consist of the following:

- Identifying situations that put a person at high risk for relapse.
- Revising plans to avoid or cope with high-risk situations (e.g., time management, relaxation training, confidence building, reducing barriers to activity).
- Correcting positive outcome expectancies for inactivity so that consequences of not exercising are placed in proper perspective. For example, people tired at the end of the work day may expect to feel refreshed if they rest rather than exercise. They actually may feel guilty, however, because the activity would likely have been invigorating.
- Expecting and planning for lapses (e.g., scheduling alternative activities while on vacation or after injury).
- Minimizing the abstinence violation effect, where a temporary lapse is catastrophized into feelings of total failure that leads to loss of confidence and complete cessation of physical activity.
- Correcting a lifestyle imbalance where "shoulds" outweigh "wants." The focus here is on optimizing the pleasure derived from activity rather than viewing exercise as another obligation.
- Avoiding urges to relapse by blocking self-dialogues and images of the benefits of not exercising. People can talk themselves out of exercise in favor of sedentary alternatives.

Knapp (1988) noted that relapse prevention was designed for reducing high-frequency undesired addictive behaviors such as smoking and substance abuse, whereas exercise is a desired but low-frequency behavior for many. Thus, the effectiveness of the relapse prevention model for increasing physical activity may require modification. Several exercise intervention studies, however, have reported increased activity rates when components of the total model, identifying high risk situations, planning for relapse and reducing barri-

ers, and minimizing the abstinence violation effect, were combined in broader cognitive-behavior modification packages (Belisle, Roskies, & Levesque, 1987; King & Frederiksen, 1984; King, Taylor, Haskell, & DeBusk, 1988; Martin et al., 1984).

A replicated and easily implemented cognitive-behavior modification technique relevant to relapse prevention has been the decision balance-sheet described by Hoyt and Janis (1975) and replicated by Wankel and Thompson (1977) and Wankel, Yardley, and Graham (1985). This technique involves a careful evaluation by the patient or client of expected or experienced benefits and costs of activity, in which the health care provider or exercise specialist can actively reinforce positive outcomes and diminish negative expectations. Activity consequences are not only considered for the patient but also for a spouse, friends, or other family members. Importantly, reinforcement of the decision to begin or resume activity is accompanied by planned strategies for overcoming perceived or real barriers to exercise. In this way the decision balance-sheet shares common aspects with the relapse prevention model.

Although behavioral interventions based in part on the principles of relapse prevention have been followed by increased exercise frequency, naturalistic studies of free-living exercise are needed to describe the incidence of relapse (e.g., Sallis et al., 1990) and the predictive validity of the processes of relapse for exercise behavior.

The Transtheoretical Model

In an early review (Dishman, 1982), I discussed the application of stage theory to understanding exercise behavior change, and I speculated on some processes of change in a subsequent paper (Dishman, 1987). Similar, but more developed and potentially more practical views are found in extensions of the transtheoretical model for behavior change in smoking, weight control, and psychotherapy (Prochaska & DiClemente, 1985). This model proposes that individuals use several common processes to move sequentially through five major stages of self-initiated change: precontemplation, contemplation, readiness for action, action, and maintenance (Prochaska & Marcus, in press).

A potential major contribution of the transtheoretical model for increasing and maintaining exercise and physical activity lies in the theory's consideration of the readiness of individuals for change, and its capacity to bridge the use of behavior modification and cognitive-behavior modification traditions with population-based approaches that influence behavior change such as health promotion and mediated persuasion and education campaigns. Recent studies have extended the stage of change component of the transtheoretical model to exercise (Prochaska & Marcus, in press). Whether or not people who have attempted to begin or maintain an exercise or physical activity routine experience the same processes of change found previously with smoking cessation, weight loss, and psychotherapy (Prochaska & DiClemente, 1985) has not been studied.

Implementable Technologies?

Table 14.2 by Donovan and Owen (in press) illustrates the use of social marketing in a population base via media within the stages of change model. Several of the processes of change proposed by the transtheoretical model require consideration of both cognitive (e.g., beliefs and values related to consciousness-raising) and behavioral (e.g., stimulus control, reinforcement management, counterconditioning) variables.

Project PACE (physician-based assessment and counseling for exercise) was developed in collaboration with the U.S. Centers for Disease Control by James Sallis and Kevin Patrick and colleagues at San Diego State University and the University of California at San Diego in response to calls for more counseling for exercise by physicians. PACE employs a triage approach to assessment of activity history and readiness for physical activity, three brief structured counseling protocols, and training manuals (Pender et al, in press). PACE is patterned after both stage theory and relapse prevention models. At entry, clients are assessed as either precontemplative (not thinking about becoming active), contemplative (never exercised or relapsed, but thinking about becoming active), or currently active. Based on this screening, clients are triaged into the following counseling protocols:

- ''Getting out of your chair,'' when expected benefits are assessed along with planning strategies to overcome expected barriers.
- ''Planning the first step,'' when expected benefits are also reinforced and barriers addressed, but more expanded exercise plans based on FITT (Frequency, Intensity, Time, Type) principles (American College of Sports Medicine, 1990), location, time, and social support are made and an activity log is kept.
- ''Keeping the pace,'' when the existing or developed plan is reviewed after implementation for safety, effectiveness, enjoyability, and so forth, and reasons and solutions for relapse are explored.

PACE is now being evaluated for effectiveness in medical settings and it also offers a practical approach for face-to-face counseling by other exercise and health professionals. Similar but unstandardized approaches have been effective in community- mediated approaches (King et al., 1988; Owen, Lee, Naccarella, & Haag, 1987).

Summary

Determinants that reside or originate in the individual are practically important because they can identify population segments that may be responsive or resistive to physical activity interventions. Smoking, occupation, ethnicity, education, income, and obesity are examples of personal attributes that can present barriers to physical activity or be sentinel markers of underlying habits

Table 14.2 Media and Stages of Change

Influences	Behavioral objective	Attitudinal / belief objective
Precontemplation	–	Raise salience and relevance
(Mass media)	–	(High)
Contemplation	Intention to try	Increase personal relevance; decrease perceived inhibitors
(Mass media)	(High)	(Moderate)
Preparation	Actual trial	Reinforcement of reasons for trial; build self efficacy
(Mass media)	(Moderate)	(Moderate)
Action	Adoption of behavior	Reinforcement of reasons for adopting; motivational and efficacy support
(Mass media)	(Low)	(Low)
Maintenance	Maintaining new behavior	Reinforcement of reasons for adoption; increase salience of rewards for maintenance; reinforcement of self efficacy
(Mass media)	(Low)	(Low)

. Application of media intervention within the Transtheoretical Model's stages of change. The behavioral and/or attitudinal/belief objectives (columns two and three) of a media campaign differ and can be high, moderate, or low depending upon influences interacting with the person's stage of readiness for change (column 1). Adapted from Donovan and Owen (in press). Copyright Rod K. Dishman.

or circumstances that reinforce sedentary living. Too few studies are available on children, the elderly, the physically challenged, ethnic and minority groups, and on direct comparisons of men and women to permit conclusions about how determinants and successful interventions in these cases may differ from general observations. Reconstructing past activity history is important for interpreting past and present determinants, designing and evaluating plausible interventions, and for predicting future activity. However, currently there is no standardized method for assessing lifetime activity history. Attitudes, beliefs and expectancies, values, and intentions are amenable to change, but they alone do not predict behavior with sufficient accuracy for practical purposes. I am unaware of validated prediction equations that combine and weigh psychological variables for use in supervised settings. Similarly, personality traits, like our self-motivation scale (Dishman, Ickes, & Morgan, 1980), will not predict exercise behavior with sufficient accuracy for practical purposes, but personality traits may help explain why cognitive and attitudinal theories offer incomplete predictions of exercise (Ajzen, 1985). Exercise programs with strong social support or reinforcement conducted in settings requiring low-frequency, low-intensity activity may offset differences in personality that might otherwise predispose a person to inactivity (Wankel, Yardley, & Graham, 1985). Physical environment variables, such as access to facilities and programs, have not been widely studied but have the potential to be as practical as altering knowledge and attitudes. Also, environmental variables may be necessary adjuvants for implementing intentions into action.

Environmental interventions have usually involved the application of behavior modification principles to individuals or small groups. However, environmental interventions can include policy and facility planning at the national and community level, and educational-behavioral applications in schools, churches, health care, and recreational settings (Dishman & Sallis, in press; King et al., 1992). They also can include the planning and monitoring of the physical activity or exercise program. However, there are practical limitations with using environmental variables assessed by self-reports. For example, objectively measured access to facilities has been related to physical activity, but perceived access usually has not been related to physical activity.

Consistent with the theme of active living, modifying traditional fitness prescriptions, so that sedentary persons pursue moderate-intensity activities such as walking, climbing, and gardening in multiple (5 to 10) bouts of short duration (e.g., 5 to 10 minutes) daily, could reduce some currently perceived barriers to participation such as time and effort. Choices of types of activities and preferred levels of exertion could increase adherence. Because there are many errors in applying traditional

fitness prescriptions in practical application, these modifications might yield comparable fitness changes in the population. Some drawbacks of the active living approach are possible, however, if it were promoted to the exclusion of traditional fitness programming. Adherence rates are lower when the prescribed frequency of exercise increases (Pollock, 1988). Also, multiple episodes of various activities might increase the behavioral complexity of physical activity for individuals whose personality or schedules better fit traditional programming. So, the overall benefit of multiple daily, short-duration sessions over current recommendations (e.g., American College of Sports Medicine, 1990) must be evaluated. While we may come to see that health outcomes do not require much time and effort, other outcomes of exercise valued by many people, such as weight loss or maintenance and improved body image, may require more time and effort than implied by active living. The population prevalence of health-oriented and fitness-oriented goals, or their relative importance among population segments, is unknown and must be determined in order to effectively plan activities for increasing adoption and maintenance of physical activity and exercise.

The success of interventions probably depends on matching the appropriate attitudinal or behavioral approach to people according to their activity history and readiness for change. Stages in physical activity include planning, adoption, maintenance, and periodicity. Decision-based theories and interventions appear helpful for increasing planning and adoption. Integrating decision theories with social marketing strategies offers an important direction for future research and applications (Donovan & Owen, in press), particularly for increasing knowledge, attitudes, and intentions to adopt physical activity. Social support, self-motivation, self-regulatory skills, and interventions such as relapse prevention, including alternative fitness programming and exercise planning, are probably necessary to maintain or resume a physical activity pattern. The origin and time for intrinsic reinforcement of physical activity remain unknown, so persistent interventions at the personal and population level, including community, school, work site, and clinical settings, are required along with national policy initiatives.

References

Ajzen, I. (1985). From intentions to actions: A theory of planned behavior. In J. Kuhl & J. Beckman (Eds.), *Action-control: From cognition to behavior* (pp. 11-39). Heidelberg: Springer.

American College of Sports Medicine. (1990). Position statement on the recommended quality and quantity of exercise for developing and maintaining fitness in healthy adults. *Medicine and Science in Sports and Exercise*, **22**, 265-274.

American College of Sports Medicine. (1991). *Guidelines for exercise testing and prescription* (4th ed.). Philadelphia: Lea & Febiger.

American Council on Exercise. (1991). *Personal trainer manual* (pp. 359-372). San Diego: Author.

Andrew, G.M., Oldridge, N.B., Parker, J.O., Cunningham, D.A., Rechnitzer, P.A., Jones, N.L., Buck, C., Kavanagh, T., Shephard, R.J., Sutton, J.R., & McDonald, W. (1981). Reasons for dropout from exercise programs in post coronary patients. *Medicine and Science in Sports and Exercise*, **13**, 164-168.

Belisle, M., Roskies, E., & Levesque, J.M. (1987). Improving adherence to physical activity. *Health Psychology*, **6**, 159-172.

Blair, S.M., Kohl, H.W., Paffenbarger, R.S., Clark, D.G., Cooper, K.H., & Gibbons, L.W. (1989). Physical fitness and all-cause mortality: A prospective study of healthy men and women. *Journal of the American Medical Association*, **262**, 2395-2401.

Cohen, J. (1977). *Statistical power analysis for the behavioral sciences*. New York: Academic Press.

Danielson, R.R., & Wanzel, R.S. (1977). Exercise objectives of fitness program dropouts. In D.M. Landers & R.W. Christina (Eds.), *Psychology of motor behavior and sport* (pp. 310-320). Champaign, IL: Human Kinetics.

Dishman, R.K. (1981). Biologic influences on exercise adherence. *Research Quarterly for Exercise and Sport*, **52**, 143-159.

Dishman, R.K. (1982). Compliance/adherence in health-related exercise. *Health Psychology*, **1**, 237-267.

Dishman, R.K. (1987). Exercise adherence. In W.P. Morgan & S.N. Goldston (Eds.), *Exercise and mental health* (pp. 57-83). Washington, DC: Hemisphere.

Dishman, R.K. (1991). Increasing and maintaining exercise and physical activity. *Behavior Therapy*, **22**, 345-378.

Dishman, R.K., Ickes, W.J., & Morgan, W.P. (1980). Self-motivation and adherence to habitual physical activity. *Journal of Applied Social Psychology*, **10**, 115-131.

Dishman, R.K., & Sallis, J. (in press). Determinants and interventions for physical activity and exercise. In C. Bouchard, R.J. Shephard, & T. Stephens (Eds.). *Physical activity, fitness, and health: International proceedings and consensus statement*. Champaign, IL: Human Kinetics.

Donovan, R.J. & Owen, N. (in press). Social marketing and mass intervention. In R.K. Dishman (Ed.), *Exercise adherence II*. Champaign, IL: Human Kinetics.

Dzewaltowski, D.A., Noble, J.M., & Shaw, J.M. (1990). Physical activity participation: Social cognitive theory versus the theories of reasoned action and planned behavior. *Journal of Sport and Exercise Psychology*, **12**, 388-405.

Ewart, C.K., Taylor, C.B., Reese, L.B., & DeBusk, R.F. (1983). Effects of early post-myocardial infarction exercise testing on self-perception and subsequent physical activity. *American Journal of Cardiology*, **51**, 1076-1080.

Friedman, H. (1968). Magnitude of experimental effect and a taste for its rapid estimation. *Psychological Bulletin*, **70**, 245-251.

Gauvin, L. (1989). An experiential perspective on the motivational features of exercise and lifestyle. *Canadian Journal of Sport Sciences*, **15**(1), 51-61.

Godin, G. (in press). Social-cognitive models. In R.K. Dishman (Ed.), *Exercise adherence II*. Champaign, IL: Human Kinetics.

Godin, G., & Shephard, R.J. (1990). Use of attitude-behavior models in exercise promotion. *Sports Medicine*, **10**(2), 103-121.

Hoyt, M.F., & Janis, I.L. (1975). Increasing adherence to a stressful decision via a motivational balance-sheet procedure: A field experiment. *Journal of Personality and Social Psychology*, **31**, 833-839.

King, A.C., Blair, S.N., Bild, D., Dishman, R.K., Dubbert, P.M., Marcus, B.H., Oldridge, M., Paffenbarger, R.S., Powell, K.E., & Yeager, K. (1992). Determinants of physical activity and interventions in adults. *Medicine and Science in Sports and Exercise*, **26**(Suppl. 6), S221-S236.

King, A.L., & Frederiksen, L.W. (1984). Low-cost strategies for increasing exercise behavior: Relapse preparation training and support. *Behavior Modification*, **3**, 3-21.

King, A.C., Taylor, C.B., Haskell, W.L., & Debusk, R.F. (1988). Strategies for increasing early adherence to and long-term maintenance of home-based exercise training in healthy middle-aged men and women. *American Journal of Cardiology*, **61**, 628-632.

Knapp, D.N. (1988). Behavioral management techniques and exercise promotion. In R.K. Dishman (Ed.), *Exercise adherence: Its impact on public health* (pp. 203-236). Champaign, IL: Human Kinetics.

Marlatt, G.A. & Gordon, J. (1985). *Relapse prevention*. New York: Guilford Press.

Martin, J.E., Dubbert, P.M., Katell, A.D., Thompson, J.K., Raczynski, J.R., Lake, M., Smith, P.O., Webster, J.S., Sikova, T., & Cohen, R.E. (1984). The behavioral control of exercise in sedentary adults: Studies 1 through 6. *Journal of Consulting Clinical Psychology*, **52**, 795-811.

Oldridge, N.B. (1979). Compliance of past myocardial infarction patients from exercise programs. *Medicine and Science in Sports*, **11**, 373-375.

Owen, N., Lee, C., Naccarella, L., & Haag, K. (1987). Exercise by mail: A mediated behavior-change program for aerobic exercise. *Journal of Sport Psychology*, **9**, 346-357.

Pender, N.J., Sallis, J.F., Long, B.J., & Calfas, K.J. (in press). Health care provider counseling to promote physical activity. In R.K. Dishman (Ed.), *Exercise adherence II*, Champaign, IL: Human Kinetics.

Pollock, M.L. (1988). Prescribing exercise for fitness and adherence. In R.K. Dishman (Ed.), *Exercise adherence: Its impact on public health* (pp. 259-277). Champaign, IL: Human Kinetics.

Prochaska, J.O., & DiClemente, C.C. (1985). Common processes of self-change in smoking, weight control, and psychological distress. In S. Shiffman & T. Wills (Eds.), *Coping and substance use* (pp. 345-363). New York: Academic Press.

Prochaska, J.O., & Marcus, B.H. (in press). The transtheoretical model: The applications to exercise. In R.K. Dishman (Ed.), *Exercise adherence II*. Champaign, IL: Human Kinetics.

Rosenthal, R. (1984). *Meta-analytic procedures for social research*. Beverly Hills, CA: Sage Publications.

Rosenthal, R., & Rubin, D.B. (1984). A simple, general purpose display of magnitude of experimental effect. *Journal of Educational Psychology*, **74**, 166-169.

Sallis, J.F., Hovell, M.F., & Hofstetter, C.R. (1992). Predictors of adoption and maintenance of vigorous physical activity in men and women. *Preventive Medicine*, **21**, 237-251.

Sallis, J.F., Hovell, M.F., Hofstetter, C.R., Elder, J.P., Faucher, P., Spry, V.M., Barrington, E., & Hackley, M. (1990). Lifetime history of relapse from exercise. *Addictive Behaviors*, **15**, 573-579.

Sallis, J.F., Hovell, M.F., Hofstetter, C.R., Elder, J.P., Hackley, M., Caspersen, C.J., & Powell, K.E. (1990). Distance between homes and exercise facilities related to frequency of exercise among San Diego residents. *Public Health Reports*, **105**, 179-185.

Sanne, H.M. (1973). Exercise tolerance and physical training of non-selected patients after myocardial infarction. *Acta Medica Scandiniavica Supplement*, **551**, 1-124.

Wankel, L.M., & Thompson, C. (1977). Motivating people to be physically active: Self-persuasion vs. balanced decision-making. *Journal of Applied Social Psychology*, **7**, 332-340.

Wankel, L.M., Yardley, J.K., & Graham, J. (1985). The effects of motivational interventions upon the exercise adherence of high and low self-motivated adults. *Canadian Journal of Applied Sport Sciences*, **10**, 147-156.

15

A Framework for Enhancing Exercise Motivation in Rehabilitative Medicine

W. Jack Rejeski
Michele Hobson

The problems with keeping clients or patients involved in formal primary prevention and rehabilitation exercise programs are well documented. One review by Dishman (1982) indicated that roughly 50% of those who initiate exercise therapy will drop out within 6 months. In response to this challenge, a number of psychologists have encouraged the use of well established clinical methods that evolved from behaviorism and cognitive science (e.g., Martin & Dubbert, 1984); a recommendation that is receiving growing empirical support (Dishman, 1991). Unfortunately, as is true of all behavioral problems, there is rarely a single best solution. Although there is wisdom in proposing interventions that include a variety of treatment options, we have found that students, exercise leaders, and program directors are frequently confused when it comes to incorporating diverse methods into practice. In fact, the dilemma of putting ideas into action was the impetus to a book which we published on fitness motivation (Rejeski & Kenney, 1988).

The purpose of the present chapter is to extend many of the ideas originally proposed by Rejeski and Kenny (1988). As a focus, we drew upon a decade of clinical experience in cardiac rehabilitation coupled with a clinical trial that was designed to examine the efficacy of exercise in treating osteoarthritis of the knee. Furthermore, the material is organized within a single conceptual model. Hopefully this framework will prove useful to others in behavioral medicine who choose to use exercise therapy as a mode of treatment.

Understanding and Intervening With Patients in Rehabilitative Exercise Programs

Chronic diseases capture the attention of their victims. This belief is based on interviews with more than 1,000 patients in cardiac rehabilitation, and on theoretical propositions that argue for perceived vulnerability as a principal motive underlying health behaviors (see Rejeski, 1992). It seems almost irrational to health professionals that people with physical dysfunction, a direct or indirect consequence of many chronic diseases, choose not to comply with exercise therapy that ostensibly will improve their quality of life. Yet, those who have hands-on experience with patients in exercise therapy know motivational problems are rampant. Why is this so? Do patients simply fail to see the connection between lack of physical activity and dysfunction, or is the problem more complex?

In developing a proactive protocol for dealing with motivational issues, we adopted a model of stress that helps us understand how people deal with the challenges and threats that occur in a physically active lifestyle (Lazarus & Launier, 1978; Rejeski, Morley, & Sotile, 1985). Such an approach is useful in understanding how and why specific intervention strategies are effective. Viewed in this manner, exercise is a potential stressor (it creates objective demands), that is, a source of harm/loss or threat/challenge that causes people to think, feel, and behave in ways that can be either productive or counterproductive (see Figure 15.1).

The critical feature of the model depicted in Figure 15.1 is appraisal. In other words, it is patients' perceptions of the demands accompanying exercise that determine their coping responses. We should add that exercise has positive consequences as well. In this respect, it deviates from negative stressors such as natural catastrophes or disease. The model also proposes that coping behavior creates a feedback loop and returns to the objective demands of physical activity. Constructive coping decreases the perceived demands of subsequent exercise behavior, whereas destructive coping increases the intensity of perceived demands. Each stage of the

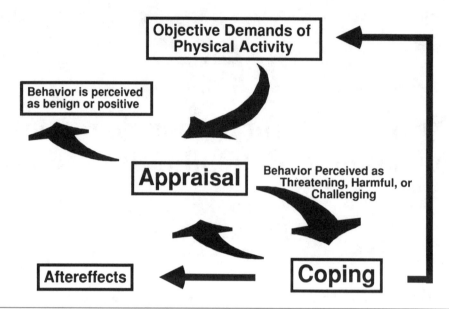

Figure 15.1 A model of stress (adapted from Lazarus & Launier, 1978).

model is discussed in greater detail in the following sections.

Objective Demands of Exercise

In order to understand how people respond to exercise therapy, it is useful to examine the demands it places on the individual. After all, the decision to approach or avoid any behavior is strongly influenced by associated costs.

A specific example could be the situation faced by elderly patients with osteoarthritis of the knee. Although these individuals confront many of the same demands with formal exercise programs as any healthy person, they are further burdened by disease-related complications. Assessing environmental, social, and personal costs is a useful way to categorize potential problems. Examples of environmental issues include the location of programs, the availability of parking, and the aesthetic features of exercise facilities. A social cost may occur if friends or spouses disapprove of a patient's involvement in exercise therapy. For example, a husband who can't understand why his wife goes all the way to the university just for a walking program. In other instances, spouses may express outright disapproval of their husbands' or wives' involvement in exercise therapy. They may ask their spouses, ''Why would you want to do something that causes pain, the very symptom you are trying to alleviate?'' Finally, examples of personal costs associated with formal exercise programs could be that the time needed for weight training or aerobic conditioning replaces valued activities at work or home, the exercise training may be boring, or the patient is forced to deal with significant discomfort.

Appraisal

As the history of cognitive psychology has shown, reality is in eye of the beholder (Neisser, 1976). Although

we certainly do not want to dismiss the objective demands inherent in exercise programs, ultimately it is an individual's construction of reality that determines any sense of threat, challenge, or loss/harm experienced. For example, research (Rejeski & Sanford, 1984) shows that it is possible to manipulate women's feelings about an exercise session so that anticipated distress leads to higher ratings of perceived exertion while performing the activity. Conversely, research also shows that teaching young women how to manage exercise discomfort is effective in enhancing positive feelings experienced during training (Kenney, Rejeski, & Messier, 1987).

Richard Lazarus (Lazarus & Folkman, 1984) has been central in showing how cognitive appraisals may influence the perceptions of various demands that accompany exercise. He proposed that there are two facets of appraisal: *primary* and *secondary*. Lazarus (1991) used primary appraisal to capture ''the stakes one has in the outcomes of an encounter'' (p. 827), whereas he used secondary appraisal to describe the perceived coping skills people have at their disposal. He also emphasized that cognitive appraisals of formal exercise programs in rehabilitative medicine change as people acquire experience with behavior and as they are forced to deal with additional demands. This component of Lazarus's model is similar to the stages of exercise discussed in Rod Dishman's and Leonard Wankel and Carol Hills's chapters (chapters 14 and 16, respectively); however, the emphasis by Lazarus is on individual perception.

Primary Appraisal

From theory and clinical experience, we have identified three major factors that influence primary appraisal in rehabilitative exercise settings.

1. The level of threat posed by disease, and the meaning (cost or benefit) associated with the various demands of exercise

2. The degree of uncertainty that accompanies exercise behavior
3. The emotional state of the patient

Meaning. Some of the most powerful determinants of patients' reactions to the demands of exercise are the perceived consequences of their disease, the value or significance of these consequences to their lives, and the meaning (cost or benefit) ascribed to the various demands of exercise (Rejeski & Kenney, 1988). This conclusion is based on several areas of research in psychology (e.g., the Health Belief Model, Becker, 1974; Social Learning Theory, Rotter, Chance, & Phares, 1972; The Theory of Reasoned Action, Fishbein & Ajzen, 1975) coupled with observations made in clinical exercise settings. For example, a recent middle-aged patient in our cardiac rehabilitation program was overwhelmed by the reduction of his physical function after by-pass surgery. He felt emasculated and vulnerable; feelings that were intensified by an ego rooted in his physical self. Although the discomfort and anxiety that accompanied vigorous physical rehabilitation were substantial, this patient approached the rehabilitative process with an aggressive attitude. His one goal in mind was to recapture his former body image.

However, people are not always rational decision makers. Janis (1984) points out that when patients perceive serious hardships in either changing or not changing their behavior, it places them in a position of conflict. This conflict can cause patients to deny the disease, to pretend that things aren't as bad as they appear, or to procrastinate. Furthermore, when the perceived costs of exercise outweigh the perceived benefits, people are prone to self-construct barriers (Rejeski, 1992). For example, patients will say that they aren't able to "steal" time from work or are unwilling to inconvenience their spouse. Although investigators in exercise science often interpret these responses as barriers, they are probably best viewed as symptoms of low commitment.

Uncertainties of physical symptoms and exercise behavior. There is little doubt that patients with cardiovascular disease or osteoarthritis of the knee will be unusually sensitive to the sensory feedback of exercise. In fact, as a general rule all patient populations have a heightened awareness of physical symptoms (Pennebaker, 1982), which makes sense when considering the role of symptom recognition as a means for survival. However, the uncertainty surrounding the significance of these physical symptoms can be responsible for dysfunctional thinking. For example, we have seen osteoarthritis patients who interpret muscular soreness and mild joint discomfort as evidence that exercise is causing the disease to spread to other joints. Obviously this conclusion, and others like it, is a deterrent to motivation and must be corrected immediately. Research has shown that some people are prone to interpret events or symptoms negatively (Peterson & Bossio, 1991); a characteristic that probably has both a biological and an experiential basis. In other words, people do not enter exercise programs with blank slates. Thus, practitioners are forced to deal with both the individual's past and present experiences.

In addition to the uncertainty of sensory cues, patients with osteoarthritis are also likely to question whether the exercise therapy will really make a difference. Motivation is weakened if people question the contingencies between their exercise behavior and desired outcomes (McAuley, 1992). Although not formally studied in exercise psychology, there is evidence that people with pessimistic explanatory styles are particularly prone to failure in environments that require persistence and effort (Peterson & Bossio, 1991). As indicated previously, some patients' cognitive styles place them at high risk for exercise drop out.

Emotional states. The patient's emotional state can also play a significant role in appraising the demands of exercise therapy. This is particularly relevant in rehabilitative medicine where sensory cues associated with exercise may be confused with disease-related symptoms. We consistently find, from both clinical interviews and psychometric testing, that patients with clinical levels of depression, anxiety, or neuroticism (i.e., negative feelings that fluctuate from anxiety, to depression, to anger, to feelings of vulnerability, and so forth) are more threatened by the demands and uncertainties they experience with exercise therapy than other patients. In fact, in other areas of health psychology, it is well recognized that neurotic patients are prone to interpret normal physical cues as a sign that "something is wrong" (Costa & McCrae, 1985). Furthermore, although negative emotional states are counterproductive, there is some evidence that positive emotional states can actually enhance people's perceptions of exercise (Kenney et al., 1987).

Secondary Appraisal

Although the initial appraisal process is extremely important to subsequent behavior, an equally important element is secondary appraisal; that is, the perceived availability of resources a person has in order to cope with either anticipated or actual demands. A core construct in psychology that is useful in understanding and investigating this process is self-efficacy, or the degree of confidence that a person has with respect to being able to perform a given behavior (Bandura, 1977). As the individual's perception of available resources or skills improves, so does the effort, persistence, and performance of various exercise behaviors (McAuley, 1992). In fact, Bandura (1991) has presented convincing evidence " . . . that much of the stress reductive effects of behavioral control stem anticipatorily from perceived capability to wield control over troublesome events rather than simply from attenuating aversive events" (p 238). However, efficacy beliefs are highly specific to the context, time, and requirements for a given behavior. Thus, exercise leaders may increase elderly patients' self-efficacy toward exercise behavior in a structured setting without increasing their self-efficacy toward exercising at home or performing other simple activities of daily living. When structuring formal interventions, this point must be considered.

Finally, patients will differ in the amount of time they need to develop efficacy beliefs. People progress at varying rates, and some are particularly reactive to minor setbacks. My experiences in cardiac rehabilitation suggest that it takes a substantial amount of time to enhance self-confidence toward exercise behavior. There are patients, who after their initial treadmill test, experience renewed confidence in their physical competencies (cf. Bandura, 1991). Yet, with other individuals it has taken anywhere from 2 to 6 months to see comparable gains in perceived behavioral control. The implication for research and clinical practice is that psychological interventions may fail simply because the dose of therapy is inadequate. Antidepressant medications are a good analagy. Someone naive to the treatment of depression with Pamelor would be disheartened by the results of the drug in the first week or two of its administration. The fact remains, however, that it can take 2 or more months before the maximum results are realized. Dosage has never been addressed in the treatment of exercise motivation with cognitive-behavioral therapy.

Coping Behavior

As seen in Figure 15.1, once the demands of physical activity are perceived as threatening, harmful, or challenging, patients initiate acts of coping. The range of responses is likely to be varied. For example, faced with pain or anxiety one patient may quit exercise training, whereas another may seek information or alternative modes of therapy (e.g., swimming as opposed to walking). Although coping frequently involves overt behavior, it also includes cognition, emotion, and even physiological arousal. Examples of cognitive coping include self-statements of defeat or determination. In a similar manner, emotional responses can be both negative and positive; that is, threats can create anger, and anxiety, or they can create pride and enthusiasm.

The important issue here is that coping can be destructive and constructive. Whereas constructive acts of coping can alleviate the adverse effects of objective demands, destructive forms of coping accelerate the level of threat accompanying a given objective demand.

A final proposition of the model is aftereffects. That is, the manner in which patients cope with the perceived demands of physical activity in specific rehabilitative contexts has meaning for long-term psychological and behavioral outcomes. For instance, when designing an exercise program it is tempting to optimize the magnitude of the treatment with the use of highly structured, vigorous activity. This may be tolerated in the short-term; however, there is some evidence with youth weight-loss programs that subjects are unwilling to persist at high levels for extended periods of time (Epstein, Wing, Koeske, Ossip, & Beck, 1982). In the investiga-

tion by Epstein and his colleagues, subjects elected to terminate structured exercise rather than lower the dose of activity.

Implications for Intervention

Existing approaches to exercise prescription rely almost exclusively on physiological criteria. For example, an exercise stimulus of 60% to 90% of heart rate reserve is a recommended target for enhanced aerobic fitness (Montoye, Christian, Nagle, & Levin, 1988). Although this may be ideal for cardiovascular benefits, it makes absolutely no sense when the exercise demand discourages people. Furthermore, as our previous discussion has shown, exercise prescription requires we consider other motivational issues such as social barriers and efficacy beliefs. Motivations are as important for the design of successful exercise therapy as the physical stimulus itself.

The model presented in this chapter provides a useful framework for developing a comprehensive, motivational plan for exercise prescription, particularly in the realm of behavioral medicine. In simple terms, there are four areas for consideration.

1. It is advisable to remove as many external barriers as possible and to reduce other negative, objective demands that may be associated with exercise.
2. It is patients' construction of reality and not our own appraisals that determine their attraction to or avoidance of exercise. When the stakes are too high or when there is no perceived benefit from exercise therapy, problems are likely to occur.
3. Patients' effort, persistence, and performance will be optimal when they believe that they possess the actual skills and/or have access to resources for dealing with perceived demands.
4. We must remember that the patients' physical condition and perceptions are dynamic and subject to constant change. There is no substitute for routine interpersonal contact and adjusting physiological prescriptions when required.

There are a number of behavioral and cognitive methods available to help design a proactive motivation plan. Also, these same techniques can be useful in treating specific problems that arise during the course of conducting a clinical trial or during day-to-day operations of a fitness facility. In the final sections of this chapter, we offer some specific examples of how a proactive motivation plan might be implemented.

Attacking Objective Demands

One strategy to motivate patients to exercise is to target environmental or social barriers and to decrease the possible personal costs, for example, joint discomfort. This might include

- providing transportation when needed,
- arranging valet parking for those who drive themselves, and
- giving careful consideration to the development of a training facility that meets the needs of the elderly.

The importance of these factors to the motivation of patients was identified in some of the earliest research on exercise compliance (e.g., Andrew & Parker, 1979).

A critical element for success is the social support or feedback that patients receive (Wankel, 1984). Thus, one strategy would be to educate spouses about the purpose and anticipated consequences of exercise therapy. Additionally, routine contact with spouses can be helpful to

- discuss progress being made,
- evaluate the attitudes and support provided by spouses, and
- give examples of or reinforce constructive interactions.

In our caridac rehabilitation program, spouses are given the opportunity to participate in the exercise therapy with their husband or wife. This has proven to be a very attactive option for some patients, and preliminary data suggest that this "team" approach has some significant benefits in terms of enhancing the quality of the rehabilitative process. Taylor, Bandura, Ewart, Miller, and Debusk (1983) conducted an interesting study in which wives went through physical stress testing with their husbands. Exposure to the graded exercise test had a clinically significant effect on enhancing the wives' perceptions of their husbands' capabilities. This is an important finding given that reactions to and recovery from chronic disease are intricately tied to the family system.

Finally, to reduce the physical demands, exercise prescriptions should be individually tailored based on electrocardiographic abnormalities and self-ratings of effort and distress. The goal should be to shape desired exercise behavior by successive approximation (sequential goals that begin at very low levels) rather than rigid external criteria (Martin & Dubbert, 1984). We encourage routinely monitoring the patient's enjoyment during exercise training, as well as levels of pain and perceived exertion. Also, it is helpful to provide visual reminders (e.g., cartoon posters) in the exercise facility that underscore the importance of gradual improvement, and the dangers of overdosing exercise therapy.

Appraisal Processes

A second line of defense concerns both primary and secondary appraisal processes. Specific objectives, derived from Figure 15.1, can be grouped into two broad categories. First, to increase the benefits and decrease the costs of exercise. Second, to instill behavioral control over the demands patients are likely to confront during their therapy.

In the early phases of center-based programs, these objectives can be achieved through interactions with personal trainers (PTs) and peers. For example, we use a procedure built around two key contacts. The first contact occurs when patients initially visit the exercise facility and meet with a PT. The second interaction occurs approximately 1 week later when patients exercise with a peer who is a seasoned veteran. During the initial exercise therapy session with the PT, there are a number of planned, semi-structured interactions. These include the following:

- The PT describes the overall exercise therapy plan and emphasizes the importance of gradual progress. Patients are encouraged to become actively involved in tailoring their exercise prescription to a tolerable level. The PT also asks each patient to list what they view as the positive and negative aspects of the program; a strategy that is similar to the decision balance sheet studied by Wankel and Thompson (1977). The purpose of acquiring this information is so valued outcomes can be converted into specific goals that are shared with each patient in the later half of the second week, and so patients have several ideas how to decrease or eliminate negative outcomes.
- During the exercise therapy, the PT educates patients about the benefits they might expect. This creates an opportunity to reinforce and broaden the positive outcomes identified by each patient. Patients are also told about the negative consequences of avoiding systematic physical activity.
- At the conclusion of the session, the PT describes some of the physical symptoms patients are apt to experience during the early stages of exercise training. Patients are also informed about the importance of following-up on any questions or concerns they may have and are given specific instructions on how to handle problems that may arise (e.g., for osteoarthritis patients you would have a specific medical procedure established to handle periodic episodes of acute inflammation).

The second interaction occurs during week 2 and involves exercising with an experienced peer. The peer tutor is trained to provide specific information that is consistent with the published work of Ajzen (1985); Belisle, Roskies, and Levesque (1987); and Wankel (1984). The peer should reinforce with the patient:

- the importance of patient interaction and fostering a group identity (monthly socials could be used to enhance relationships that are initiated in the exercise therapy sessions),

- the value of sticking with the program despite minor setbacks and the availability of support if problems do occur,
- the temporary nature of most aches and pains,
- the misconceptions of myths associated with exercise therapy,
- the solutions for anticipated barriers, and
- the benefits that they and other patients have experienced.

These early contacts are reinforced by periodic interactions from both the PT and the peers throughout the first 3 months of the program. The specific goals of each patient are reinforced and re-evaluated at 1 month intervals. Furthermore, newsletters can highlight unique achievements, and monthly lists can be posted in the exercise facility to acknowledge outstanding attendance rates.

If you are working with patients in home-based programs, we advise the PT conduct home visits to help patients organize and maintain an exercise program at their house. Additionally, it is very helpful to phone the patient biweekly. In phone conversations, PTs discuss patient progress and offer support and guidance for relapse prevention (King, Taylor, Haskell, & Debusk, 1988).

Summary

This chapter describes a model that can be used to understand exercise motivation and provides some specific examples of how a structured motivational plan can be implemented in a rehabilitative exercise setting. There are a number of different strategies that can be used in designing an exercise intervention program (Rejeski & Kenney, 1988). Our approach is to implement the strategies before an individual starts a program, as opposed to restricting treatment to patients who are struggling to maintain prescribed behavior. It is our belief that exercise prescriptions should be made on psychosocial as well as physiological considerations.

References

Ajzen, I. (1985). From intentions to actions: A theory of planned behavior. In J. Kuhl & J. Beckman (Eds.), *Action-control: From cognition to behavior* (pp. 11-39). Heidelberg: Springer.

Andrew, G.M., & Parker, J.O. (1979). Factors related to dropout of post-myocaridal infarction patients from exercise programs. *Medicine and Science in Sports and Exercise, 11*, 376-378.

Bandura, A. (1977). Self-efficacy: Toward a unifying theory of behavioral change. *Psychological Review, 84*, 191-215.

Bandura, A. (1991). Self-efficacy mechanism in physiological activation and health-promoting behavior. In J. Madden IV (Ed.), *Neurobiology of learning, emotion, and affect*. New York: Raven Press.

Becker, M.H. (Ed.) (1974). The health belief model and personal health behavior. *Health Education Monograph, 2*.

Belisle, M., Roskies, E., & Levesque, J.M. (1987). Improving adherence to physical activity. *Health Psychology, 6*, 158-172.

Costa, P.T., & McCrae, R.R. (1985). Hypochondriasis, neuroticism, and aging. *American Psychologist, 40*, 19-28.

Dishman, R.K. (1982). Compliance/adherence in health-related exercise. *Health Psychology, 1*, 237-267.

Dishman, R.K. (1991). Increasing and maintaining exercise and physical activity. *Behavior Therapy, 22*, 345-378.

Epstein, L.H., Wing, R.R., Koeske, R., Ossip, D., & Beck, S.A. (1982). Comparison of lifestyle change and programmed aerobic exercise on weight and fitness changes in children. *Behavior Therapy, 13*, 651-665.

Fishbein, M., & Ajzen, I. (1975). *Beliefs, attitude, intention, and behavior: An introduction to theory and research*. Reading, MA: Addison-Wesley.

Janis, I.L. (1984). The patient as a decision maker. In W.D. Gentry (Ed.), *Handbook of behavioral medicine*. New York: Guilford.

Kenney, E.A., Rejeski, W.J., & Messier, S. (1987). Managing exercise distress: The effect of broad spectrum intervention on affect, RPE, and running efficiency. *Canadian Journal of Sport Science, 12*, 97-105.

King, A.C., Taylor, C.B., Haskell, W.L., & Debusk, R.F. (1988). Strategies for increasing early adherence to and long-term maintenance of home-based exercise training in healthy middle-aged men and women. *American Journal of Cardiology, 61*, 628-632.

Lazarus, R.S. (1991). Progress on a cognitive-motivational-relational theory of emotion. *American Psychologist, 46*, 819-834.

Lazarus, R.S., & Folkman, S. (1984). *Stress, appraisal, and coping*. New York: Springer.

Lazarus, R.S., & Launier, R. (1978). Stress-related transactions between person and environment. In L.A. Pervin & M. Lewis (Eds.), *Perspectives in interactional psychology* (pp. 287-327). New York: Plenum.

Martin, J.E., & Dubbert, P.M. (1984). Behavioral management strategies for improving health and fitness. *Journal of Cardiac Rehabilitation, 4*, 200-208.

McAuley, E. (1992). Understanding exercise behavior: A self-efficacy perspective. In G.C. Roberts (Ed.),

Understanding motivation in sport and exercise (pp. 107-127). Champaign, IL: Human Kinetics.

Montoye, H.J., Christian, J.L., Nagle, F.J., & Levin, S.M. (1988). *Living fit*. Menlo Park, CA: Benjamin/Cummings Publishing Co.

Neisser, U. (1976). *Cognition and reality: Principles and implications of cognitive psychology*. New York: W. H. Freeman.

Pennebaker, J.W. (1982). *The psychology of physical symptoms*. New York: Springer-Verlag.

Peterson, C., & Bossio, L.M. (1991). *Health and optimism*. New York: The Free Press.

Rejeski, W.J. (1985). Perceived exertion: An active or passive process? *Journal of Sport Psychology, 7*, 371-378.

Rejeski, W.J. (1992). Motivation for exercise behavior: A critique of theoretical directions. In G.C. Roberts (Ed.), *Understanding motivation in sport and exercise* (pp. 129-157). Champaign, IL: Human Kinetics.

Rejeski, W.J., & Kenney, E.A. (1988). *Fitness motivation: Preventing participant dropout*. Champaign, IL: Human Kinetics.

Rejeski, W.J., & Sanford, B. (1984). Feminine-typed females: The role of affective schema in the perception of exercise intensity. *Journal of Sport Psychology, 6*, 197-207.

Rotter, J.B., Chance, J.E., & Phares, E.J. (1972). *Applications of a social learning theory of personality*. New York: Holt Rinehart & Winston.

Taylor, C.B., Bandura, A., Ewart, C.K., Miller, N.H, & Debusk, R.F. (1983). Exercise testing to enhance wives' confidence in their husbands' cardiac capabilities soon after uncomplicated acute myocardial infarction. *American Journal of Cardiology, 55*, 635-638.

Wankel, L.M. (1984). Decision-making and social support strategies for increasing exercise involvement. *Journal of Cardiac Rehabilitation, 4*, 124-135.

Wankel, L.M., & Thompson, C. (1977). Motivating people to be physically active: Self-persuasion vs. balanced decision making. *Applied Social Psychology, 7*, 332-340.

16

A Social Marketing and Stage of Change Perspective of Interventions to Enhance Physical Activity: The Importance of PRs

Leonard M. Wankel

Carol Hills

Recent research has clearly indicated that regular physical activity can contribute positively to physiological and psychological health (Bouchard, Shephard, Stephens, Sutton, & McPherson, 1990). At the same time, surveys show a large portion of the general population in most developed countries is not active enough to obtain many of the potential health benefits (Bauman, 1987; Stephens & Craig, 1990; Stephens, Jacobs, & White, 1985; Wankel, 1988). Of those individuals who do initiate activity programs, 50% or more do not maintain regular involvement (Dishman, 1987, 1990a; Sallis & Hovell, 1990). These observations stress the importance of understanding how interventions might help regular activity involvement.

A number of reviews of physical activity interventions are available. Martin and Dubbert (1984, 1985) and Taylor and Owen (1989) have reviewed behavioral-medicine approaches in largely clinical populations. Dishman (1987, 1990a, 1991; Dishman, Sallis, & Orenstein, 1985) and Wankel (1987, 1988) have reviewed determinants or interventions in different contexts. Promotional or educational approaches to fostering activity in the general population, or in specific communities or specific workplace contexts have been reviewed by Cox (1984), Dishman (1990b), Godin and Shephard (1983), and Iverson, Fielding, Crow, and Christenson (1985). An examination of these reviews, together with more recent research published in the area, leads to the conclusion that a variety of different interventions (e.g., behavior prompting, goal-setting, self-control training, relapse prevention counseling, as well as positive reinforcement and the decision balance-sheet) can increase physical activity involvement. No one intervention has

been found to be consistently superior to others, nor has one intervention, or combination of interventions, been effective for all individuals. Prochaska and associates (Prochaska & DiClemente, 1983, 1984; Prochaska & Marcus, in press) have argued that an intervention's effectiveness depends on its appropriateness for the client group or individual. They developed a behavior change model that targets the appropriate process of change to the client's stage of change. This is parallel to marketing a product where product development and promotion is targeted to a specific market segment. In each case, behavior change is viewed as an ongoing, dynamic process.

We advocate such a process-oriented approach to interventions for helping physical activity involvement. In this chapter, we combine basic concepts from social marketing with the behavior change stages discussed in Prochaska and associates' transtheoretical model of behavior change (Prochaska & DiClemente, 1984; Prochaska & Marcus, in press), to provide a two-dimensional framework for considering interventions. The four Ps of the market mix (product, place, price, and promotion) are combined with Prochaska and Marcus's (in press) five R's of the activity involvement process (resistance, recruitment, retention, relapse, and recovery) to form a PR matrix for physical activity promotion.

A Marketing Approach

A marketing approach to service delivery implies the philosophy that products or services are developed to satisfy consumer needs or wants. It is essential to research the needs of pertinent market groups so appropriate products or services can be developed and provided. In contrast, a product-based selling approach is where an agency develops a product that is considered desirable and then attempts to sell it to various potential client groups. Of central importance in following any marketing approach are the four Ps of the market mix—product, place, price, and promotion. These four factors symbolize critical considerations for developing appropriate products and making them available and attractive to potential customers.

Product

The first step is to analyze the product to be marketed. In the era of fitness promotion, the product was clearly better health gained through exercise. A selling approach was adopted that prescribed a particular type of exercise (e.g., that recommended by the American College of Sports Medicine, 1978) for a certain type of outcome, for example, aerobic fitness. An attempt was made to sell this "desirable product" to the general population, but as indicated by activity and fitness trends over the years, only a minority of the population "bought into this product." Furthermore, the sedentary population, who would most benefit from an increase in activity level, were least affected by such campaigns.

Segment-specific market research is fundamental to successfully marketing physical activity to hard-to-reach market groups. It is necessary to decide what concepts are marketable. It may be that exercise, fitness, and health are hard to sell, whereas physical activity, active living, enjoyment, lifestyle, and quality of life are more readily accepted. The more accepted concepts have the potential to cater to broader needs and may have a greater appeal. Attitudinal research on "physical activity" indicates that this concept has multiple meanings to different individuals and groups (Kenyon, 1968). Moreover, research in both Australia and Canada has shown that the concept of "physical activity" has more positive public acceptance than does "exercise" (Becker, 1977; Nielson, Borsdorf, & Corbin, 1987). Although for simplicity it is desirable to have a uniform product that can easily be recognized across the whole population, this is unrealistic from a product acceptance perspective. For widespread success, it is likely that specific products will have to be identified, developed, and targeted at specific population segments. For example, it is necessary to provide a diverse array of physical activity products all congruent with an active, high quality lifestyle. This does not mean that the products, the actual activities themselves, must differ markedly. Rather, it is the needs or interests the activities address that differ. Therefore, it is the presentation of the activity that is important. The same activities can have many different meanings and functions. Once the

nature of the product is clear, then steps can be taken to market the product in terms of place, price, and promotion.

Place

A well researched and perfectly designed product will not receive widespread acceptance unless it is made available to the target population groups. Availability, or distribution of opportunities to participate, is a key. Leisure surveys consistently indicate that although television viewing is one of the most pervasive leisure activities, satisfaction ratings are much lower for it than for less popular activities. Much leisure activity is of a habitual nature, simply reflecting accessibility and convenience factors. This should be considered in attempting to promote widespread physical activity involvement. Research has identified the importance of geographical location and time constraints to physical activity participation (Dishman et al., 1985; Stephens & Craig, 1990). However, although some activities are readily accessible, they may not be as appealing as more facility-demanding activities. Walking may not have the same appeal as tennis or basketball for many individuals. Facility and program schedulers must consider how their plans affect the opportunities of different market groups.

Physical activity through regular daily living is more available both in terms of location and time than segmented leisure time exercise workouts. For example, walking or cycling as routine forms of transportation are readily accessible activities. Further, such environmentally friendly activities contribute to not only individual healthy lifestyles but also environmental well-being. Urban planners should place a priority on how their plans for city development can influence active and healthy living.

Price

The price placed on a product influences its popularity. Although expensive activities (e.g., alpine skiing, sailing, or golf) restrict the participation of lower economic groups, it doesn't follow that the lowest price is always the best one for promoting involvement in an activity. The optimal price, in terms of making an activity attractive, varies from one group to another. Psychological considerations and market research is required when setting the price for a product (Crompton, 1981, 1982). It is a serious mistake to spend considerable time and expense to develop a top-notch program or product and then simply attach an arbitrary price to it.

Promotion

Promotion entails all the efforts made to inform potential consumers about the positive attributes of the products and services, and to indicate how an individual could participate in them. A key component of a marketing approach is gearing the message about the product and its purpose to the needs of the individual or market segment. Different general promotion messages as well as specific audience messages may be used. The work of Prochaska and associates (Prochaska & DiClemente, 1983; Prochaska & Marcus, in press) provides valuable information concerning the stages that individuals go through in making health-related behavior changes. This stage approach can provide useful information for altering the market mix to effectively meet the changing needs of a specific population's particular segment. Different information is required depending upon which stage an individual is at in shifting from a sedentary to an active lifestyle.

In their transtheoretical model of behavior change, Prochaska and DiClemente (1984) describe six stages of change: precontemplation, contemplative, preparation, action, maintenance, and termination. Precontemplation refers to a preliminary stage wherein individuals do not intend to change their behavior in the foreseeable future. In the contemplation stage, individuals are seriously considering changing their behavior within the next 6 months, but have not yet made a commitment. Individuals at the preparation stage intend to take action in the near future, usually within 1 month. They typically have developed a plan of action and may have taken some action to initiate the desired activity but not yet at the desired level. The action stage occurs when individuals have initiated the desired change, at the specified criterion level, within the past 6 months. When the desired behavior change has been maintained longer than 6 months the maintenance stage is reached. This lasts until termination, when there is no longer any danger of relapse to the undesirable behavior. With respect to changing from a sedentary to an active lifestyle, however, it is questionable whether a true termination point is ever reached.

The PRs Approach to Facilitating Physical Activity

Stages are conceived as the midway point between stable traits and transient states; they are considered to be stable but still open to change. Prochaska and Marcus (in press) reformulated the six stage model in terms of five Rs for physical activity involvement: resistance, recruitment, retention, relapse, and recovery. A notable feature of the model is that any given attempt to change a lifestyle behavior is not a simple dichotomous success or failure situation. Rather, an individual typically passes through the successive stages. Prochaska and Marcus observe that commonly, five or six attempts are required before a relatively stable condition of successful change is reached. Further, they suggest that the

change process may be even more dynamic for the adoption of physical activity than has been observed in their research on smoking.

Combining the 4 Ps of marketing with the 5 Rs of the behavior change process provides a 4 × 5 matrix for considering interventions that foster increased physical activity (see Figure 16.1). We will use this matrix to discuss approaches that facilitate active living. This will be done by considering the successive stages of change.

Resistance and Recruitment

Thirty-two percent of the sedentary people surveyed in the 1981 Canada Fitness Survey (Fitness and Amateur Sport Canada, 1983) indicated that nothing would influence them to be more active. This has led some observers to say that resources should not be wasted on convincing this hard-to-reach group to be active. Such a conclusion, however, probably reflects a selling philosophy. A differentiated product approach may be more successful in assisting these individuals to be active.

Most attempts to promote physical activity have used a general media or educational approach. Although these approaches have not been subjected to extensive systematic study, in general the results have been unimpressive. Such promotional campaigns as *ParticipACTION* in Canada and *Life Be In It* in Australia have succeeded in increasing awareness; however, there is little evidence they created significant behavior change (Donavon & Owen, in press; Wankel, 1988).

In large part these promotion campaigns have focused on the general desirability and availability of activity. However, the PR matrix suggests greater precision is required to find what physical activity product interests resisters. Data from the Campbell Survey of the Well-Being of Canadians (Stephens & Craig, 1990) shows

R Stage of the Process of Involvement	P (Market-Mix Variable)			
	Product	Place	Price	Promotion
Resistance (pre-contemplation)				
Recruitment (pre-contemplation)				
Retention (contemplation; preparation)				
Retention (action; maintenance)				
Relapse				
Recovery				

Figure 16.1 The PR matrix for interventions to facilitate physical activity involvement.

there may be identifiable subgroups within the overall group. Different activity groups reported different leisure time goals. Those who were inactive (i.e., resisters and lapsers) scored higher than active people (adherers) on leisure goals—relaxing and socializing. Inactive people scored lower on such goals as feeling better mentally, feeling better physically, getting outdoors, and improving fitness. In assessing how much involvement in physical activity would contribute to these goals, inactive respondents scored lower than active respondents on relaxing, but they scored the same on socializing. This may indicate that for the resisters in general, the physical activity product that might be most effectively promoted would initially promote socializing and would not be overly demanding (e.g., relaxation). A larger proportion of the inactive respondents, in contrast to the active respondents, indicated that a number of such internal factors as perceived energy, ability, and self-discipline. Financial cost was not a particular deterrent for the inactive group, but lack of a partner was. The national survey data suggests certain approaches to resisters, but more in-depth market research is required to develop specific guidelines for this market group. Local agency-specific information based on the client group is likely to be the most valuable. Such a marketing approach will require more attention on needs assessment and customer satisfaction research.

Prochaska and Marcus (in press) wrote that continually prodding individuals in the contemplative stage to try a major behavior change (e.g., stop smoking for 24 hours) can produce greater resistance to change. A more effective strategy is to help an individual to make small behavioral changes (e.g., reduce daily total number of cigarettes slightly). A broadened perspective of physical activity will benefit such an approach. For example, outreach events to involve sedentary individuals in innovative and enjoyable activities where convenience (place) and reasonable cost (price) are emphasized might overcome the inertia of resisters. By contrast, only a small portion of the inactive are likely to write or call a facility in response to an advertisement or announcement. On the spot personal invitations, or community on-site activity demonstrations where people are actively recruited to participate, may stimulate initial involvement.

Retention

Most intervention techniques have addressed retention of program participants. Typically, interventions have been studied over relatively short time periods (e.g., less than 6 months). Information garnered from this research is briefly reviewed here in terms of the four Ps.

Product

Although there is little systematic research on the key attributes of physical activity that effect involvement,

there is evidence that participation patterns are relatively similar across a variety of activity types. Personal preference appears to be the key, and no one activity will be most popular with all. Differences reflect socialization, cultural, environmental, and current situational influences. Research shows that simple, easily available activities such as walking, gardening, and cycling are the most popular activities (Stephens & Craig, 1990). In terms of mass appeal, these lifetime activities are probably easier to market than facility-based sport programs or formal exercise programs. However, individual choice is an essential aspect to remember when promoting activity. This is important because coercion and loss of freedom produce reactance and resistance to behavior change (Brehm, 1972).

Intensity of the activity is related to retention. High intensity, high frequency activity results in an increase in injuries and a decrease in activity adherence (Pollock, 1988). In addition, perceived effort or exertion is negatively associated with participation (Dishman, 1990a). Again, individual differences must be considered, however, as individuals who seek a high intensity workout will be dissatisfied by a less strenuous approach (Morgan, Shepard, Finucane, Schimmelfing, & Jazmaji, 1984).

Place

Convenience is important to involvement. This has been one of the strong arguments, together with the importance of social support, for the provision of work-site physical activity programs (Cox, 1984). Similarly, convenient community recreation centers are important for accessibility from residential areas. Although definitive evidence is not available on the optimal location of exercise sites for different groups, poor accessability becomes a large barrier for less mobile groups, especially the young or the elderly (Alberta Recreation & Parks, 1981).

Price

There is little systematic evidence to document the relevance of price to physical activity involvement. The association of socioeconomic status with levels of involvement in different activities, however, supports the common sense view that cost, at least for some activities, is a significant barrier to lower income groups. Although some activities may not be available to all income groups, it is nevertheless true that activity in some form is available to all. The perception that certain activities are more acceptable or desirable than others, however, works against the unrestricted substitution of one activity for another. Nevertheless, the Campbell Survey of Well-Being indicated that although cost was a barrier to increased activity for about 15% of the Canadian population, it was equally important to the active and the inactive (Stephens & Craig, 1990).

Another aspect to consider is the price of a product as an important factor influencing consumer demand. A price that is too low or too high can affect a consumer's perceptions. For example, a low price, or no charge, may lead to a perception that a product is of inferior quality, hence causing the demand to decrease. Customary practices, local conventions, and product information all influence the perception of fair price. It is important that involvement agencies conduct their own market research to establish appropriate price levels for their services.

Promotion

Our review of the literature and other recent reviews (Dishman, 1991; Sallis & Hovell, 1990) conclude that a number of interventions may enhance physical activity involvement. A variety of behavior modification techniques (e.g., self-monitoring, reinforcement, contracting), cognitive behavior modification techniques (e.g., goal-setting, decision balance-sheet, self-talk), and health-education approaches have been shown to help increase the frequency of involvement, at least over relatively short time periods. Although the majority of this research has been devoted to structured exercise class settings, limited research also has indicated the viability of some techniques in naturalistic or home-based settings. Cognitive-based, self-control oriented interventions have been shown to assist home-based activity as much as personal interventions in structured settings (Bocksnick, 1991; Owen, Lee, Naccarella, & Haag, 1987).

Data from the Campbell Survey of Well-Being (Stephens & Craig, 1990; Wankel, Sefton, & Mummery, 1991) indicated that a number of social-psychological variables were related to previous activity involvement as well as intentions for future participation. The more active participants reported more positive attitudes toward activity, stronger social support from significant others, and greater perceived behavioral control over their regular activity schedule. To predict intentions to be physically active, these three variables were placed within the context of the theory of planned behavior (Azjen, 1985). Perceived behavioral control was the most important predictor (B = 0.32), followed by attitude (B = 0.25), and social support or social norm (B = 0.11) (Wankel et al., 1991). Although these overall population patterns held true for most subgroups, there were some differences that have implications for promotional efforts. For example, attitude was a strong predictor of activity intention in young adults but was less important in older adults. Perceived behavioral control was a stronger predictor in older adults than in younger adults.

Educational programs could use the specific beliefs underlying these composite variables to promote activity to different groups. For example, programs for young adults might emphasize the potential for obtaining enjoyment, making new friendships, and developing new skills through physical activity. Programs for older groups (e.g., 60 years of age or older) might emphasize opportunities for safe physical activities without fear of injury, contributions of appropriate activities to health and well-being, and interactions in a positive social environment with friends.

However, the available evidence does not strongly support the relation between psychological variables (e.g., beliefs, values, attitudes) and continued activity involvement (Dishman, 1991). This may reflect that general measures have been used to assess these psychological variables and that people who are active are already convinced of the general values of activity. Although they may have an overall knowledge of the benefits of activity and of the desirability of leading an active lifestyle, they may not know the optimal intensity, duration, and frequency for particular benefits (Casperson, Christenson, & Pollard, 1985). Information should be provided about the benefits of specific activities, how to do these activities, and opportunities for doing them.

One specific technique which has consistently enhanced activity involvement, at least over a relatively short period (e.g., 12 weeks), is a decision balance-sheet procedure (Wankel, 1985; Wankel, Yardley, & Graham, 1985). The individual completes a balance-sheet grid considering the anticipated gains and losses, to oneself and significant others, of participating in regular physical activity. The responses on the completed grid are read aloud to the counselor who selectively reinforces the desired responses. The procedure effectively combines self-reinforcement, self-disclosure, and planning to maximize success and minimize failure.

Self-efficacy training has been another effective means of fostering greater activity involvement. Consistent with survey studies indicating that self-efficacy distinguishes between those who are active and those who are not (Sallis et al., 1989), self-efficacy intervention programs have been shown to facilitate participation (Ewart, Taylor, Reese, & DeBusk, 1983; Kaplan, Atkins, & Reinsch, 1984). Performance feedback on fitness tests can be an effective method of enhancing self-efficacy for physical activity. Verbal persuasion can also be effective as long as the source is credible and does not contradict behavioral information. Efficacy training is especially valuable for those who have suffered physical injury or have been debilitated through illness, or have had a negative early experience in sport or physical activity. Efficacy training would be particularly relevant for older people whose fear of injury becomes a significant barrier to activity (Stephens & Craig, 1990).

It is important to note that the relative importance of different exercise goals generally changes over time with continued involvement. Whereas various health benefits are the principal reason that adults join activity programs, they continue involvement because of enjoyment of the program and social considerations (Sallis et al., 1989; Wankel, 1985, 1988). Despite this evidence indicating the importance of enjoyment to continued involvement, little attention has been given to what leads to enjoyment of physical activity. Research in the area of youth sports, as well as research on intrinsic motivation, has documented the importance of competence and challenge. Csikszentmihalyi (1990) has developed the concept of "flow" to account for situations where individuals are intrinsically motivated to do an activity in the absence of any apparent external rewards. The key to reaching a flow state is to match an individual's perceived competencies with the perceived challenge of the task. This element of self-challenge and skill development is an important part of physical activity involvement. The sense of personal meaning and self-identity obtained through testing one's capabilities is self-affirming. This is especially true for older citizens, and those whose continued independence is threatened because of sickness or injury. For some individuals an activity itself will be sufficient for engendering positive motivation, for others the physical surroundings or the social context may be a more meaningful challenge. The key is to identify those elements that are meaningful and stimulating to the given individual.

For long-term involvement, physical activity must virtually become an aspect of one's self-identity. Kendzierski (1988) has reported that individuals who participate regularly in exercise tend to have a self-schemata for exercise. They see themselves as exercisers, and identify with exercisers. On the other hand, nonschematic people, those who don't see activity as an important part of their self-image, have difficulty maintaining regular activity involvement. As with the development of self-efficacy, perhaps trial programs, persuasive communication, and general encouragement can help foster the development of self-schemata for activity in more individuals.

Relapse and Recovery

Similar to the stage perspective of behavior change, relapse and recovery are not outcomes but rather are parts of a process. Relapse is a return to an earlier stage of change and can occur at any stage in the process. The particular strategy that will be most appropriate for assisting return (recovery) to an action or retention phase will depend on the individual's current stage. Understanding his or her exercise history will help design an appropriate intervention. There are no longitudinal studies to address what interventions may best ease a return to regular activity. It would seem general strategies used during recruitment would be appropriate, but they could be more quickly faded into retention strategies than in initial recruitment. Caution must be exercised so that participants don't "tune out" customary messages; this suggests that novel and stimulating approaches must be adopted.

Conclusion

In summary, we have argued that the adoption of an active lifestyle is an ongoing, dynamic process. It is not simply a matter of being active or not. Accordingly, professionals and volunteers working to promote active living should consider the ongoing process when attempting to help individuals or groups become regularly active. It has been argued that no one intervention technique or strategy ensures a desired behavior change. Rather, there are a variety of techniques that may be helpful. To use these techniques appropriately, the counselor must adopt a problem-solving stance and ask, how might the individual or group be assisted to make the desired change? To design an effective intervention, attention must be paid to the essential aspects of the target behavior. In other words, the counselor should consider the market mix for physical activity—the product, place, price, and promotion as they pertain to the specific individual or group. These considerations can be assisted by assessing the individual's stage of change (resistance, recruitment, retention, relapse, or recovery). The result is a 4 × 5 PR matrix. Hence, this strategy for behavior change might be summarized as follows: "For success in promoting physical activity involvement, you must attend to your PRs!"

References

Ajzen, I. (1985). From intentions to actions: A theory of planned behavior. In J. Kuhl & J. Beckman (Eds.), *Action-control: From cognition to behavior* (pp. 11-39). Heidelberg: Springer.

Alberta Recreation & Parks. (1981). *Barriers to participation. A look at leisure.* Edmonton, AB: Author.

American College of Sports Medicine. (1978). Position statement on the recommended quantity and quality of exercise for developing and maintaining fitness in healthy adults. *Medicine and Science in Sports and Exercise*, **10**, vii-x.

Bauman, A. (1987). Trends in exercise prevalence in Australia. *Community Health Studies*, **9**, 190-196.

Becker, R. (1977). *Introduction and development of "Life Be In It" campaign. Minister's paper, Government of Victoria, Melbourne.* Paper presented at the International TRIMM Conference, Paris.

Bocksnick, J.G. (1991). *Effectiveness of a physical activity adherence counselling program with older females.* Unpublished doctoral dissertation, University of Alberta, Alberta, Canada.

Bouchard, C., Shephard, R.J., Stephens, T., Sutton, J.R., & McPherson, B.D. (Eds.) (1990). *Exercise, fitness and health: A consensus of current knowledge.* Champaign, IL: Human Kinetics.

Brehm, J.W. (1972). *Responses to loss of freedom: A theory of psychological reactance.* Morristown, NJ: General Learning Press.

Casperson, C.J., Christenson, G.M., & Pollard, R.A. (1985). Status of the 1990 physical fitness and exercise objectives—evidence from HHIS 1985. *Public Health Reports,* **101,** 587-592.

Cox, M.H. (1984). Fitness and lifestyle programs for business and industry: Problems in recruitment and retention. *Journal of Cardiac Rehabilitation,* **4**(4), 136-142.

Crompton, J.L. (1981). How to find the price that's right. *Parks & Recreation,* **16**(3), 32-39, 64.

Crompton, J.L. (1982). Psychological dimensions of pricing leisure services. *Recreation Research Review,* **9**(3), 12-20.

Csikszentmihalyi, M. (1990). *Flow: The psychology of optimal experience.* New York: Harper Collins.

Dishman, R.K. (1987). Exercise adherence and habitual physical activity. In W.P. Morgan & S.E. Goldston (Eds.), *Exercise and mental health* (pp. 57-83). Washington, DC: Hemisphere Publishing Corporation.

Dishman, R.K. (1990a). Determinants of participation in physical activity. In C. Bouchard, R.J. Shephard, T. Stephens, J.R. Sutton, & B.D. McPherson (Eds.), *Exercise, fitness and health: A consensus of current knowledge* (pp. 75-102). Champaign, IL: Human Kinetics.

Dishman, R.K. (1990b). Physical activity in medical care. In J.S. Torg, R.P. Welsh, & R.J. Shephard (Eds.), *Current therapy in sports medicine–2* (pp. 122-129). Philadelphia: B.C. Decker Inc.

Dishman, R.K. (1991). Increasing and maintaining exercise and physical activity. *Behavior Therapy,* **22,** 345-378.

Dishman, R.K., Sallis, J.F., & Orenstein, D. (1985). The determinants of physical activity and exercise. *Public Health Reports,* **100,** 158-171.

Donavon, R.J., & Owen, N. (in press). Social marketing and mass interventions. In R.K. Dishman (Ed.), *Exercise adherence II.* Champaign, IL: Human Kinetics.

Ewart, C.K., Taylor, C.B., Reese, C.B. & Debusk, R.F. (1983). Effects of early post myocardial infarction exercise testing on self-perception and subsequent physical activity. *American Journal of Cardiology,* **51,** 1076-1080.

Fitness and Amateur Sport Canada. (1983). *Fitness and lifestyle in Canada: The Canada fitness survey.* Ottawa, ON: Author.

Godin, G., & Shephard, R.J. (1983). Physical fitness promotion programmes: Effectiveness in modifying exercise behavior. *Canadian Journal of Applied Sport Sciences,* **8,** 104-113.

Iverson, D.C., Fielding, J.E., Crow, R.S., & Christenson, G.M. (1985). The promotion of physical activity in the United States population: The status of programs in medical, worksite, school and community settings. *Public Health Reports,* **100,** 212-224.

Kaplan, R.M., Atkins, C.J., & Reinsch, S. (1984). Specific efficacy expectations mediate exercise compliance in patients with COPD. *Health Psychology,* **3,** 223-242.

Kendzierski, D. (1988). Self-schemata and exercise. *Basic and Applied Social Psychology,* **9,** 45-61.

Kenyon, G.S. (1968). A conceptual model for characterizing physical activity. *Research Quarterly,* **39,** 96-105.

Martin, J.E., & Dubbert, P.M. (1984). Behavioral management strategies for improving health and fitness. *Journal of Cardiac Rehabilitation,* **4,** 200-208.

Martin, J.E., & Dubbert, P.M. (1985). Adherence to exercise. In R.L. Terjung (Ed.), *Exercise and sport sciences reviews* (pp. 137-167). Syracuse, NY: MacMillan.

Morgan, P.P., Shephard, R.J., Finucane, R., Schimmelfing, L., & Jazmaji, V. (1984). Health beliefs and exercise habits in an employee fitness programme. *Canadian Journal of Applied Sport Sciences,* **9,** 87-93.

Nielsen, A.B., Borsdorf, L.L., & Corbin, C.B. (1987, April). *Attitude assessment and term variation in physical education.* Paper presented at the convention of the American Alliance of Health, Physical Education, Recreation and Dance, Las Vegas, NV.

Owen, N., Lee, C., Naccarella, L., & Haag, K. (1987). Exercise by mail: A mediated behavior-change program for aerobic exercise. *Journal of Sport Psychology,* **9,** 346-357.

Pollock, M.L. (1988). Prescribing exercise for fitness and adherence. In R.K. Dishman (Ed.), *Exercise adherence: Its impact on public health* (pp. 259-277). Champaign, IL: Human Kinetics.

Prochaska, J.O., & DiClemente, C.C. (1983). Stages and processes of self-change of smoking: Toward an integrative model of change. *Journal of Consulting and Clinical Psychology,* **51**(3), 390-395.

Prochaska, J.O., & DiClemente, C.C. (1984). *The transtheoretical approach: Crossing traditional boundaries of therapy.* Pacific Grove, CA: Brooks-Cole.

Prochaska, J.O., & Marcus, B.H. (in press). The transtheoretical model: Applications to exercise. In R.K. Dishman (Ed.), *Exercise adherence II* . Champaign, IL: Human Kinetics.

Sallis, J.F., & Hovell, M.F. (1990). Determinants of exercise behavior. In K.B. Pandolf & J.O. Holloszy (Eds.), *Exercise and sport sciences reviews, Volume 18* (pp. 307-330). Baltimore, MD: Williams & Wilkins.

Sallis, J.F., Hovell, M.F., Hofstetter, C.R., Faucher, P., Elder, J.P., Blanchard, J., Casperson, C.J., Powell, K.E., & Christenson, G.M. (1989). A multivariate study of determinants of vigorous exercise in a community sample. *Preventive Medicine*, **18**, 20-34.

Stephens, T., & Craig, C.L. (1990). *The well-being of Canadians: Highlights of the 1988 Campbell's Survey*. Ottawa, ON: Canadian Fitness and Lifestyle Research Institute.

Stephens, T., Jacobs, D.R., & White, C.C. (1985). The descriptive epidemiology of leisure-time physical activity. *Public Health Reports*, **100**, 147-158.

Taylor, C.B., & Owen, N. (1989). Behavioral medicine: Research and development in disease prevention. *Behavioral Change*, **6**, 3-11.

Wankel, L.M. (1985). Personal and situational factors affecting exercise involvement: The importance of enjoyment. *Research Quarterly for Exercise and Sport*, **56**(3), 275-282.

Wankel, L.M. (1987). Enhancing motivation for involvement in voluntary exercise programs. In M.

Maehr & D. Kleiber (Eds.), *Advances in motivation and achievement: Enhancing motivation* (pp. 239-286). Greenwich, CT: JAI Press Inc.

Wankel, L.M. (1988). Exercise adherence and leisure activity: Patterns of involvement and interventions to facilitate regular activity. In R.K. Dishman (Ed.), *Exercise adherence: Its impact on public health* (pp. 369-396). Champaign, IL: Human Kinetics.

Wankel, L.M., Sefton, J., & Mummery, K. (1991). *Testing the theory of planned behaviour and developing physical activity promotion strategies for specific target groups with data from the Campbell Survey of Well-Being (CSWB)* (Research report to Canadian Fitness and Lifestyle Research Institute). Ottawa, ON.

Wankel, L.M., Yardley, J.K., & Graham, J. (1985). The effects of motivational interventions upon the exercise adherence of high and low self-motivated adults. *Canadian Journal of Applied Sport Sciences*, **10**(3), 147-156.

17

Fostering Active Living for Children and Youth: The Motivational Significance of Goal Orientations in Sport

Joan L. Duda

The woods would be silent if only the birds with the most beautiful voices were allowed to sing.

Author unknown

One popular arena among children and youth for participation in physical activity is sport. Although the degree of physical activity experienced while playing some youth sports is questionable, sport can play a critical role in fostering present and future active living for boys and girls. I suggest that youth sport participation should lay the groundwork for lifetime physical activity when

- such participation results in enjoyment and a sense of competence among young people,
- success in the athletic domain is considered to be primarily a function of trying hard rather than possessing superior talent, and
- sport involvement is linked to a belief in the efficacy of physical activity in promoting wellness throughout the lifespan.

When sport is experienced in this way, boys and girls should then be more willing to continue engagement in sport and exercise activities both while they are young and when they move into the adult years.

In this paper I propose that the promotion of active living through youth sport participation is dependent on the goal perspective emphasized by young people in that setting. My thesis is based on contemporary motivation work in the academic domain (Ames, 1992; Dweck, 1986; Nicholls, 1989) and the sport context (Duda, 1989a, 1992, 1993). This literature suggests that the personal goals that people adopt influence how they interpret and respond to achievement activities. It is assumed that the determinants of continued and maximal investment in academic or athletic pursuits are best

understood when we consider variations in goal perspectives.

The Goal Perspective Theory of Motivation

Differences in personal goals relate to how people judge their levels of ability and subjectively define success in performance-oriented situations (Nicholls, 1989). There are two major goal perspectives, task orientation and ego orientation, and these perspectives have been found to be independent (individuals can be high or low in both orientations or high in one and low in the other). When people are primarily task oriented, they tend to base their perceived competence on and view success as personal improvement and task mastery. When ego orientation predominates, perceptions of one's ability are based on social comparison. Perceiving oneself as able means that the person sees herself or himself as better than relative others. Among ego-oriented individuals, subjective success results when superior competence is demonstrated.

Classroom-based research has clearly shown that the adoption of task-oriented goals relates to positive achievement strivings and an adaptive approach toward achievement activities (Ames, 1992; Dweck, 1986; Nicholls, 1989). In contrast, a strong ego orientation (particularly when the person in question perceives his or her competence to be lacking) has been found to correspond to maladaptive achievement patterns. From this work has sprung a push for creating a more task-oriented classroom environment so that young people will assume a task-oriented goal perspective (Ames, 1992), which it is presumed will impart a lifelong love of learning.

123

In light of the objective of enhancing active living among boys and girls, the research to date calls for the reinforcement of task-oriented goals and the downplaying of ego-oriented goals in the sport realm as well. To support this claim, I review several lines of inquiry. In particular, I will highlight research on the relationship of goal orientations to boys' and girls' enjoyment of sport, perceived sport competence, beliefs about the causes of sport success, and views about the purposes of sport involvement. Extrapolating from this literature, I conclude with suggestions for fostering young people's endorsement of adaptive personal goals in the physical activity domain.

Goal Orientations and Sport Enjoyment

Investigations of the motives for participation in and dropping out of sport among U.S. and Canadian youth have shown that "fun" is an important dimension of sport involvement (Wankel & Kreisel, 1985). In general, reported enjoyment has been found to be a positive correlate of persistence in sport.

A consistent finding in the goal perspective literature has been the positive association between task orientation and sport enjoyment. In studies of U.S. college students enrolled in sport classes (Duda, Chi, Newton, Walling, & Catley, in press), high school–age athletes and nonathletes (Duda & Nicholls, 1992), young basketball players (Hom, Duda, & Miller, 1993), and adolescent tennis players (Newton & Duda, 1992), a tendency to emphasize task-oriented goals was linked to greater enjoyment of and interest in athletic activities. Similar results were reported in a recent investigation of British children (Duda, Fox, Biddle, & Armstrong, 1992).

Taking a different approach to this issue, Walling and her colleagues examined the relationship of goal orientations and competitive outcome to children's pregame and postgame responses to a sport competition (Walling, Duda, & Crawford, in press). The subjects were 238 youths (12 to 17 years old) competing in a soccer, swimming, track and field, bowling, wrestling, basketball, or volleyball tournament or meet. The results indicated that, regardless of who won or lost, highly task-oriented children tended to report that they enjoyed their sport more before they competed. Further, among those who lost, a positive association was revealed between task orientation and postcompetition ratings of the degree of fun experienced.

Rather than focus on the correlates of individual differences in goal perspective, Seifriz, Duda, and Chi (1992) determined the interdependencies between perceived situational goal structure (i.e., the degree to which the atmosphere on a sport team is characterized as task- or ego-involving) and high school male basketball players' reported enjoyment of their sport. In this study,

a task-oriented motivational climate was characterized by a focus on hard work, an acceptance of mistakes as part of the learning process, and a belief that every player has an important role to fill. Conversely, an emphasis on outdoing others (even one's own teammates) and a coach's tendency to reward only the best players were viewed as the hallmarks of an ego-oriented team climate. Players who perceived that the predominant goal structure on their team was task oriented indicated a greater enjoyment of basketball.

In sum, past work has indicated that having fun is relevant to the quality and quantity of young people's involvement in athletic activities. Sport research stemming from goal perspective theory tells us that enjoyment is more likely to be the rule than the exception when a task orientation prevails.

Goal Orientations and Perceived Sport Competence

An abundance of studies (from a multitude of theoretical perspectives) have found perceived ability to be a positive predictor of performance and participation among youngsters in the physical domain. Goal perspective theory suggests that the goals emphasized in achievement situations mediate people's perceptions of ability in those environments. Specifically, perceptions of competence are expected to be "heartier" when one is task oriented—because perceived ability is construed in terms of one's own performance, it is expected that youngsters are less likely to feel incompetent when participating in sport. Further, it is predicted that viewing oneself as not exceptionally able in sport is not a motivational handicap if the focus is on task-oriented goals.

When predominantly ego oriented, perceptions of sport ability are presumed to be more fragile. The adoption of such a goal perspective means that young sport participants are prone to compare themselves to others when judging their ability. In this case, one's competence is typically on one's mind while performing. Therefore, given the highly competitive nature of sport, there is a greater probability that children will believe their competence to be insufficient when high ego orientation exists. An emphasis on ego-oriented goals coupled with questions about one's ability are expected to lead to decreased performance and lack of persistence.

Recent sport-related research (Chi, 1993; Roberts, Kleiber, & Roberts, 1981; Treasure, 1993) has supported these predictions, providing another rationale for the promotion of a task orientation. That is, it appears that active living is more likely when boys and girls feel capable in the physical domain. Further, the literature suggests that there is a greater chance for youngsters to perceive themselves as capable when they have internalized a task-oriented goal perspective in sport.

Goal Orientations and Beliefs About Success

It is assumed that boys' and girls' sport motivation would vary according to their beliefs about what leads to sport success. Drawing from the tenets of goal perspective theory as well as other well-accepted motivation frameworks (e.g., cognitive evaluation theory, attribution theory of achievement motivation), one expects that youth sport participants are more prone to work hard and to invest in sport when they perceive that the determinants of success are within their control. When the perceived causes of success are considered external to the individual or less controllable, one predicts diminished interest and motivation.

According to Nicholls (1989), people's goal orientations correspond in a conceptually coherent manner to their beliefs about the causes of success. Nicholls considers these belief systems to reflect an individual's ideas about how an achievement activity (such as sport) operates. His work in education has shown that such ideas are consistent with what a person perceives to be important in the activity (i.e., one's personal goal).

Recent sport research has examined the relationships between goals and beliefs. Studies of U.S. high school students (Duda & Nicholls, 1992), U.S. and British youth (Duda et al., 1993; Hom et al., 1993; Newton & Duda, 1992), Canadian disabled adolescent athletes (White & Duda, 1992), and collegiate athletes (Duda & White, 1992) have revealed an interdependence between task orientation and the beliefs that hard work, motivation, and collaboration with others result in success. In contrast, ego orientation was associated with the belief that high ability determines sport achievement.

The belief that ability is the primary cause of achievement is less self-determining than the view that individual and collective effort are precursors to sport success. Youngsters have less influence over their level of athletic ability than over how hard they try. Further, when doubts about competence exist, the view that ability is the major antecedent of achievement is even more disconcerting—if one feels like he or she lacks ability and being highly able is considered necessary for success, why stay involved?

The research has also indicated that ego orientation is associated with the perceptions that sport success stems from external factors (e.g., having the right equipment, knowing how to impress the coach); deceptive tactics (e.g., cheating); and, among high level competitors, performance enhancement drugs (Duda & White, 1992). This link between the latter two beliefs and an ego-oriented goal perspective is compatible with past work that has found a negative relationship between ego orientation and sportsmanship attitudes (Duda, Olson, & Templin, 1991).

In general, these perceived causes of sport success are also problematic. Young athletes who believe that external elements play an important role in achievement do not think that sport success is predominantly under their control. Moreover, with respect to both ethics and health, it is not desirable that young people perceive taking an illegal advantage (such as by breaking the rules or using steroids) to be advantageous in the athletic domain. If legitimate means to sport success (such as working hard and utilizing one's ability) appear ineffective to a youngster, a child holding an ego-oriented perspective might be more likely to try something that is against the rules or potentially harmful to himself or herself.

The existing literature on goals and beliefs in sport provides an additional argument for fostering young people's orientation to task-focused goals. Active living seems more likely when young sport participants view success as an experience they can take credit for achieving. We want children and adolescents to feel that *they* are the major reasons for their accomplishments—and such a viewpoint is more likely if they are task oriented than if they are ego oriented.

Goal Orientations and Views About the Purposes of Sport

According to Nicholls (1989, p. 102), different goal orientations "involve different world views." In other words, the way a child or adolescent defines success in sport is assumed to be compatible with her or his views concerning the wider purposes of athletic activities.

Among a sample of high school athletes, I examined the interdependencies between dispositional goal perspectives and perceptions of the overall purposes of sport involvement (Duda, 1989b). The athletes held several beliefs about the purpose of sport participation. Specifically, it was considered that sport should

- teach people about the importance of trying hard and working with others,
- promote active living across the lifespan,
- encourage good citizenship,
- enhance competitiveness,
- set the stage for a high-status career,
- increase an individual's self-esteem and sense of self-importance, and
- make people popular.

The results indicated a logical relationship between goal orientations and high school athletes' views about the wider purposes of sport. Athletes who were high in task orientation were more likely to report that through sport we should learn the value of hard work and cooperation. Highly task-oriented athletes tended to disagree that an important purpose of sport was to enhance participants' social status. The belief that involvement in sport should foster an active lifestyle positively related to the emphasis placed on task-oriented goals.

In contrast, ego orientation was associated with perceived purposes of sport that were more extrinsic and focused on personal gains. High school athletes who were strongly ego oriented tended to believe that sport should make people more competitive and popular and feel more important. These youngsters were less likely to perceive that sport ought to help people become better citizens.

The findings of the Duda (1989b) study suggest that sport is considered a vehicle for learning to keep trying and keep active when the athletic experience is interpreted in a task-oriented fashion. An ego-oriented perspective on sport success suggests that athletics is a road to personal glory and gains that are outside the intrinsic facets of physical activity itself. Thus, once again, the preeminence of a task orientation is warranted.

Fostering Active Living for Children and Youth

The reviewed research suggests that young people's goal orientations are predictive of a variety of meanings in terms of how sport is experienced. Dependent on their degree of task and ego orientation (and the degree to which the sport environment is task- or ego-involving), boys and girls are more or less likely to enjoy sport and feel competent in this context. Personal goals also have been linked to youngsters' beliefs about the antecedents of athletic success and to their opinions concerning what sport should do. It is suggested that these interpretations and responses are critical to maximizing youth sport and having physical activity be a salient, rewarding, and continuing part of young people's lives.

Whether a person is focused on task- or ego-involved goals in any particular situation is a function if dispositional or individual differences (i.e., the degree of task and ego orientation), developmental differences, and situational influences. In most studies referenced in this paper, dispositional goal perspectives were assessed via the Task and Ego Orientation in Sport Questionnaire (Duda, 1989b; Duda et al., 1991). It is assumed that people develop their proneness for emphasizing a task- or ego-involved goal (or individual differences in goal perspectives) through childhood socialization experiences. Goal orientations appear to be a product of children's interactions with significant others (such as parents and coaches) and the goal structure evident in sport as they move through the athletic system. Indeed, past work has revealed a correspondence between children's personal sport goals and their perceptions of the goal orientations of their parents (Duda & Hom, 1993). Sport participants at higher competitive levels (e.g., collegiate or high school) also have been found to be higher in ego orientation than athletes competing at lower levels (Chaumeton & Duda, 1988; White & Duda, in press).

Research on the socialization of goal orientations in the physical domain is in its infancy. Because dispositional goal perspectives have emerged as a significant predictor of the different ways that people process sport, more investigations in this area are clearly needed.

With regard to situational determinants of goal perspectives, goal perspective theory and related studies in the academic (Ames, 1992) and athletic (Chaumeton & Duda, 1988; Seifriz et al., 1992) domains have provided a foundation for the promotion of adaptive conceptualizations of success in sport. Although further research is necessary, practitioners seem to be advocating an ego-involved goal perspective when they create a sport environment for young people that

- is highly competitive and results in only one "winner,"
- entails constant and overt evaluation of and comparison among youngsters,
- stresses that "winning is the only thing" and reinforces children on the basis of outcome rather than effort,
- informs children that mistakes and weaknesses are to be avoided,
- brings recognition only to the talented,
- makes children think that only the best have something to contribute, and
- tells children that success comes to only those who "can do" rather than those who "do try."

On the other hand, the literature suggested that task-involved goals would be stressed when children's sport encounters emphasize:

- how you play is at least as important as winning and losing,
- being the best is doing your best,
- mistakes are part of learning and improving,
- all children, regardless of their ability, have something to offer and receive from sport, and
- working with, rather than trying to always outdo, others is a valuable dimension of the sport experience.

Conclusion

One forum in which many North American children are exposed to the potential joys of being active is youth sport. For active living to be a reality for youngsters in the present and future, sport participation needs to get boys and girls moving and keep them moving. A goal perspective analysis of children's sport motivation provides insight into how these aims can be met.

References

Ames, C. (1992). Achievement goals, motivational climate, and motivational processes. In G. Roberts (Ed.), *Motivation in sport and exercise* (pp. 161-176). Champaign, IL: Human Kinetics.

Chaumeton, N., & Duda, J. (1988). Is it how you play the game or whether you win or lose? *Journal of Sport Behavior, 11,* 157-174.

Chi, L. (1993). *The prediction of achievement-related cognitions and behaviors in the physical domain: A test of the theories of goal perspectives and self-efficacy.* Unpublished doctoral dissertation, Purdue University.

Duda, J.L. (1989a). Goal perspectives and behavior in sport and exercise settings. In C. Ames & M. Maehr (Eds.), *Advances in motivation and achievement* (Vol. 6, pp. 81-115). Greenwich, CT: JAI Press.

Duda, J.L. (1989b). The relationship between task and ego orientation and the perceived purpose of sport among male and female high school athletes. *Journal of Sport and Exercise Psychology, 11,* 318-335.

Duda, J.L. (1992). Motivation in sport settings: A goal perspective approach. In G. Roberts (Ed.), *Motivation in sport and exercise* (pp. 57-91). Champaign, IL: Human Kinetics.

Duda, J.L. (1993). Goals: A social cognitive approach to the study of achievement motivation in sport. In R.N. Singer, M. Murphey, & L.K. Tennant (Eds.), *Handbook on research in sport psychology* (pp. 421-436). St. Louis: Macmillan.

Duda, J.L., Chi, L., Newton, M., Walling, D., & Catley, D. (in press). Task and ego orientation and intrinsic motivation in sport. *International Journal of Sport Psychology.*

Duda, J.L., Fox, K.R., Biddle, S.J.H., & Armstrong, N. (1992). Children's achievement goals and beliefs about success in sport. *British Journal of Educational Psychology, 62,* 313-323.

Duda, J.L., & Hom, H.L. (1993). Interdependencies between the perceived and self-reported goal orientation of young athletes and their parents. *Pediatric Exercise Science, 5.*

Duda, J.L., & Nicholls, J.G. (1992). Dimensions of achievement motivation in schoolwork and sport. *Journal of Educational Psychology, 84,* 1-10.

Duda, J.L., Olson, L.K., & Templin, T. (1991). The relationship of task and ego orientation to sports-manship attitudes and the perceived legitimacy of aggressive acts. *Research Quarterly for Exercise and Sport, 62,* 79-87.

Duda, J.L., & White, S.A. (1992). The relationship of goal perspectives to beliefs about the causes of success among elite skiers. *The Sport Psychologist, 6,* 334-343.

Dweck, C.S. (1986). Motivational processes affecting learning. *American Psychologist, 41,* 1040-1048.

Hom, H.L., Duda, J.L., & Miller, A. (1993). Correlates of goal orientations among young athletes. *Pediatric Exercise Science, 5,* 168-176.

Newton, M.L., & Duda, J.L. (1992). *The relationship of goal orientations to motivation-related processes among adolescent tennis players.* Manuscript submitted for publication.

Nicholls, J.G. (1989). *The competitive ethos and democratic education.* Cambridge, MA: Harvard University Press.

Roberts, G.C., Kleiber, D.A., & Duda, J.L. (1981). An analysis of motivation in children's sport: The role of perceived competence in participation. *Journal of Sport Psychology, 3,* 206-216.

Seifriz, J.J., Duda, J.L., & Chi, L. (1992). The relationship of perceived motivational climate to intrinsic motivation and beliefs about success in basketball. *Journal of Sport and Exercise Psychology, 14,* 375-391.

Treasure, D. (1993). *A social-cognitive approach to understanding children's achievement behavior, cognitions, and affect in competitive sport.* Unpublished doctoral dissertation, University of Illinois at Urbana-Champaign.

Walling, M.D., Duda, J.L., & Crawford, T. (in press). Goal orientations, outcome, and responses to youth sport competition among high/low perceived ability athletes. *International Journal of Sport Psychology.*

Wankel, L., & Kreisel, P. (1985). Factors underlying enjoyment of youth sport motivation research: Sport and age group comparisons. *Journal of Sport Psychology, 7,* 51-64.

White, S.A., & Duda, J.L. (1992). Dimensions of goal beliefs about success among disabled athletes. *Adapted Physical Activity Quarterly, 10,* 125-136.

White, S.A., & Duda, J.L. (in press). The relationship of gender, level of sport involvement, and participation motivation to goal orientation. *International Journal of Sport Psychology.*

Part III

Active Living for Specific Populations and Settings

The promotion of physical activity, fitness, health, and active living in the population has been enthusiastically pursued by tireless and creative professionals in our field. In Part III, the inherent value of focusing on the idiosyncrasies of specific populations and settings will be underscored through an examination of the promotion of active living in pregnant women, children and youths, older persons, and persons with disabilities, and in the workplace.

Mottola and Wolfe discuss the results of a survey of physical activity practices in women during pregnancy and address the delicate issue of exercise prescription during pregnancy. Mottola and Wolfe conclude that extant evidence and information allow for the safe prescription of physical activity during this important stage of a woman's life. Campbell focuses on the promotion of active living in children and youths through a historical survey of milestones in the promotion of physical activity in the Canadian school system. Campbell concludes that active living reflects the direction that physical education may take in the school system but that there is a need for continued teacher training, research, and marketing of the concept.

Through his personal experience and vast knowledge of the scientific literature, Åstrand dispels selected myths about exercise and aging. Åstrand offers principles and ideas that can be widely disseminated to promote physical activity and fitness, specifically in the aging population. Orban reviews a number of key factors that influence physical activity and fitness as people grow older. Orban then integrates this information into a comprehensive model. Watkinson addresses the special considerations that must be given to persons with mental disabilities. Watkinson emphasizes the prerequisite knowledge and skills that persons with mental disabilities must acquire if they are to effectively integrate into culturally normative physical activity settings.

Steadward documents the considerable progress that has been made in the field of sport for persons with a disability. However, Steadward also identifies the need for more effective community-based sport programs for persons with disabilities and expresses concern with the fact that elite athletes with disabilities have not been fully integrated into the Olympic games. Cox and Miles examine how physical activity and fitness may be promoted in the workplace through an examination of the emerging concepts of total quality management and workplace active living. Cox and Miles conclude that the time is right to examine the integration of these two concepts in current corporate culture.

Fielding and Knight conduct a systematic analysis of the costs and benefits of workplace active living programs, presenting data available from analyses conducted by companies. Fielding and Knight conclude that, given the data and methods available, the final decision to invest funds into such programs is ultimately subjective rather than objective.

18

Active Living and Pregnancy

Michelle F. Mottola
Larry A. Wolfe

The effects of pregnancy on maternal physical performance and the impact of chronic exertion on maternal and fetal health are subjects of considerable importance in contemporary Canada. In recent years, increasing numbers of women have been employed in physically demanding occupations, including military service, police work, fire fighting, carpentry, and plumbing (Alegre, Rodriguez-Essudero, Cruz, & Prada, 1984; Creasy, 1991; Fox, Harris, & Brekken, 1977; Homer, Beresford, James, Siegal, & Wilcox, 1990; Manschande, Eckels, Manschande-Desmit, & Vlietinek, 1987; McDonald et al., 1988; Murphy, Dauncey, Newcombe, Garcia, & Elbourne, 1984; Naeye & Peters, 1982; Ramirez, Grimes, Annegers, Davis, & Slater, 1990; Saurel-Cubizolles & Kaminski, 1986; Tafari, Naeye, & Gobeze, 1980). Thus, it is important to know the effects of frequent occupational physical activity on work performance and on pregnancy outcome. A closely related issue is the effect of prenatal exercise programs and other leisure-time physical activity on maternal health and fitness and pregnancy outcome.

It seems clear that Canadian women are adopting more active lifestyles and that many women are interested in maintaining or improving their prepregnancy level of physical fitness. As a result, the traditional view that pregnant women should rest is being challenged and the concept that pregnancy is a good time to adopt healthy lifestyle habits (including regular exercise) is gaining support based on recent scientific evidence (Brenner, Monga, Webb, McGrath, & Wolfe, 1991; White, 1992; Wolfe, Ohtake, Mottola, & McGrath, 1989).

Effective promotion of active living during pregnancy depends on the availability of two types of information. First, it is important to know the extent and nature of physical activity during pregnancy among typical Canadian women, to survey their attitudes and those of their physicians toward such participation, and to determine the influence of regular exercise participation

on pregnancy outcome. Second, scientifically valid information must be available to aid physicians in the process of preparticipation health screening and to guide exercising women, their physicians, and prenatal fitness leaders in designing individualized programs for active living during pregnancy. Accordingly, in the first part of this chapter we will present the results of a survey conducted in Ontario in which occupational and leisure-time physical activity patterns of pregnant women were assessed and related to pregnancy outcome. In the second part of this chapter we will discuss implications of the study results and other recent research findings for the processes of preparticipation health screening and exercise prescription during pregnancy.

Survey Methods

Approximately 10 physician or obstetrician offices were contacted in Toronto, Hamilton, Guelph, Kitchener, Windsor, Ottawa, Kingston, Thunder Bay, Sudbury, and London. Each office was requested to distribute self-contained, self-explanatory, self-addressed questionnaires to 10 pregnant patients. The survey given to each pregnant woman contained 45 questions on health behavior, lifestyle, and activity patterns both prior to (recall) and during pregnancy, and a consent form to permit evaluation of birth record information. The questions were adapted from the Canadian Fitness Survey (1981). Each questionnaire was coded to maintain confidentiality. Of the initial contacts, physicians in Hamilton, Kingston, Thunder Bay, Kitchener, Sudbury, and London agreed to participate. The contacts were then expanded to include Niagara Falls, St. Catharines, Sarnia, Clinton, Brantford, Chatham, Palmerston/Harriston, Woodstock, Tillsonburg, and Ingersol. Of the 200 questionnaires given out to pregnant patients, 100 were returned, and birth record information was recorded for 78 women. Medical records on pre- and postbirth information were examined with permission of the volunteers and their attending physicians.

Survey Results

Of the 78 respondents, 12.8% were in their first trimester, 43.6% were in their second trimester, and 43.6% were in their third trimester. Thus, about 87% were at least 4 months pregnant at the completion of the survey. In addition, approximately 22% were age 35 or older (see Table 18.1).

Of the total sample, 76.9% were employed outside the home; the others identified themselves as homemakers. The occupations reported most were clerical, teacher/ social worker/student, and investigator/lab worker. In addition, 6.4% worked as factory/farm laborers or fitness instructors (see Table 18.2).

When the women were asked to rate themselves on fitness compared to women of the same age, 37.2% were more fit, 12.8% were less fit, 43.6% were the same fitness, and 6.4% were not sure. When asked whether they participated in regular exercise (defined as at least 3 times/week) prior to pregnancy, 52.6% said yes and 47.4% said no. Of those women who said they participated in regular exercise prior to pregnancy, 82.9% planned to continue regular exercise during pregnancy,

Table 18.1 Respondents by Age

Age (years)	Percent
20–25	9.0
26–30	34.6
31–34	34.6
35 and over	21.8

Table 18.2 Occupation of Respondents

Occupation	Percent
Communications	6.4
Teacher/student	17.9
Homemaker	23.1
Factory/laborer/fitness instructor	6.4
Administration	3.8
Clerical	23.1
Driver	1.3
Investigator/lab	10.3
Nurse	3.8
Cashier/cook	3.8

and 17.1% said they would not continue regular exercise. Of those women (47.4%) who did not participate in regular exercise prior to pregnancy, 37.8% planned to start regular exercise during pregnancy.

When asked what activities were part of their weekly routine prior to pregnancy, 64.1% identified walking/ biking for leisure as the most popular activity. The next most popular activity was walking for exercise (44.9%); 33.3% of the women participated in "working out." In addition, 25.6% of the sample engaged in recreational activities such as bowling and curling. The most popular "other" activity was swimming (10.3%) and 5.1% of the women lifted weights (see Figure 18.1). When women were asked what activities they engaged in during pregnancy as part of their weekly routine, the same activities were most prominent, but the frequency of participation decreased slightly. Walking/biking for leisure was the most popular activity with 51.3% of the sample engaged in this during pregnancy. Participation in walking for exercise decreased to 41.0%. Only 19.2% of the women still "worked out," and 16.7% were involved in recreational activities. Prenatal classes were also cited as part of the "other" category, and the number of women who lifted weights during pregnancy was reduced to 1.3% (see Figure 18.2).

Self-reported frequency (number of times per week) and duration (minutes per session) of exercise prior to pregnancy is shown in Figure 18.3. We found it interesting that 62.8% of the sample exercised at least 20 minutes per session, and 14.1% of the population was active for more than 60 minutes. In addition, approximately 50% of the sample exercised at least 3 times per week. This indicates that prior to pregnancy more than 50% of the sample were maintaining fitness levels by exercising at least 15 minutes per session, at least 3 times per week (American College of Sports Medicine [ACSM], 1991). Self-reported frequency and duration of exercise during

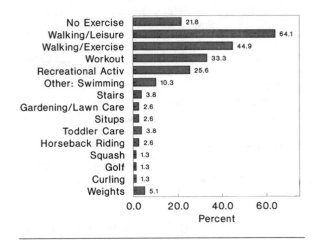

Figure 18.1 Activities of weekly routine prior to pregnancy. Values are presented as percentages. Activ - refers to activities.

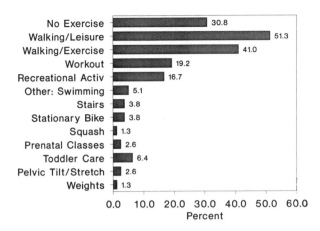

Figure 18.2 Activities of weekly routine during pregnancy. Values are presented as percentages. Activ - refers to activities.

pregnancy are presented in Figure 18.4. The number of women exercising at least 20 minutes per session decreased to approximately 45% of the sample; 24.4% exercised between 31 and 60 minutes per session; and 9% exercised for more than 60 minutes. During pregnancy, the number of women who exercised at least 3 times per week was reduced to approximately 35%. The ACSM *Guidelines for Exercise Testing and Prescription* (1991) suggest the appropriate frequency of exercise is three to five times per week. A duration of 15 to 30 minutes of exercise per session seems well tolerated by most pregnant women. It is interesting to note that more than 30% of this sample indicated that they exercised at a level more strenuous than that recommended for pregnant women by ACSM.

The birth outcome data were obtained from pre- and postbirth medical records from the office of the physician. A low frequency of births at less than 37 weeks gestation (5.1%) occurred compared to births at 37 weeks and older (94.8%). Infant sex was evenly distributed between male (53.8%) and female (46.2%) babies. APGAR scores at 1 minute and 5 minutes after birth were grouped as 7 or less and 8 or above. At 1 minute after birth, 20.5% of the sample had APGAR scores of 7 or less; 79.5% had scores of 8 or above. At 5 minutes after birth, the number of babies with scores of 7 or less decreased to 2.6%; those with scores of 8 or above increased to 97.4%. Mode of delivery was divided into vaginal births (including induced) and Caesarean sections (C-sections, including repeats). Of the 78 women, 83.3% had vaginal deliveries and 16.7% had C-sections. Maternal complications (9.0%) included gestational diabetes and borderline hypertension. Fetal complications (16.7%) included bradycardia and fetal heart rate deceleration. Birth weight was grouped as less than 2,500 g (6.4%) and 2,500 g or more (93.6%).

The Ontario Ministry of Health (Campbell, in press) has recently released a report that analyzed births (approximately 13,000) in the province in 1987. This report showed that the incidence of low birth weight (<2,500 g) was approximately 5.7%, and the rate of prematurity (<37 weeks gestation) was about 6.3%. Therefore, the low birth weight percentage of 6.7% and the prematurity percentage of 5.1% in the present study suggest that this data set conforms to the normal distribution for this province.

When maturity and birth weight were stratified by self-reported fitness of the mother, no patterns emerged. This sample included four women who gave birth to babies less than 37 weeks and five women who gave birth to babies weighing less than 2,500 g. When occupation was recoded to correspond to the occupational groupings of McDonald et al. (1988), who used classifications according to the Standard Occupational Classifications of Statistics Canada (1980), our data fit into three of the authors' six occupational classifications: managerial, health, and, clerical. McDonald et al. (1988) did not

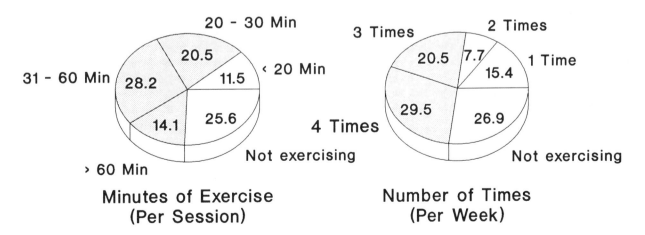

Figure 18.3 Self-reported duration and frequency of exercise prior to pregnancy. Values are reported as percentages. The shaded area represents duration and frequency of exercise required to maintain fitness.

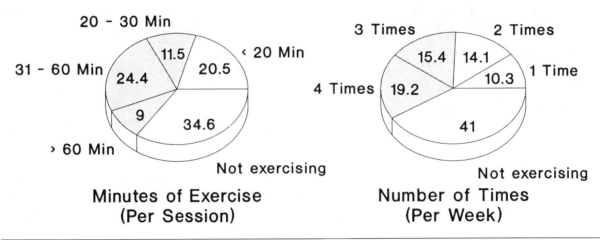

Figure 18.4 Self-reported duration and frequency of exercise during pregnancy. Values are reported as percentages. The shaded area represents duration and frequency of exercise required to maintain fitness.

include "homemaker" as a distinct occupation, as we did. When maturity and birth weight were stratified by these four occupational classifications, again no pattern emerged, possibly because of the small sample size and because the data are normally distributed.

In the literature, employment and effects on pregnancy outcome are controversial with respect to preterm delivery, small birth weight babies, and spontaneous abortion. Despite an increasing number of women who are employed during pregnancy, the overall incidence of preterm delivery has not changed (Creasy, 1991). However, other studies have reported decreased mean fetal weight in women who continue to work past the last 6 weeks of pregnancy (Alegre et al., 1984); an association between physical load and structural birth defects (Nurminen, Lusa, Ilmarinen, & Kurppa, 1989); an increased risk in delivering preterm, low birth weight infants in women who work in jobs characterized by high levels of physical exertion (Homer et al., 1990); and an increased risk of spontaneous abortion in women who engage in heavy lifting (McDonald et al., 1988). In contrast, Ahlborg, Bodin, and Hogstedt (1990) showed that heavy lifting during pregnancy did not increase the risk of fetal death. Clearly, more research on occupation and pregnancy is warranted.

Two questions from the survey were used to determine the role of the physician or obstetrician in giving advice on activity during pregnancy. The first question determined whether the pregnant patient approached her doctor about exercise during pregnancy or whether the physician approached the patient. The results are shown in Table 18.3. There was no discussion between patient and doctor in 46.2% of the sample. In 39.7% of the cases, women asked their doctor about exercise, and 14.1% of the physicians initiated the topic. This is an important observation considering that more than 80% of this sample were in their second or third trimester. In addition, more than 80% of those women who exercised before

pregnancy planned to continue, and more than 37% of those who did not exercise before pregnancy planned to start an exercise program.

The second question determined the patient's perception of the physician's feelings about exercise and her pregnancy. The results are shown in Table 18.4. The physicians made no comment to 38.5% of the women. In 32.1% of the sample, the physician encouraged exercise but with moderation; in 6.4% the physician encouraged exercise with no restrictions; in 15.4% the physician encouraged exercise to the same level as before pregnancy but with no increases; and in 3.8% the physician discouraged exercise. Exercise was discouraged for medical reasons and because the physician never encourages exercise during pregnancy.

In summary, it appears that many women are physically active before and during pregnancy, but the frequency of participation in activities decreases slightly during pregnancy. The most popular activities appear to be walking/biking for leisure or for exercise, although many women participate in work-outs and recreational activities during pregnancy. A segment of the population of pregnant women exercise more than 3 times per week or are active for more than 30 minutes per session, some for more than 60 minutes. In addition, many women are

Table 18.3 Patient-Reported Information About Physician and Exercise During Pregnancy

Patient-reported information	Percent
No discussion	46.2
Patient asked doctor	39.7
Doctor initiated	14.1

Table 18.4 Patient-Reported Information About Physician, Exercise, and Her Pregnancy

Patient-reported information	Percent
No comment	38.5
Encourages in moderation	32.1
Encourages no restrictions	6.4
Encourages same	15.4
Discourages	3.8
Don't know	3.8

employed outside the home in various occupational roles. It is encouraging that in this population of active women, birth outcome values are normally distributed. However, it appears that many women are not receiving information about exercise during pregnancy from their physician or obstetrician and participate in activities on their own.

Practical Implications for the Promotion of Active Living

The survey results support the validity of a number of logical but previously unsubstantiated assumptions that form a rational basis for promotion of active living during pregnancy:

- Many women of childbearing age in Ontario participate in regular occupational or leisure-time physical activity; the majority of these women wish to remain physically active during pregnancy.
- Many women who have not been physically active prior to pregnancy have an interest in starting a new fitness program during pregnancy.
- The pregnancy outcomes of women engaged in regular moderate physical activity are similar to those of the general population in Ontario.
- As a rule, physicians and obstetricians hold widely varying opinions concerning the advisability of promoting active living during pregnancy; many hesitate to advise their patients concerning physical activity during pregnancy. Presumably, this is the result of lack of information or fear of the medical and legal consequences of giving unsubstantiated or incorrect advice.

Our findings verify the practical rationale for two recent initiatives funded by the Ontario Ministry of Tourism and Recreation. In this regard, the final report of Ontario's Fitness Safety Standards Committee (Fitness Safety Standards Committee, 1990) included a chapter on "Special Exercising Populations and Concerns." A subsection devoted to pregnant women deemed it essential (identified

as a "standard") that pregnant women receive individual medical advice concerning the safety of exercise participation. To facilitate this process, the Physical Activity Readiness Examination for Pregnancy (PAR-X for Pregnancy) was formulated as the first section of a two-part form for promoting exercise safety in pregnancy. This questionnaire was included as a guideline for physicians and obstetricians and strongly recommended for use in providing medical clearance for prospective participants in prenatal exercise programs.

The PAR-X for Pregnancy is a completely revised version of the standard Physical Activity Readiness Examination (Chisholm, Collis, Kulak, Davenport, & Gruber, 1975), which has been used successfully across Canada for many years. Based on the individual's health and obstetrical history, lifestyle information provided by the participant, and medical examination (if needed), the physician completes a checklist to determine whether an individual has absolute or relative contraindications to exercise during pregnancy. Pregnant women with absolute contraindications to exercise (Table 18.5) should definitely not participate in strenuous exercise. For individuals with relative contraindications (Table 18.6), the risks of exercise may exceed the expected benefits, and the decision whether to participate should be made in accordance with careful medical judgment. Questionnaire items were selected in accordance with a thorough review of available scientific literature (Wolfe, Hall, Webb, Goodman, & McGrath, 1989) and direct advice from obstetricians, fitness specialists, and exercise physiologists working in this area of study. Preliminary versions of this questionnaire have also been used successfully over a 6-year period in the Exercise/Pregnancy Research Program at Queen's University (Brenner et al., 1991).

The second part of this form is called the PARχ for Pregnancy (Physical Activity Prescription for Pregnancy). Guidelines are provided for the prescription of both muscular and aerobic conditioning. Advice for muscular conditioning was adapted, updated, and summarized from prenatal fitness leadership manuals published by Fitness Canada (1982) and the Fitness Ontario Leadership Program (1983). These manuals have been used successfully for nearly a decade in Ontario and across Canada.

Guidelines for aerobic exercise prescription are based on two recent scientific reviews (Wolfe, Hall et al., 1989; Wolfe, Ohtake et al., 1989) and the results of two large-scale studies of aerobic conditioning during pregnancy conducted at Queen's University. These guidelines are also consistent with recent recommendations from ACSM (1991). Important highlights of these guidelines are the following:

- Participation in non-weight-bearing or low impact weight-bearing activities (e.g., walking, stationary cycling, aquatic exercise) is encouraged.
- Aerobic exercise should be done regularly (3 to 5 sessions/week); a minimum duration of 15 min and

Table 18.5 Absolute Contraindications for Strenuous Exercise in Pregnancy: Checklist To Be Completed by a Qualified Physician*

Does the patient have:	Yes	No
1. Clinically significant valvular or ischemic heart disease?	___	___
2. Type I diabetes mellitus, peripheral vascular disease, thryoid disease or uncontrolled hypertension, other serious systemic disorder (hepatitis, mononucleosis, etc.)?	___	___
3. An incompetent cervix (usually diagnosed in an earlier pregnancy)?	___	___
4. A history of two or more spontaneous abortions?	___	___
5. Bleeding or placenta previa?	___	___
6. Reptured membranes, premature labor?	___	___
7. Toxemia or preeclampsia (current pregnancy)?	___	___
8. Evidence of fetal growth retardation (current pregnancy)?	___	___
9. Very low % body fatness, eating disorder (anorexia, bulimia)?	___	___
10. A multiple pregnancy (e.g., triplets)?	___	___

*A "yes" answer to any of these questions strongly suggests that it is medically unwise to begin or continue a strenuous exercise program. Data from American College of Obstetricians and Gynecologists (1985); Wolfe et al. (1989); Fitness Ontario Leadership Program (1992).

Table 18.6 Relative Contraindications for Strenuous Exercise in Pregnancy: A Checklist To Be Completed by a Qualified Physician*

	Yes	No
1. History in previous pregnancies of premature labor, intrauterine growth retardation?	___	___
2. Anemia or iron deficiency (Hb < 10 g/dl)?	___	___
3. Clinically significant pulmonary disease (e.g., COPD)?	___	___
4. Mild valvular or ischemic heart disease, significant cardiac arrhythmia?	___	___
5. Very low physical fitness prior to pregnancy?	___	___
6. A prescription of drugs that can alter cardiac output or blood flow distribution?	___	___
7. Obesity and/or Type II diabetes prior to pregnancy?	___	___

Note. Aerobic conditioning may be benefical to prevent or treat gestational diabetes.

*A "yes" answer to any of these questions indicates that risks of participation in strenuous exercise may exceed the expected benefits; a decision to exercise or not should be made by a qualified physician based on a thorough medical evaluation. Data from American College of Obstetricians and Gynecologists (1985); Wolfe et al. (1989); Fitness Ontario Leadership Program (1992).

a maximum of 30 min/session is appropriate for most women (Brenner et al., 1991).

- Exercise intensity should be prescribed by combining the methods of pulse rate targeting (modified for pregnant women, Table 18.7) and rating of perceived exertion (Ohtake, Wolfe, Hall, & McGrath, 1988b; Wolfe, Van Raay, Dumas, & McGrath, 1992); the "talk test" should be used as a final check to avoid overexertion (Fitness Canada, 1982; Ohtake, Wolfe, Hall, & McGrath, 1988a; Walker, Wolfe, Dumas, & McGrath, 1992).
- Following medical clearance, previously sedentary women can begin a new aerobic exercise program and gradually increase exercise quantity and quality during the second trimester, when the discomforts of pregnancy and risks of exercise are lowest (Brenner et al., 1991; Wolfe, Ohtake et al., 1989).
- Additional advice for exercise safety is provided (Table 18.8), and pregnant exercisers are encouraged to be familiar with symptoms that indicate that they should discontinue exercise and seek medical advice (American College of Obstetricians and Gynecologists, 1985; Fitness Canada, 1982; Wolfe, Ohtake et al., 1989).

The PAR-X/PARχ for Pregnancy has other important design features. First, using this form will help familiarize

Table 18.7   Modified Heart Rate Target Zones for Aerobic Exercise in Pregnancy*

Maternal age	Heart rate target zone
Less than 20 years	140–155 beats/min
20–29 years	135–150 beats/min
30–39 years	130–145 beats/min
Greater than 40 years	125–140 beats/min

*Values apply to most healthy pregnant women. Exercise at the lower part of the recommended heart rate target ranges at the beginning of a new exercise program and in late gestation. Data from Wolfe (in press); Fitness Ontario Leadership Program (1992).

Table 18.8   Additional Advice for Safe Exercise Participation During Pregnancy

- Obtain medical clearance before starting or continuing a strenuous exercise program in pregnancy.
- Avoid prolonged or strenuous exertion during the first trimester.
- Avoid exercise for more than a few minutes while lying on your back.
- Avoid isometric exercise or straining while holding your breath.
- Avoid activities that involve physical contact or danger of falling (e.g., footall).
- Avoid exercise in warm, humid environments.
- Periodic rest periods may help to minimize possible hypoxic or temperature stress to the fetus.
- Maintain adequate nutrition and hydration (drink liquids before and after exercise).
- Know reasons to stop exercise and consult a qualified physician immediately if they occur.

Data from Wolfe et al. (1989); Fitness Ontario Leadership Program (1992).

physicians with current methods for medical screening and exercise prescription in pregnancy. Because pregnant women are usually very health conscious, an opportunity is created for physicians and obstetricians to encourage their patients to adopt healthy lifestyle habits, including regular exercise.

Use of the PAR-X/PARχ for Pregnancy will also help to promote three-way communication among the pregnant exercise participant, her obstetrician, and the prenatal fitness instructor. The instructor provides a copy of the form to prospective program participants. The woman fills out the part of the form related to her past and current health history, current lifestyle habits, and the instructor's

name and telephone number. She then gives it to the physician monitoring her pregnancy. The physician checks the information provided and then completes brief checklists concerning the presence or absence of contraindications to exercise in pregnancy (Tables 18.5 and 18.6). If none exists, he or she informs the woman that she has been medically cleared to participate. The woman then fills out a detachable section of the PARχ for Pregnancy that confirms that medical clearance has been obtained and lists the name, address, and telephone number of her physician. This is returned to the prenatal fitness instructor who can then admit the women to exercise classes. The physician retains the remainder of the form and is encouraged to withdraw medical clearance by informing the woman and calling the prenatal fitness instructor if contraindications to physical activity develop. In addition to promoting this three-way communication, the process encourages responsibility on the part of the pregnant participant.

A closely related initiative by the Ontario Ministry of Tourism is the recent production of a manual titled *Fitness and the Childbearing Year* (Fitness Ontario Leadership Program, 1992). The manual will be used as the main textbook for workshops sponsored by the Fitness Ontario Leadership Program. Its content was designed in accordance with guidelines published by the National Fitness Leadership Advisory Committee (1989) for the training of specialty fitness leaders, and it replaces an earlier manual titled *Pre/Post Natal Fitness* (Fitness Ontario Leadership Program, 1983).

Fitness and the Childbearing Year is divided into five teaching units. Unit 1 provides both a practical rationale and philosophical basis for the promotion of active living during pregnancy. Anatomic, physiologic, and psychological effects of pregnancy are discussed in Unit 2, with a specific emphasis on the implications of these changes for the design of prenatal fitness classes. Unit 3 describes procedures for medical screening and the design and monitoring of muscular and aerobic conditioning programs as listed on the PAR-X/PARχ for Pregnancy form. A detailed rationale is provided for each subsection of the form (a copy of the PAR-X/PARχ for Pregnancy questionnaire is included as an appendix). Unit 4 includes helpful guidelines for the overall design of prenatal fitness classes. Unit 5 is devoted to procedures to aid in the return to active living following childbirth. This manual was written and edited by researchers from the Exercise/Pregnancy Research Program at Queen's University with input from a special advisory committee composed of experienced pre- and postnatal fitness instructors from across Ontario.

Summary and Conclusions

This chapter included original survey data that confirm that pregnant women are adopting more active lifestyles. Data related to pregnancy outcome in the population sample also support the view that regular, moderate physical activity does not alter pregnancy outcome. The study results also suggested that many physicians are either reluctant or lack essential information needed to advise pregnant patients concerning safe levels of activity. Thus, there is an urgent need to inform pregnant women, fitness leaders, and physicians about optimal methods for medical screening and exercise program design during pregnancy.

Recent collaborative projects funded by the Ontario Ministry of Tourism and Recreation have provided important educational materials that can be used for the safe and effective promotion of active living in pregnancy. Specifically, the PAR-X/PARχ for Pregnancy form originally designed by members of the Fitness Safety Standards Committee (1990) provides a simple, inexpensive method for use by physicians to clear women for exercise participation in pregnancy. Valid procedures for the safe prescription of aerobic and muscular conditioning exercise are also summarized. A manual published by the Fitness Ontario Leadership Program provides a complete curriculum for conducting workshops to train pre- and postnatal fitness leaders. Use of these new materials should be promoted actively by the Ministry of Tourism and Recreation. It is also recommended that these materials be revised as new scientific information becomes available.

Acknowledgments

The survey of physical activity patterns during pregnancy was performed in the Exercise and Pregnancy Research Laboratory under Dr. M.F. Mottola, director, with financial support from the Canadian Fitness and Lifestyle Research Institute.

We also received financial support for exercise/pregnancy research from the following agencies: Health and Welfare (Canada), Canadian Fitness and Lifestyle Research Institute, Ontario Ministry of Tourism and Recreation, Ontario Ministry of Health, Ontario Respiratory Diseases Foundation, and N.S.E.R.C. (Canada).

We wish to thank Michele C. Amey for expert typing of the final manuscript.

A copy of the PAR-X/PARχ for Pregnancy can be obtained by writing Dr. L.A. Wolfe, School of Physical and Health Education, Queen's University, Kingston, Ontario, K7L 3N6, Canada.

References

Ahlborg, G., Bodin, L., & Hogstedt, C. (1990). Heavy lifting during pregnancy—A hazard to the fetus? A prospective study. *Journal of Epidemiology* **19**, 90-97.

Alegre, A., Rodriguez-Essudero, F., Cruz, E., & Prada, M. (1984). Influence of work during pregnancy on fetal weight. *Journal of Reproductive Medicine,* **29**, 334-336.

American College of Obstetricians and Gynecologists. (1985). Pregnancy and the postnatal period. *ACOG home exercise programs* (pp. 1-5) Washington, DC: Author.

American College of Sports Medicine. (1991). *Guidelines for exercise testing and prescription* (4th ed.). Philadelphia: Lea & Febiger.

Brenner, I.K.M., Monga, M., Webb, K., McGrath, M.J., & Wolfe, L.A. (1991). Controlled prospective study of aerobic conditioning effects on pregnancy outcome (abstract). *Medicine and Science in Sports and Exercise,* **23**, S169.

Campbell, M.K. (in press). *Perinatal mortality in Ontario in 1987: Time trends, major determinants of mortality and directions for the future.* Toronto: Ontario Ministry of Health.

Canada Fitness Survey. (1981). Ottawa: Canada Fitness Survey.

Chisholm, D.M., Collis, M.L., Kulak, L.L., Davenport, W., & Gruber, N. (1975). Physical activity readiness. *British Columbia Medical Journal,* **17**, 375-378.

Creasy, R.K. (1991). Lifestyle influences on prematurity. *Journal of Developmental Physiology,* **15**, 15-20.

Fitness Canada. (1982). *Fitness and pregnancy: A leader's manual.* Ottawa: Fitness and Amateur Sport Canada.

Fitness Ontario Leadership Program. (1983). *Pre/post natal fitness.* Toronto: Ontario Ministry of Tourism and Recreation, Sports and Fitness Branch.

Fitness Ontario Leadership Program. (1992). *Fitness and the childbearing year.* Toronto: Ontario Ministry of Tourism and Recreation, Toronto.

Fitness Safety Standards Committee. (1990). *Final report to the Minister of Tourism and Recreation on the development of fitness safety standards in Ontario (Canada).* Ontario: Ontario Ministry of Tourism and Recreation.

Fox, M.E., Harris, R.E., & Brekken, E.L. (1977). The active military duty pregnancy: A new high risk category. *American Journal of Obstetrics and Gynecology,* **129**, 705-707.

Homer, C., Beresford, S., James, S., Siegel, E., & Wilcox, S. (1990). Work-related physical exertion and risk of preterm, low birthweight delivery. *Paediatric & Perinatal Epidemiology,* **4**, 161-174.

Manschande, J.P., Eckels, R., Manschande-Desmit, V., & Vlietinek, R. (1987). Rest versus heavy work during the last weeks of pregnancy: Influence on fetal growth. *British Journal of Obstetrics and Gynaecology,* **94**, 1059-1067.

McDonald, A., McDonald, J., Armstrong, B., Cherry, N., Cote, R., Lavoie, J., Nolin, A., & Robert, D.

(1988). Fetal death and work in pregnancy. *British Journal of Industrial Medicine, 45*, 148-157.

Murphy, J.E., Dauncey, M., Newcombe, R., Garcia, J., & Elbourne, D. (1984). Employment in pregnancy: Prevalence, maternal characteristics, perinatal outcomes. *Lancet, 1*, 1163-1166.

Naeye, R.L., & Peters, E.C. (1982). Working during pregnancy: Effects on the fetus. *Pediatrics, 69*, 724-727.

National Fitness Leadership Advisory Committee. (1989). *Fitness and the childbearing year specialty module.* Ottawa: Fitness and Amateur Sport Canada (Promotions and Communications).

Nelson, P.S., Gilbert, R.D., & Longo, L.D. (1983). Fetal growth and placental diffusing capacity in guinea pigs following long-term maternal exercise. *Journal of Developmental Physiology, 5*, 1-10.

Nurminen, T., Lusa, S., Ilmarinen, J., & Kurppa, K. (1989). Physical workload, fetal development and the course of pregnancy. *Scandinavian Journal of Work Environment and Health, 15*, 404-414.

Ohtake, P.J., Wolfe, L.A., Hall, P., & McGrath, M.J. (1988a). Physical conditioning effects on exercise heart rate and perception of exertion in pregnancy (abstract). *Canadian Journal of Sport Sciences, 13*, 71P-73P.

Ohtake, P.J., Wolfe, L.A., Hall, P., & McGrath, M. (1988b). Ventilatory responses to physical conditioning during pregnancy (abstract). *Physiologist, 31*, A158.

Ramirez, G., Grimes, R., Annegers, J., Davis, R., & Slater, C. (1990). Occupational physical activity and other risk factors for preterm birth among U.S. Army primigravidas. *American Journal of Public Health, 80*, 728-730.

Saurel-Cubizolles, M.J., & Kaminski, M. (1986). Work in pregnancy: Its evolving relationship with perinatal outcome (a review). *Social Science and Medicine, 22*, 431-442.

Statistics Canada. (1980). *Standard occupational classification.* Ottawa: Author.

Tafari, N., Naeye, R.L., & Gobeze, A. (1980). Effects of maternal undernutrition and heavy physical work during pregnancy on birth weight. *British Journal of Obstetrics and Gynaecology, 87*, 222-226.

Walker, R.M.C., Wolfe, L.A., Dumas, G.A., & McGrath, M.J. (1992). Plasma lactate responses of pregnant women to acute and chronic exercise (abstract). *Medicine and Science in Sports and Exercise, 24*, S170.

White, J. (1992). Exercising for two: What's safe for the active pregnant woman? *Physician and Sportsmedicine, 20*(5), 179-184, 186.

Wolfe, L.A. (in press). Pregnancy. In J.S. Skinner (Ed.), *Exercise testing and prescription for special cases: Theoretical bases and practical application* (2nd ed.). Philadelphia: Lea & Febiger.

Wolfe, L.A., Hall, P., Webb, K.A., Goodman, L.S., & McGrath, M.J. (1989). Prescription of aerobic exercise in pregnancy. *Sports Medicine, 8*, 273-301.

Wolfe, L.A., Ohtake, P.J., Mottola, M.F., & McGrath, M.J. (1989). Physiological interactions between pregnancy and aerobic exercise. *Exercise and Sport Sciences Reviews, 17*, 295-351.

Wolfe, L.A., Van Raay, A.M., Dumas, G.A., & McGrath, M.J. (1992). Perception of exertion in pregnancy: Aerobic conditioning effects (abstract). *Medicine and Science in Sports and Exercise, 24*, S170.

19

The School System and Active Living Programs for Children and Youth

Warren C. Campbell

The 1986 Canadian Summit on Fitness defined fitness as "a state of total well-being of the individual—physical, mental, emotional, spiritual and social" (Fitness Canada, 1986b, p. 7). This, then, was the origin of the concept of active living, "a way of life in which physical activity is valued and integrated into daily life" (Fitness Canada, 1991, p. 16).

The Ontario Ministry of Education's most recent physical education curriculum guideline defines fitness as "the term used to collectively define the moving and living skills knowledge, and behaviours essential to reaching the goal of a physically active, healthy lifestyle" (1988, p. 145). This definition correlates with the definition of fitness by the fitness summit members and subsequently labeled active living.

Background

Although the concept of physical fitness has changed over the years, the educational environment has consistently projected, or perhaps reflected, the current concept of fitness held by the Canadian public. Fitness has evolved from a strictly physical concept of the ability to generate energy—"Physical fitness is the ability of an individual to have the energy to get through a normal day's work, to be involved in leisure time pursuits and to have a reserve of energy for emergencies" (Scarborough Board of Education, 1956, p. 2)—to a much broader definition encompassing "a state of total well-being of the individual—physical, mental, emotional, spiritual and social" (Fitness Canada, 1986b, p. 7). What brought about this change?

The conclusions of the Canada Fitness Survey of 1981 precipitated a series of events resulting in the current focus recommended by professionals. The Canada Fitness Survey stimulated three important areas of involvement with children and youth:

1. a focus by the Federal Government on a Federal–Provincial/Territorial Task Force on Youth and the formation of a Youth Secretariat;
2. the sponsoring of the Canadian Symposium on Youth Fitness in 1985; and
3. the organization and initiation of the Canadian Summit on Fitness in 1986.

It was at this summit on fitness that experts from all provinces and territories, representing every aspect of the profession, looked at the concept of fitness in Canada and projected it to the year 2000. All levels of education participated in this conference, representing the interests and beliefs of the current school systems with respect to fitness and active living. The outcome of the summit was a much broader, more inclusive definition of fitness. It provided a more realistic and reachable set of goals for the population, including those students who felt excluded from the traditional concept of fitness. The new set of goals demands that the schools assume a more significant role in the active living cycle.

The Current Situation in Canadian Schools

Traditionally, the elementary school physical education program has been taught by the classroom teacher, regardless of his or her qualifications. A possible exception to this is in Manitoba, where closer attention has been paid to the problem of the classroom teacher and physical education. In the past, very little training, curriculum, and assistance has been available to the classroom teachers. Fortunately, over the last 10 years, Canadian students have benefited from a greater use of physical education specialists, improved teacher training programs, and a strong emphasis on curriculum development. In some provinces larger school boards have improved program development and delivery, although smaller districts must struggle to find sources of curriculum materials. In other provinces, education departments have developed curricula, identified resources, and initiated inservice programs.

In 1986 the Quality, Daily, Physical Education (QDPE) program was launched by the Canadian Association of Health, Physical Education and Recreation (CAHPER), together with Fitness Canada. This program has had a significant effect on increasing the time and quality of the elementary school physical education program. Secondary schools, on the other hand, have traditionally hired professional physical educators and have worked independently with their curricular and cocurricular program.

After universities started to deemphasize the teacher-oriented physical education programs of the 1950s and '60s, physical education teachers studied more scientific and generalized subjects in their undergraduate work, subjects not specifically oriented to teaching. Some observers believe that the new emphasis has preempted the importance of the classroom program and that it is a factor in fewer students selecting physical education.

Other factors have reduced physical education enrollments in secondary schools. Most provincial and territorial education departments have changed physical education programs in our secondary schools from compulsory to optional. Research indicates that students select more "important" subjects in lieu of physical education. The concern about declining enrollments in secondary school programs has been heightened by the lack of status these programs have with education decision makers. The QDPE program, however, has made a significant impact on the school program, as documented in a 1991 Gallup poll:

- 36.6% of Canadian schools (about 5,500 schools) are currently providing daily physical education for at least a portion of their student population (p. 2).
- 31.4% of those schools (about 1,725) provide daily physical education for all of their students (p. 5).
- 18.2% of the schools in Canada (about 2,730) have a plan in place to increase the amount of daily physical education being provided (p. 7).

Although no baseline figures are available, these figures indicate a significant improvement since the early 1980s in the time allocated to physical education in Canadian schools. The significance of the CAHPER and Fitness Canada's efforts through the QDPE program are obvious—Gallup showed that 49.4% of the schools in Canada (about 7,410 schools) indicate that they are aware of the QDPE program and 43.1% of the schools involved have initiated their program since 1986, the year the QDPE program was begun.

Community support is growing. Many provincial and national organizations have prepared position papers supporting QDPE. The Canadian Medical Association, the Heart and Stroke Foundation of Canada, the Canadian Chiropractic Association, and the Canadian Home and School Association are among the many provincial and national groups that support the concept of quality, daily physical education. Education decision makers are responding to the overwhelming influx of supportive information and professional commitment.

School physical and health education programs are on a roll; change is starting to occur. The task now is to direct this activity to "instill in learners the knowledge, skills and attitudes necessary to embrace active living," that is, to take advantage of the opportunities available in the current educational environment for a balanced physical and health education program that will meet the needs of all children. These goals of physical education in Canadian schools are representative of the philosophy and concepts declared at the fitness summit and conceptualized in the active living movement. However, some questions remain unanswered: Are school physical education programs addressing all the current objectives (i.e., the development of knowledge, skills, and attitudes necessary to embrace active living) or are they addressing only some of them? Have we evaluated our school physical education programs to ensure that they are designed to include all students? Do these programs include those whose activity choices differ from the norm? In support of our current programs, it should be noted that some teachers have, in part, responded to student feedback and have adapted their curricula over the years. Team-oriented programs still influence our choices, most of the students who are currently involved in physical education like these programs and wish to continue. But we must now provide alternatives for those students who do not accept the current syllabus and are looking for other activities to experience the fitness adventure.

What Challenges Face School Physical Educators?

"The epidemic of lifestyle related diseases is an educational failure, not a medical failure" (Bailey, 1989, p. 4). The model adapted from Godbout and colleagues (1991), and presented by Gauvin, Wall, and Quinney (in chapter 1) provides the foundation from which to outline the challenges that face physical educators in Canadian schools.

The Practitioners

Many teachers involved in physical education will have to change their mind-set. Generalist teachers at the elementary level will continue to face the current dilemma. In the immediate future, they will learn on the job, desperate to acquire some semblance of expertise in physical education. Positive changes are occurring: Some school boards, such as Hamilton's, have used teachers' class preparation time for a specialist to teach physical education or assist the classroom teachers' efforts. Secondary school programs are changing, but they must change more quickly to avoid a mass exodus of students to more "important" subjects. There is a need for women and visible minorities to become more involved.

Certainly, a broader selection of physical activity alternatives will accommodate all students but such a proposal precipitates additional queries. Many school practitioners are concerned with how the interpretation of active living might affect physical education curriculum development. Because various levels of government can be flexible in their interpretation, there is a fear of a watered down program, void of challenges, lacking in structure and direction, and deprived of specifics. The strength of the active living concept may be viewed by some as its weakness. These critics believe that active living must be directed at discrete stages of an individual's development. CAHPER has responded to this concern and is currently drafting a foundations document to clarify its concept of active living and its position with respect to physical education in our schools.

> Active Living is a way of life in which physical activity is valued and integrated daily. Quality, Daily Physical Education means a planned program of instruction and activity for all students on a daily basis throughout the entire school year. QDPE provides learners with the knowledge, skills, and attitudes that enables them to embrace active living. QDPE is the key to Active Living in schools and the means by which it is fully achieved (Robins, 1987, p. 16).

Program Managers

The physical education department head, chairman, or contact teacher in a school assumes the responsibility of the program manager whose primary function is to promote program development, delivery, and evaluation. Presently, our settled teaching population does not lend itself to experimentation and innovation. It does, however, serve as a starting point to look at the immediate future and seek out creative and innovative supervisory personnel.

Executives

Perhaps the most significant challenge facing physical education practitioners rests with the executives (i.e., trustees and administrators), in the model adapted from Godbout and colleagues (1991). We must convince them to be proactive. "Imagine that public-health authorities had an immunizing agent that was effective against a variety of degenerative diseases that was withheld or applied sporadically and haphazardly. The outrage would be widespread and justifiable" (Pipe, 1989, p. B-4). Physical educators deal with three levels of government that may be reluctant to communicate among themselves and are, in many cases, developing policies and making decisions based on political realities rather than research or advice from professionals. Knowledge of the outcome of physical activity, or a lack of it, does not penetrate the political shield of these executives. School trustees and senior administrators are more susceptible to fads. Provincial decision makers are tuned in to larger lobbies and federal spokespersons are refused entry into this predetermined provincial jurisdiction. All too often, a philosophy of "pay me now or pay me later" allows policy makers to direct their priorities to a more politically astute audience. As educators, we must enlist the powers of science and the scholars in our field to react to these decisions and delineate the long-term solutions.

The Consultants

The study conducted by Robins (1987) indicated that consultants have an important role to play in increasing physical education time and in improving the quality of the programs. The strong cadre of consultants developed over the 1970s and '80s has been quietly diluted. Physical education consultants involved in curriculum development, implementation, and problem solving are being eliminated or replaced with generalists responsible for a wide range of educational curriculum. For example, the Calgary Board of Education has eliminated its physical education department, which produced resources presently found in most Canadian school districts. Its *Basic Skill Series* has sold more than 60,000 copies and provided a professional foundation for many programs.

The demise of such programs results in a vacuum in problem solving. Many permanent consultants are being replaced with term appointments, which tends to deplete the current practical knowledge and resource base. In Ontario, attendance at the Ontario Association for the Supervision of Physical and Health Education (OASPHE) conference in 1992 was half the attendance of 10 years earlier. Some school boards have delegated responsibility to current teaching staff. In many cases, their reward or remuneration is the designation of "super teacher."

What Are the Solutions?

The school provides the most important environment in which to instill the values and concepts of active living. It can be the environment where all of the positive (and, unfortunately, negative) social, psychological, and physiological dimensions flourish. We have a captive audience. All areas of society are aware of this fact and, as a result, there is a tremendous demand on the time available during the school day. Therefore, we must promote the importance of physical education and its relationship to the concept of active living. This will not be easy. In general, the public has a misconception of what physical education in the schools is or should be; many people associate the physical education program solely with interschool sports programs and gauge its effectiveness by the win–loss record. This misconception complicates any vision of what can be and what should be. We must therefore take advantage of every possible opportunity to promote physical education and its relationship to the active living concept.

Many of our teachers across the country, particularly in our elementary schools, are ill prepared to teach physical education in the classroom. This lack of preparation adds to the difficulty of advancing the concept of active living in our schools and highlights the need for more professional development and a greater emphasis on school physical education. This situation, coupled with the fact that policy setters and change agents (trustees and senior administrators) are ill prepared to develop creative policies with respect to physical education, demands immediate response. The time is right for a significant change.

Teacher Training

The teacher cycle has run its course, and within the next 5 to 8 years there will be a revolution in teacher recruitment that may parallel or surpass that of the early 1960s. With retirements at an all-time high, young professionals will once again play a significant role in program enhancement. The key then is more knowledgeable change agents and increased emphasis and time spent on teacher training in physical education. Some teacher training programs, such as those of UBC and York, have partially addressed this lack and have increased their emphasis on school physical education pedagogy.

Every problem we have with school physical educators is prevalent to some degree among teacher educators. This is an appropriate time for program revision in teacher training, because many of our university staffs are entering a similar period of turnover and change. An in-depth training program is needed that focuses on school physical education, that will convince teachers in training that such programs are important to all students, and that will instill in these young teachers a vitality that demands success. Too often our current teachers direct tremendous energy to one aspect of the program at the expense of other areas. It is in their professional training that young physical education teachers will be influenced and provided with the incentives to promote the concept of active living through a sound physical education program. It is important that universities improve their communication and efforts

to share ideas. As a result, teachers of teachers will better understand the concept of active living and be better able to apply it to school physical education. To this end, a national conference, Active and Healthy Living: A Dialogue on Teacher Preparation, was held in March 1990 (Shannon & McCall, 1990). It is hoped that this conference will stimulate greater understanding and better communication among provincial education teacher training programs.

Marketing

We must take advantage of the current and future community marketing programs that are associated with active living. Nationally and provincially, professional organizations must be aggressive in their interest and involvement. A good example of this is the inclusion of QDPE information on two Body Break public service announcements produced by ParticipACTION and cosponsored by CAHPER and Fitness Canada. As educators, we should welcome involvement with and support from other agencies. In a marketing strategy prepared by ParticipACTION for the Ontario Ministry of Tourism and Recreation, the schools have been clearly invited to be involved. All too often, education lags behind other ministries or departments or divorces itself from programs initiated by other government agencies. It is important for physical educators to be a part of local marketing programs and to use this involvement to integrate, enhance, and promote school programs.

Research

Physical education researchers must address the school as a valuable research environment. As practitioners we must collaborate with our colleagues in the sport sciences and do more research in our classrooms. We have the laboratories, subjects, and longevity to pursue important questions. The process will enhance and promote our programs in the school and the community. We must remember that research results are not good or bad in themselves but rather are information that can be useful in supporting or improving our physical education curriculum.

Professional Organizations

Recently we have experienced a rise in the popularity and prestige of provincial professional organizations. Memberships have increased, organization has improved, and professional development programs and local conferences have flourished, often surpassing national memberships and conferences. National organizations have a significant role to play, but they do it best in concert with the provincial groups. For example, for the past 5 years CAHPER has provided the opportunity for provincial organizations to meet and share ideas. Its effort in promoting QDPE through provincial organizations is an excellent example of national and provincial cooperation. CAHPER also plays an important yet difficult role in bringing together theory and practice. CAHPER and the Canadian Intramural Recreation Association (CIRA) are playing an important role in the development of active living programs in schools. It appears that although national organizations can draw on vast resources and expertise, they must also rely on grassroots contact with school physical educators, as provincial organizations do. National and provincial organizations must work together to be effective. In addition, provincial organizations have developed a close association with provincial recreation departments over the years. It is this network, together with the key position of provincial–territorial physical education associations, that will help implement the concept of active living.

Conclusion

The Canadian Summit on Fitness provided a unique opportunity for Canadian professionals to look at the concept of fitness in the future. The concept of active living, although not entirely new, more clearly reflects the directions our school programs will take. Many of our teachers across the country are ill prepared to teach this comprehensive program. In addition, policy setters and educational change agents lack the proper mindset and motives to set policies with respect to school physical education. Physical education in Canadian schools is much different today from what it was 25 years ago, and we have the opportunity to reach every one of our children and youth. We must continue to improve our own professional network, taking advantage of the current popularity of activity in the community and the efforts of other organizations and institutions. Most important, teacher training at all levels will provide the foundation from which school programs can evolve. My own professional training included many of the concepts encompassed in the active living philosophy. Although I enjoyed my experiences in crafts, oil painting, recreational activities, skiing, and camping, I must confess, at the time I was a little tentative in admitting to them as part of an undergraduate program. This was a mistake and I hope others can find the secrets to achieving wisdom with youth. How many times have we come to realize that those "loonies" of the past were in fact the "prophets" of the future?

References

Bailey, D. (1989). *R. Tait McKenzie Address*, CAHPER Conference, Halifax, Nova Scotia.

Canadian Youth Foundation. (1990, March). *Youth views on physical activity*.

Dahlgren, W. (1988). *Young females and physical activity*. Internal report. Ottawa: Fitness Canada.

Edwards, P. (1990). *A healthy city is an active city: A strategic framework for promotion of active living at the community or city level*. Internal report.

Fitness Canada. (1985). *Choices and challenges: A status report on youth physical activity programs in Canada*. Ottawa: Author.

Fitness Canada. (1986a). *Fitness fits! The Canadian Symposium on Youth Fitness*. Ottawa: Author.

Fitness Canada. (1986b). *Fitness . . . the Future—The Canadian Summit on Fitness*. Ottawa: Author.

Fitness Canada. (1989). *Because they're young: Active living for Canadian children and youth*. Ottawa: Author.

Fitness Canada. (1990). *From blueprints to action: An invitation to act*. Ottawa: Author.

Fitness Canada. (1991). *Active living: A conceptual overview*. Ottawa, Ontario: Government of Canada.

Focus on Active Living '92 Secretariat. (1992). *Building active living in your community: A research kit*. Toronto: Ministry of Tourism & Recreation.

Gagan, M. (1985). *Marketing fitness to Canadian youth*. Ottawa: Fitness Canada.

Gallup. (1991). *A survey of daily physical education in Canadian schools*. Ottawa: CAHPER.

Godbout, P., Samson, J., & Bérubé, G. (1991). The service component of the physical activity sciences. In C. Bouchard, B.D. McPherson, & A.W. Taylor (Eds.), *Physical activity sciences*. (pp. 131-138). Champaign, IL: Human Kinetics.

Ontario Ministry of Education. (1988). *Curriculum guideline—Physical and health education, validation draft*. Toronto: Ontario Ministry of Education.

Ontario Ministry of Tourism & Recreation. *Active living for kids*. Toronto: Author.

ParticipACTION Ontario. (1991). *Active living '92 . . . and beyond: An implementation strategy for the Government of Ontario Ministry of Tourism and Recreation*.

Pipe, A. (1989, September 14). Time for our children to get (and stay) fit. *Globe and Mail*, p. L1.

Posterski, D., & Bibby, R. (1989). Canada's youth "ready for today." Ottawa: Youth Secretariat.

Robins, S.G. (1987). A survey of schools with a Quality, Daily, Physical Education Program. *CAHPER Journal*, **53**(6).

Scarborough Board of Education. (1956). *W.A. Porter C.I.—Health education curriculum guide*. Scarborough, ON: W.C. Campbell & Associates.

Shannon & McCall Consulting Ltd. (1990). *Active and healthy living: A dialogue on teacher preparation. A national status report*. Ottawa: Fitness Canada.

Zitzelsberger, L. (1989). *Physical activity and the child: Review and synthesis*. Ottawa: Fitness Canada.

20

Age Is Not a Barrier: A Personal Experience

Per-Olof Åstrand

There is unanimous agreement that regular physical activity is essential for optimal function of the human body. In a recent review I summarized positive effects of such activities, mainly based on research in physiology and medicine (Åstrand, 1992).

Children and Adolescents

We tend to make age a barrier, there is too much emphasis on chronological age, and this is actually a recent strategy in human history. The fact that children and adolescents mature with a wide range in chronological age complicates education, particularly in sports, because we usually classify students according to age. Tanner (1981) established the framework of biological age. By regular measurements of physical characteristics such as height and weight at least twice a year, and observations on the development of secondary sex characteristics and skeletal maturity, the maturity of the young individual may be followed. A longitudinal recording of height, which is easy to do, gives a good picture of the onset of puberty. Figure 20.1 shows the distribution of chronological age at peak height velocity age (PHVage) for 357 girls and 373 boys followed from age 9 up to ages 16 and 18, respectively (Lindgren, 1978). In average, the increase in height at PHVage was 8 cm for girls and 10 cm for boys. The girls' first menstruation normally occurs soon after this accelerated growth spurt, with a time lag of about 1 year. In this group, PHVage occurred as early as age 9.5 years for some girls but not until the age of 15 years for others.

In boys the range was from 11 to 17 years of age. With regard to sexual maturity, the girls were approximately 2 years ahead of the boys. From a biological viewpoint, data on physical performances, lung functions, maximal aerobic and anaerobic power, muscle strength, and effects of training should, when possible, be evaluated with biological age as a baseline (i.e., with PHVage as a midpoint). A prolem is that we cannot predict when a child will reach PHVage (see Malina & Bouchard, 1991).

How important are habitual physical activities during childhood and adolescence for optimal development, for prevention of various diseases during that time, and for the person's health in the future? Which educational system is optimal to create a positive attitude and life-long interest in sports? We know very little. One problem in physical education classes is the wide range in fitness and interest. It has been pointed out that maturation age differs markedly. At chronological age 13 years we can find a boy with a weight 30 kg and a height 130 cm, and his classmate may weigh 80 kg and be 180 cm tall. Leg strength can be 150 N and 850 N, respectively. Because of such differences, it is a challenge to be a physical education teacher.

How physically active are children and adolescents in the educational system and during leisure time? In many industrial countries compulsory time for physical education in schools and colleges is being reduced. I find this trend very unfortunate, particularly for individuals who do not choose sports and outdoor activities

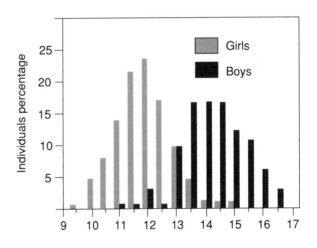

Figure 20.1 Distribution of age at peak height velocity age (PHVage) for girls ($n = 357$) and boys ($n = 373$) (adapted from Lindgren, 1978).

147

during their leisure time. It is interesting to note that when I attended "gymnasium" (at age 16 to 19 years) some 50 years ago, we had compulsory physical education four times per week for 40 min per session plus 12 full days reserved per year for recreational activities dominated by sports. Today students attend physical education classes two or three times per week, for 40 to 60 min, or less, and only a few days are available for recreational activities per year. I would prefer a curriculum with daily physical education.

Engström (1990) used questionnaires to map out frequency of recreational physical activities in random samples in various areas of Sweden, including a group of approximately 2,000 females and males. The study was longitudinal starting at age 15. Strenuous exercise was defined as sports and keep-fit activities performed at least once a week with a level of strain comparable to that of jogging, aerobics, swimming, or playing ball games. The results are presented in Figure 20.2. For both men and women there is a quite dramatic downhill slope from age 15 to 20 years. Then men reach a plateau with 50% exercising at least once a week. For the women there is an increase from 30% to 40% from ages 25 to 30. If the level of effort is increased to involve engagements several times a week at a relatively high level of strain, the proportion of participants decreases from approximately 70% in the 15-year-old male group to 20% and from 45% to about 3% at the age of 30 years for women (Engström, 1986). These figures do not support the general conception that Swedes devote much time to keeping physically fit. One excuse for the women can be that many of them were mothers with young children.

In my opinion it is an advantage that competitive sports in Sweden are organized by clubs within the Swedish Sports Federation. Therefore, physical education in the schools is basically "sports for all" with little emphasis on competition. Engström (1990) found that between 1968 and 1984 there was an impressive increase in the percentage of 15-year-olds who belong to sports clubs; the percentage of boys increased from 50% to 70%, and the percentage of girls increased from approximately 17% to 50%. However, the total number of active young people has diminished. The explanation is that in 1984 almost none were involved in sports during leisure time unless they were members of a sports club (see Figure 20.3).

The curriculum in physical education is quite different in different countries, but the drop in sports participation after high school/college is relatively universal. Therefore, the key factor behind this reduced physical activity is probably not the experiences during lectures in physical education but simply a consequence of human nature.

Training: How to Find Talent for Competitive Sports

Rowland (1992) recently summarized the literature related to effects of training with emphasis on aerobic

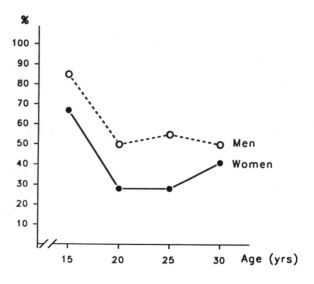

Figure 20.2 The proportion of regularly active females and males age 15 to 30 years, as found in a longitudinal study. The lowest acceptable level of strain was defined as jogging or corresponding activities once a week (adapted from Engström, 1990).

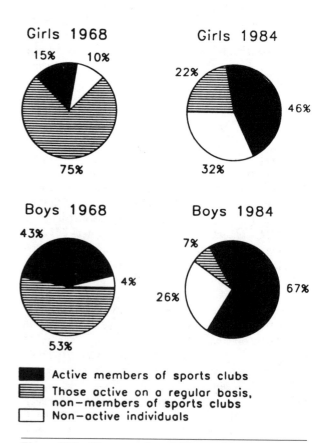

Figure 20.3 The proportion of 15-year-old sports participants within and outside sports clubs in 1968 and 1984. The lowest acceptable level of strain was defined as walking once a week (qdapted from Engström, 1990).

responses in children. He concluded that prepubertal children appear to be capable of responding to endurance training with improvements in maximal aerobic power. Such adaptations are qualitatively similar to but probably quantitatively less than those of adults. Froberg, Anderson, and Lammert (1991) reported that the period extending from 2 years to 1 year before PHVage is one in which intense high-volume training can increase relative maximal aerobic power to the same degree as seen in adults.

In this context it should be mentioned that the five best Swedish male tennis players (of 1985) were engaged in many sports before age 14, at which age they started to specialize in tennis. At the time of the study they ranked among the top 15 players in the world. They were compared with a control group who were as good or better at tennis when 12 to 14 years old. The control players specialized much ealier in tennis, trained more, and matured earlier. Therefore, the controls performed well but apparently they were not gifted enough to reach world class (Carlson, 1988). It is best if children and young teenagers try many sports and do not concentrate on one event until after PHVage. In my opinion, competition in marathons and triathlons should not be allowed before age 18. This is one case in which age should be a barrier.

One conclusion from the mentioned study of tennis players is that performance at ages 12 to 14 is not a good predictor of future elite achievements. Malina (1990) pointed out that with few exceptions, interage correlations for indicators of growth, fitness, and cardiovascular status are generally moderate to low and thus have limited predictive utility. A boy who starts specializing in high jump or basketball and stops growing when 170 cm tall has picked the wrong event.

Human Aging:
Usual and Successful

Rowe and Kahn (1987) stated that

> research in aging has emphasized average age-related losses and neglected the substantial heterogeneity of older persons. The effects of the aging process itself have been exaggerated, and the modifying effects of diet, exercise, personal habits, and psychosocial factors underestimated. Within the category of normal aging a distinction can be made between usual aging in which extrinsic factors heighten the effects of aging alone, and successful aging, in which extrinsic factors play a neutral or positive role. Research on the risks associated with usual aging and strategies to modify them should help elucidate how a transition from usual to successful aging can be facilitated.

Relevant to this point are cross-sectional data indicating that maximal oxygen uptake peaks in the late teenage years and then gradually declines (see Åstrand and Rodahl, 1986). Data on maximal stroke volume and cardiac output follow a similar pattern. In cross-sectional studies, maximal strength in isometric and dynamic activations peaks around 25 years of age; then it drops and the slope is similar as for maximal oxygen uptake. The key question is to what extent functional impairments with age beyond the 2nd to 3rd decade are inevitable consequences of the individual's innate genetic composition (i.e., intrinsic factors) and to which extent the individual's lifestyle (i.e., extrinsic factors) can modify the picture. The same reasoning can be applied to analysis of morbidity and mortality. A decline in maximal oxygen uptake of 10% per decade is considered normal. However, it is well documented that training can improve this maximum from a few percent up to 100% depending on the individual's initial fitness, his or her potential to respond to training, and intensity and duration of training (see Åstrand & Rodahl, 1986, chapter 10). In this regard, one longitudinal study reported by Åstrand and Rodahl (1986) is enlightening. Maximal oxygen uptake was measured here in a group of subjects. At the first occasion the subjects were students in physical education. At the second occasion, 21 years later, the maximal aerobic power was on average 20% less. However, 12 years later the women had maintained their maximum. For the men there was an average decline of 4%. There were marked individual variations, however, in both groups. In 1949 two subjects had both $4.0 \text{ L} \cdot \text{min}^{-1}$ as maximal oxygen uptake. In 1982 one of them had, at age 61 years, the same maximum but his colleague, age 65, only attained $2.0 \text{ L} \cdot \text{min}^{-1}$. The latter was gradually forced into a relatively sedentary lifestyle due to rheumatoid arthritis. The 4-L man was very active and ran marathons. These two cases illustrate how critical lifestyle can be for the aging effect on the potential of the oxygen transport system. The percentage improvement in maximal oxygen uptake in elderly individuals is the same as in young people when both groups undergo similar training regimes (see Åstrand, 1992).

Åstrand and Rodahl (1986) examined maximal oxygen uptake values as a function of years of age. To underscore the role of age in training regimens, we can consider the fact that the oxygen demand during walking at a speed of $5 \text{ km} \cdot \text{hr}^{-1}$ for persons with weights of 75 and 100 kg are $1.0 \text{ L} \cdot \text{min}^{-1}$ and $1.5 \text{ L} \cdot \text{min}^{-1}$, respectively. It is evident that the margin between maximal oxygen uptake and the demand during walking is reduced with aging. It should be emphasized that the data on maximal oxygen uptake were based on measurements of relatively well-trained subjects. Even so, for people who are overweight, just walking can tax the oxygen transport system to its maximum at age 50 years for a woman or age 70 years for a man (mean values minus 2 *SD*). Six weeks of training at a power that only demands submaximal oxygen uptake can improve the maximal aerobic power some 15% to 20%, which may decrease biological age 15 to 20 years.

In a recent study, nine frail, institutionalized women and men, mean age 90, range 86 to 96 years, undertook 8 weeks of high-intensity resistance training (Fiatarone et al., 1990). Strength gain averaged 174% ± 31% and midthigh muscle area increased 9.0% ± 4.5%. Apparently the functional response to training is positive up to very high ages.

There is a dramatic increase in the proportion of the population age 80 years and over. As mentioned, aging is "normally" associated with reduced maximal aerobic power and reduced muscle strength (i.e., with reduced physical fitness). Being overweight in addition to these handicaps is unfortunate because these factors taken together make walking, climbing stairs, getting up from bed or a chair, or entering a bus or train more difficult and fatiguing and eventually impossible. The ability to lift and carry weights becomes reduced. The aging person will lose her or his independence and autonomy. As a consequence of diminished exercise tolerance, a large and increasing number of elderly persons live below, at, or just above "thresholds" of physical ability to render them completely dependent.

Now we are back to the question of intrinsic and extrinsic factors in the deteriorations typical for aging. Again, training can readily produce a profound improvement of functions essential for physical fitness in old age and thus effectively postpone physical deterioration for some 10 to 20 years. In a sense, retired people have all the time they need to keep themselves physically fit. Unfortunately, various diseases and handicaps can prevent exercise. Rowe and Kahn (1987) argued that "a direct-assistance treatment is typical of approaches to older people that do for them what they could do or learn to do for themselves. The effect is infantilizing; the lesson is learning helplessness." The body will quickly adapt to reduced demands on muscle activities, resulting in an accelerated rate of functional impairment and reduced physical fitness. In addition, a sedentary lifestyle is a risk factor for coronary heart disease, high blood pressure, unfavorable blood lipid profile, reduced glucose tolerance, hyperinsulinemia, and osteoporosis (see Åstrand, 1992).

Life Expectancy

In the United States life expectancy increased from 47 years of age in 1900 to approximately 75 years of age in 1988. What about upper limits to human longevity? It has been calculated that eliminating ischemic heart disease would only increase life expectancy at birth by 3.0 years for females and 3.5 years for males (see Figure 20.4). Eliminating all forms of cancer (22.5% of all

death in 1985) would increase life expectancy by 7.0 years for females and 8.1 years for males (see Figure 20.4) (Olshansky, Carnes, & Cassel, 1990). In other words, the effects of eliminating major diseases on life expectancy are not dramatic. Advances in medical treatment more than improvements in risk factors may be allowing elderly persons who are frail and who suffer from fatal degenerative diseases to survive longer after the onset of the disease than was the case in the past. Current research efforts by the medical community are focused on prolonging life rather than preserving the quality of life. An obvious conclusion, therefore, is that the time has come for a shift toward ameliorating the quality of life for people with nonfatal diseases of aging (Olshansky et al., 1990). One may conclude that the relationship between aging and various diseases—and physical fitness—has become abnormal in our modern society. Over millions of years the older person was very important and respected in society because she or he was credited with experience essential for the well-being and survival of the people. Therefore, the aging individual was still an important member of the group. A compulsory retirement at a given age is also a new invention in human history.

I grew up in the countryside. At that time, when the farmer could not continue to work full-time, one of the farmer's children would take over the farm. The old farmer was the teacher, providing generations of experiences and practices and still working behind the plough, chopping firewood, and swinging the scythe. The elderly person was still important and active. Then modern techniques, tools, machines, and fertilizers appeared on the market and the old farmer's knowledge became useless. Again, this is a new situation in human history.

Active Recreation

By *active recreation* I mean a kind of hobby that involves some form of muscular exercise. Examples of passive recreation are watching TV, attending a concert or opera, playing cards or chess, and collecting stamps. Both active and passive recreation should be something to look forward to with joy and expectation every day. Recreational activities in the open air are well anchored in our biological heritage; education in "flora and fauna" was once very essential. A similar education today, unfortunately much neglected, could create a lifelong interest and promote excellent hobby activities. There are those who do not like walking just for the sake of walking, but a hobby like bird-watching might spur them to walk. In addition, knowledge in biology in a broad sense can teach us how to help our planet, endangered by human behaviors, to survive. Humanity is exposed to situations that millions of years of ancestors' experiences do not help.

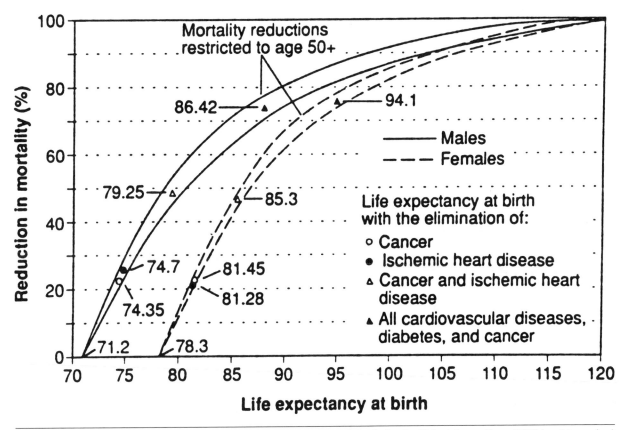

Figure 20.4 Percentage of reduction in the conditional probability of death for the United States (from 1985 levels) required to produce a life expectancy at birth from 80 to 120 years (adapted from Olshansky, Carnes, & Cassel, 1990).

In the 1950s we launched the idea that simple training tracks should be built. In Sweden they have sprung up like mushrooms. They are located in parks or other suitable areas, have smooth surfaces that are often covered with a mixture of sand and sawdust, and are 2 to 3 km or more long and a good 1 m wide. The winding cross-country track is frequently illuminated, since the Swedish winter is dark, and provides excellent facilities for cross-country skiing. With the Swedish climate it would be tough to rely exclusively on outdoor activities. All facilities for physical activities connected with schools and universities are available for the public after ordinary school hours. In other words, the administration and maintenance of sport grounds, swimming pools, and sport buildings are joint efforts between state, school, and community.

My 15-km trip from home to work in the center of Stockholm is often taken on bicycle. Most of the ride is on a separate lane free from motor vehicles! In Sweden the laws are quite generous to those who love outdoor activities. By law, forests, beaches, and non-cultivated territories are available for everyone, independent of ownership. Picking berries and mushrooms is free. Most trade unions organize major sport programs and various outdoor actvities (games, skating, bicycling,

and walking, often as family activities). Such activities are subsidized by the company.

How Important Is a Medical Examination Before Training Starts?

I remember conferences and symposia in the 1960s devoted to sports medicine, fitness, health, and well-being. Usually experts in exercise physiology were first on stage presenting positive effects of habitual physical activity. Then came epidemiologists and cardiologists. There were many reports of physical inactivity being a risk factor for ischemic heart disease. The conclusion was, however, that a "stress test," with recordings of electrocardiograms (ECG) and so forth, must be conducted before participation in a training program could be permitted. I eventually raised the question whether there were enough qualified physicians available to do the stress testing and analyze the ECG and test results, particularly if a drive for more exercise was successful. Of course, anyone who is in doubt about her or his health should consult a physician.

However, my conclusion was that a medical examination is more urgent for those who intend to remain sedentary than for those who want to get into good physical shape by training. I also remember that I was taken by the police in Chicago, I think it was in 1963, because I was out jogging . . .

Concluding Remarks

Physicians in general have been quite passive in promoting the effects of lifestyle on fitness and health. One explanation can be that few pages in standard textbooks of physiology and medicine are devoted to discussions of the effects of exercise on different functions and structures. It is time for a change.

Jogging is now accepted as a quite normal behavior. I am afraid that hope for remodeling cities to permit safe play for children, to allow safe walking and bicycling, and to provide inexpensive access to facilities for recreational activities indoors and outdoors for all ages will just be a dream.

References

Åstrand, P.-O. (1992). Why exercise. *Medicine and Science in Sports and Exercise.* **24**, 153-162.

Åstrand, P.-O., & Rodahl, K. (1986). *Textbook of work physiology.* New York: McGraw-Hill.

Carlson, R. (1988). The socialization of elite tennis players in Sweden: An analysis of the players' backgrounds and development. *Sociology of Sport Journal,* **5**, 241-256.

Engström, L.-M. (1986). The process of socialization into keep-fit activities. *Scandinavian Journal of Sports Sciences,* **81**, 89-97.

Engström, L.-M. (1990). Sports activities among young people in Sweden—trends and changes. In R. Telema, L. Laakso, M. Piéron, I. Ruoppila, & V. Vihko (Eds.), *Physical activity and life-long physical activity* (Report of physical culture and health 73) (pp. 11-23). Jyväskylä.

Fiatarone, M.A., Marks, E.C., Ryan, N.D., Meredith, C.N., Lipitz, L.A., & Evans, W.J. (1990). High-intensity strength training in nonagenarians. *Journal of the American Medical Association,* **263**, 3029-3034.

Froberg, K., Anderson, B., & Lammert, O. (1991). Maximal oxygen uptake and respiratory function during puberty in boy groups of different physical activity. In R. Franke & I. Szmodis (Eds.), *Pediatric work physiology: XV. Children and exercise* (pp. 265-280). Budapest: National Institute for Health Promotion.

Lindgren, G. (1978). Growth of school children with early, average and late ages of peak height velocity. *Annals of Human Biology,* **5**, 253-267.

Malina, R.M. (1990). Growth, exercise, fitness, and later outcomes. In C. Bouchard, R.J. Shephard, T. Stephens, J.R. Sutton, & B.D. McPherson (Eds.), *Exercise, fitness, and health: A consensus of current knowledge* (pp. 637-653). Champaign, IL: Human Kinetics.

Malina, R.M., & Bouchard, C. (1991). *Growth, maturation, and physical activity.* Champaign, IL: Human Kinetics.

Olshansky, S.J., Carnes, B.A., & Cassel, C. (1990). In search of Methusalah: Estimating the upper limit to human longevity. *Science,* **250**, 634-640.

Rowe, J.W., & Kahn, R.L. (1987). Human aging: Useful and successful. *Science,* **237**, 143-149.

Rowland, T.W. (1992). Aerobic responses to physical training in children. In R.J. Shephard & P.-O. Åstrand (Eds.), *Endurance in sports* (pp. 381-389). London: Blackwell Scientific.

Tanner, J.M. (1981). *A history of the study of human growth.* Cambridge, UK: Cambrdige University Press.

21

Active Living for Older Adults: A Model for Optimal Active Living

William A.R. Orban

The purpose of this paper is to examine the interaction between physical activity and the older adult as it relates to quality of life. Because quality of life is dependent on energy capacity, the focus will be on the energetics of physical activity. The relationship between volume, duration, and intensity of physical activity and the impact of activity on the older adult will be examined in relation to the concept of optimal active living.

Because a satisfactory age-adjusted active living model could not be found, one is mathematically formulated and graphically illustrated. This serves as the conceptual model in the discussion about optimal active living, assists in the examination of the distance and velocity curves of the aging process, and allows a comparative analysis of age-specific energetics, disabilities, morbidity, and mortality.

Basic Laws of Physical Activity

Power and Intensity

For a given volume, power is a linear function of the intensity of physical activity. Volume is the total physical work accomplished or the energy expended. Intensity is measured either by the rate of work performed or by power output (rate of energy expenditure); the duration of a given volume determines the intensity. These relationships are illustrated in Figure 21.1.

The power required to run a distance, for example, increases linearly with intensity (mean speed) until maximal power is attained for this distance. Because performance and energy capacity of each individual for each type of physical activity are determined by genetic and environmental factors, the slope and the length of the vector are unique to each individual for each type of activity.

Volume and Intensity

For a given physical activity the energy cost is independent of the duration or intensity with which it is performed, and the duration is inversely related to intensity. Neither the duration nor the intensity of an activity changes the volume. This is illustrated in Figure 21.1.

Because power output is a limited capacity, it is exhaustible. Kennelly (1906) proposed the "law of approximate fatigue," which states that the mean speed (intensity) decreases as the distance (volume) and duration (performance time) increase. That is, approximate fatigue occurs as maximal performance intensity for a given volume is approached. Although the law was proposed for running, it applies to any physical activity composed of a repetitive or constant resistance element.

Power Capacity and Intensity

The corollary of the fatigue law is the power capacity law, which states that the maximal power for a specific activity, of different volumes (e.g., running different distances), is an exponential function of the maximal performance intensity. The polar coordinates of power and exercise intensity (mean speed) produce a unique vector for each volume, as illustrated in Figure 21.1. The tangent or slope of the vector reflects the economy of the performance, that is, work output/energy expenditure that has also been defined as partial efficiency. The polar coordinates of the radius vectors representing different volumes yield a second-degree polynomial curve. Maximal power accelerates rapidly as intensity (mean speed) increases and volume (distance) diminishes.

As stated, the power–intensity relationship is unique to, and dependent on, the physical economy of each individual. Physical economy, however, is not a constant. Because of sustained interaction between genetic and environmental influences, a change in age or fitness level, for example, influences the economy and therefore the power–intensity relationship (the tangent of the vector).

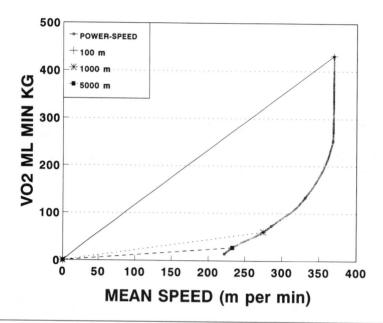

Figure 21.1 The functional-performance relationship of a 70-year-old male running three distances. Each radius vector represents the maximal intensity capacity for that volume (distance). The polar coordinates of all the maximal distance vectors generate the power-speed capacity curve (heavy line). The ordinate values represent the oxygen requirement rate, i.e., the sum of the exercise and recovery oxygen uptake rate.

Age and Physical Economy

It is universally accepted that performance and power capacity decline with age. The older one gets the less physical work (volume) one can do and the longer it takes to do a given volume. One reason for this is the loss of physical economy.

Reported studies provide evidence that cardiovascular and respiratory functional efficiency decreases with increased age (deVries et al., 1989; Shephard, 1990). Consequently, as the supportive functional cost proportionally increases it reduces the net energy available for the activity. The result is a decreased cost-effective power to perform a given volume and intensity of activity.

Furthermore, not only does the caloric cost increase for a given volume as one ages, but the maximal intensity to perform a given volume of activity decreases as well. For example, more energy is expended to run the same distance at a decreased mean speed.

The Aging Process

Age-Associated Functional Decline

Functional capacity decline with age is universal, progressive, irreversible, and unique. Figure 21.2 shows relative age-specific mean values of 18 reported functions. The functions include creatinine clearance, achlorhydria, glucose tolerance, aerobic capacity, and nerve conduction velocity, among others (Goldman & Rockstein, 1975; Harris & Frankel, 1977; Rockstein, 1974; Smith & Bierman, 1973; Strehler, 1977). The boxed line is the plot of Master's world records plotted by age class, and the dotted line illustrates the decline in the 18 functions with age.

Analysis of the effect of physical activity on functional capacity decline is impossible due to the lack of adequate physical activity indicators in the data. If the cause–effect relationship between active living and the aging process is to be analyzed, a model with bench marks for physical activity is essential.

Uniqueness of Aging

The onset and the rate of decline of each function in each organism are different. Consequently each individual ages in a unique way. A universal active living model related to general functional capacity and life cycle is needed. The concept ought to be based on data from large age-specific populations. Age class world records provide such data. These records are reliable, valid, and represent a large sample base. Furthermore, the different events provide a full range of energy capacity from both aerobic and anaerobic sources.

Two assumptions are made for the formulation of the model:

- There is an age-specific decline of general performance and functional capacity.
- The population frequency distribution of the running performance of each event for each age-specific population is Maxwellian.

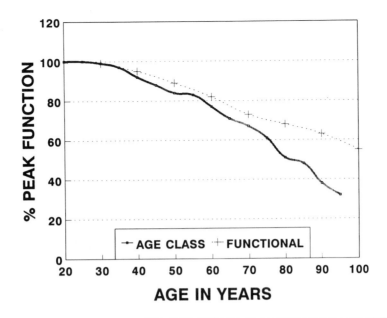

Figure 21.2 The age-specific relative functional-performance decline. The age class curve shows relative world age class running performances, and the functional curve shows the relative functional capacity of 18 different functions. The decline is expressed as the age-specific percent of the peak value.

Age-Adjusted Functional Capacity Model

Age Shift of Normality

The frequency distributions of a standard physical performance score for each age-specific population ought to show a shift of the mean from right to left corresponding to the mean performance. Age class world records provide support for such a model. Instead of the means, however, the highest values (the right tail) of each distribution are used.

One hundred eighty-seven records of 12 events ranging from the 100-m to the 50-mile event and from 19 to 98 years of age (Burfoot, 1981) provide the basic data for analysis. When each performance is transformed into the percentage of the world record for each event, all events are comparable. The means of the relative performances for each age class are graphically shown by the line in Figure 21.2.

Whereas the general functional curve lacks any indicators of health ahd fitness level, the age class curve is based on physical performance capacity. Because function is linearly related to performance, the age class curve also provides the benchmark of upper limits of the age-adjusted functional and energy capacity.

In order to smooth the curve and adjust for the unequal number of cases in the 9th and 10th decades, I have calculated and mathematically corrected the means for each decade. I used the mathematical solution to generate the upper limits (potential) of the model (Figure 21.3).

Age Decline Rate

The rate of decline accelerates with increasing age. Although a rate of 1% per year decline is generally accepted, the possibility of acceleration after 65 has been speculated by Shephard (1991). The model shows that the rate of decline, although less than 0.25% per year in the 4th decade, increases to about 1% per year in the 7th decade and to more than 2% per year in the 10th decade. With some confidence, therefore, I can say that the model does not disagree generally with the current reported trends.

Although the model provides an age-related upper limit of active living, a lower limit is required to complete the theoretical concept.

A Universal Age-Adjusted Energy Capacity Model

The baseline of active living is generally described as a "normal-sedentary" individual who is without impairment and not engaged in any occupational or leisure physical activity.

A consensus of this baseline benchmark for performance or functional capacity was not found. Therefore, a model by Simonson, (1977) of comparative age-specific samples was arbitrarily selected. This showed that the aerobic capacity of a normal-sedentary sample is approximately 36% below that of active athletes. And 36% is used as the baseline for the model of optimal active living, shown in Figure 21.3. The dark line in Figure 21.3 represents decline in performance

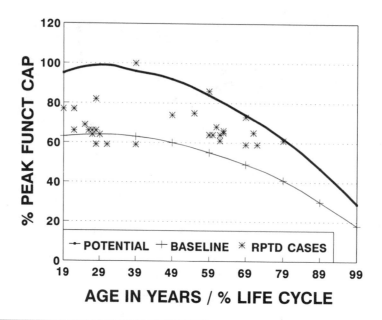

Figure 21.3 Age-adjusted optimal active living model. The potential curve is the mathematically generated human upper activity limit (world age class records). The baseline curve is the lower activity limit (normal-sedentary). The RPTD cases are randomly selected cases with reported appropriate indicators. The *x* values can be read as years or as percent of the life cycle.

with age as reflected in the Master's world records. In other words, it is assumed that this plot represents the performance potential at each age level. If it is assumed that one can improve only approximately 20%, then the lower line represents the inactive population's performance in relation to the performances of those who meet their optimal potential based on world records. Figure 21.3 is presented in percentage of functional capacity to facilitate its use.

When adequate indicators are available, the model provides individual and universal age–active living benchmarks for comparison and analysis (Figure 21.3). Although the model is based on performance capacity, it expresses the functional synergy required to generate energy (Niinimaa & Shephard, 1978). Because the wide range of events used for the model requires a synergy of the maximal aerobic and anaerobic capacity, the model represents a normative standard of life-cycle energy capacity (Figure 21.4). It is presented in relative terms, that is, percentage of peak power. It could be presented in absolute terms by ml/kg · min of VO_2 or any other unit of energy rate.

Not only does energy capacity decline with age but the incremental age-specific capacity diminishes as well. The decade-specific increment indicates the possible potential energy gain that may be acquired through active living.

Benefits of Active Living

Age-Specific Energy Capacity

Exercise physiologists unanimously agree that regular exercise is essential for optimal function of the human body (Åstrand, 1986). The positive benefits of habitual physical activity are well documented. Most reported evidence supports a positive effect on specific and general functions of the organism (Åstrand, 1991). Moreover, it is arguable that habitual physical activity enhances and extends age-specific functional and energy capacity and that the benefits are limited only by dosage.

The extent of the gain can be determined through comparison of the baseline at any age to the upper limit at a later age in the model (Figure 21.3). Life cycle gains of potential capacity may be expressed in years, and functional gains may be expressed as a relative capacity increase at a given age.

For example, an 80-year-old who leads an optimal active lifestyle has the same functional capacity as a normal-sedentary 40-year-old. This is a 40-year gain, or, if the gain is viewed vertically, the 80-year-old has gained a 20% higher capacity.

Increased capacity enables one to fulfill and extend the quality of life. Increased functional and energy capacity protects one against chronic disability and morbidity and perhaps even increases life expectancy.

Compressed Impairment and Morbidity

Age-added functional capacity reduces the risk of or protects against the impact of certain age-associated impairments. For example, chronic airway obstruction, arthritis, and musculoarthrodynia decrease or are perceived to decrease physical performance and can even inhibit performance.

The inhibitory effects of such disabilities may be overridden or suppressed by active living even though

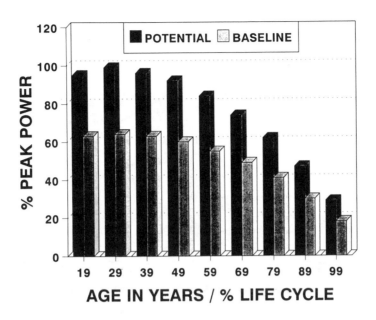

Figure 21.4 Life cycle energy model, with relative potential and baseline energy capacity for each decade or percent of life cycle. The difference between the two illustrates the possible capacity gain through optimal active living.

the impairment is not eliminated. Increased functional demand produces physiological adaptive and self-regulating mechanisms. The resultant increased performance and functional capacity may evoke feelings of well-being and self-efficacy.

Ankylosing spondylitis is an example of this type of functional-induced impairment. Although a person with this condition has a restricting spinal and chest wall mobility, aerobic capacity can be increased with supple mentary exercise without any measurable improvement in the impairment (Fisher, Cawley, & Holgate, 1990). One study has shown that physical activity significantly improved maximal work capacity in subjects with chronic airway obstruction but did not significantly change expiratory flow rates (Lake, Henderson, Briffa, Openshaw, & Musk, 1990). In spite of the absence of any measurable impairment reduction, subjects showed a greater performance and functional capacity and had increased self-confidence and self-esteem.

The probable general effects of improved functional capacity on disability and impairments are illustrated in Figure 21.5. The dark line represents functional potential of optimally active individuals, and the thin line represents the decline with age of the functional potential of inactive individuals. The starred line shows the possible exponential increase of the incidence of impairments with age for the inactive population. The boxed line reflects the shift to later onset of the incidence of impairments with age, as well as the less steep predicted increase in such incidence of impairment.

The benefits, physical or mental, of active living may be viewed as (a) a gain in years, through either a compression of impairments or a shifting of their effects to

a later period, or (b) a higher performance and functional capacity at a specific age (Figure 21.5). Both provide a higher quality of life.

Compressed Morbidity

Active living increases the possibility of a longer, healthier life by compressing the age-associated chronic disease period at the end of the life cycle. There is compelling evidence that active living significantly reduces the risk and incidence of certain common degenerative cardiovascular diseases. Furthermore, due to increased adaptive and compensatory mechanisms, if such disease does occur it is less serious and allows a more rapid recovery (Jette & Landry, in press).

There is also persuasive evidence that active living has a positive effect on infectious disease. Optimal active living probably increases the natural killer-cell activity just as effectively in the elderly as in the young (Fiatarone et al., 1989). Other studies have shown that although the immune system shows an age-related decrement, age-impaired responsiveness can be improved by deep sleep stimulation associated with habitual active living. Because the age-related morbidity curve is very similar to the impairment curves, similar comparisons and observations about the protective effects of active living against degenerative and infectious disease can be made.

Although advances in health care and other factors are more significant in the prevention of infectious disease, a persuasive argument can be made that active living increases the possibility of a longer, healthier life.

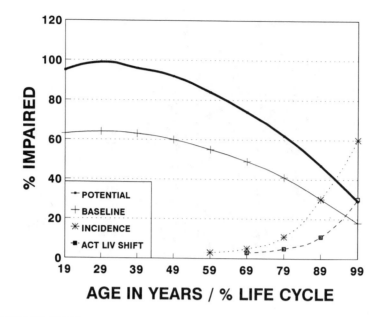

Figure 21.5 The age-specific disability and morbidity incidence curve (Emerson, 1990) and its possible shift due to optimal active living (ACT LIV SHIFT) curves, superimposed on the active living model. The y-axis values represent percentage age-specific population afflicted with age-associated disabilities. The abscissa values are in years or percentage of life cycle.

Not only does it add life to one's years but may also add years to one's life.

Longevity

Current evidence indicates that active living has a positive effect on longevity. An active person has greater adaptability and a higher potential energy capability than an inactive person. The greater the functional capacity the greater the possibility of survival (Snowdon, Ostwald, Kane, & Keenan, 1989). Blair et al. (1989) have shown that "higher levels of physical fitness appear to delay all-cause mortality" (p. 2395) in both men and women. The effect of active living on longevity is illustrated in Figure 21.6.

To the extent that functional capacity benefits survival, active living increases longevity. One can argue, therefore, that living in the state of optimal functional capacity maximizes one's life expectancy with the possibility of aborting the inevitable frailty at the end of the life cycle. It is generally accepted that in addition to one's normal daily non-occupational activity some supplemental activity is required to bring about the full benefits of physical activity.

Optimal Exercise Dosage

To develop and maintain potential energy capacity a person needs an adequate dosage of regular supplemental physical activity. This may be through occupational or leisure activities. Although a consensus exists on the minimal amount (volume or duration) and type of

physical activity required for such benefits, much ambiguity remains regarding the optimal prescribed dosage, particularly for the older adult. In the following paragraphs dosage is examined in detail.

The Quantitative Component (Volume)

An exercise dosage is made up of three interdependent elements: volume, duration, and intensity. There is general consensus that a minimum weekly volume of 2,000 kcal is required for a positive influence on a number of coronary and heart diseases (Jette & Landry, in press). A greater volume, however, may be required for other types of benefits (Dearman & Francis, 1983).

The Durative Component (Duration)

It is acknowledged that training for competition requires a greater duration than that necessary for a high level of fitness or optimal living. However, most agree that a duration of 20 to 30 min three times per week is minimal to maintain a high level of fitness.

In order to satisfy both minimal durative and volume requirements one must do a volume of 650 kcal of work in 30 min three times a week. This would be dangerous if not impossible for an older sedentary adult. The intensity to meet the minimal volume and duration requirement would be beyond a beginner's capacity. Obviously, the intensive component becomes the critical element (Stamford, 1973).

Furthermore, it is important to note that in runners at the Master's level the durative component declines 1.3 times more rapidly than aerobic capacity (Shephard,

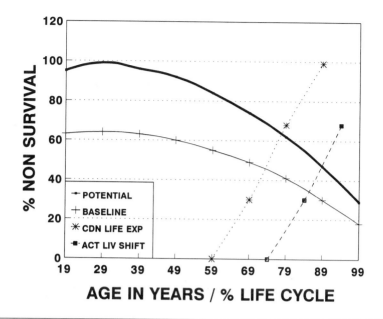

Figure 21.6   The percentage of age-specific mortality of the population, surviving to age 60 (CDN LIFE EXP) (Emerson, 1990) and the possible shift due to active living (ACT LIV SHIFT) curves, superimposed on the active living model. The abscissa values are in years or percentage of life cycle.

1991). The volume and duration decrease more rapidly with age than the intensive component. Thus it can be arguably concluded that intensity is the critical component in optimal activity dosage for older adults.

The Intensive Component (Rate of Work)

The intensive component—the energetics of activity—with a given volume has been shown to be critical in the degree of benefits derived from supplemental activity (Blair et al., 1989; Jette & Landry, in press; Paffenbarger, Wing, Hyde, & Jung, 1983). The implication is that the more vigorously supplemental physical activity is performed, the greater are the benefits. Figure 21.7 illustrates the interdependency of the quantitative, durative, and intensive components of physical activity and the relative positive benefits for any dosage.

Minimal Intensity Threshold

Energy capacity can be increased only by expending energy. And only an adequate total energy expenditure can stimulate an adaptive change to increased energy capacity. Energy expenditure is limited by one's current energy and habitual performance capacity (fitness level). Consequently, the relative minimal intensive threshold depends upon the individual's functional capacity state, which is determined by age and fitness level.

Figure 21.8 illustrates the practical application of the dosage model to a specific case. The volume of activity is 5,000 m or approximately 635 kcal for a 70-year-old male. A daily run at 75% of aerobic capacity lasts 35 min, slightly over the minimal duration dosage. Only

an all-out run of approximately 97% of his maximal aerobic capacity would decrease the duration to 30 min at a 635-kcal volume and a 30-min duration dosage. Obviously, for a normal-sedentary older adult beginner such an exercise dosage is unrealistic.

Therefore, because volume and duration determine the intensive component of physical activity, and because the minimal volume is beyond the beginner's capacity, the initial volume (of any aerobic activity) is determined by the subject's initial volume and duration capacity. The beginner must first increase the volume to the required amount before attempting to reduce the duration (increase intensity) in order to be able to perform at 75% of maximum available capacity. This agrees with the minimal threshold generally recognized for an effective training intensity.

Standard Threshold Targets

The dosage models (Figures 21.7 and 21.8) are based on the caloric values for a specific activity and individual. Although similar models can be constructed for any given individual and any specific activity, they are not readily available.

Simpler, more general models using functional response to activity are more commonly used. For example, target heart rate models can provide guidance concerning the dosage of exercise for beginner older adults. These models, however, may greatly underestimate the threshold for a more fit older adult and thus deprive her or him of the optimal active living benefits.

For example, the heart rates corresponding to the actual power-performance levels in Figure 21.8 for a

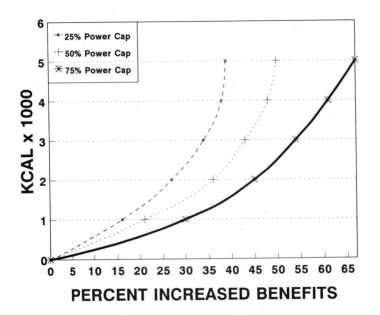

Figure 21.7 General dosage-benefit model. The interdependence of volume in kilocalories, relative intensity (percentage of power capacity), and relative increased benefits are illustrated. The percent increased benefits represent possible relative age and functional gains from active living (adapted from Jette & Landry, in press).

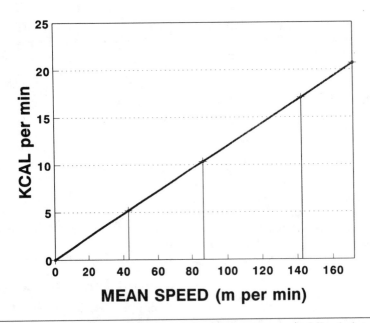

Figure 21.8 Specific dosage model, which illustrates the relationship between power (kilocalorie per minute) and mean speed required by a 70-year-old male in running 5,000 m. The vertical lines indicate the relative intensities of 25%, 50%, and 75% of maximal energy and performance capacity. The volume (total cost) is independent of the intensity (mean speed) and duration.

70-year-old subject are 100, 120, and 168. It should be noted that this a very active individual with relatively high age-specific VO_2 for a trained 70-year-old person. The implication of using a standard heart rate target zone model of 102-132 for this 70-year-old is obvious. On the other hand the fact that this subject does the equivalent of a 1,900-kcal volume of physical activity for a total duration of 105 min per week at a heart rate

of 168 or 17-kcal per min intensity to maintain his optimal functional capacity is significant.

Summary

This paper has focused on the development and maintenance of optimal activity by supplemental physical activity. However, evidence suggests that regular periodic energy stimulation throughout the day is increasingly important for the older adult. Intermittent normal activity vigorously performed throughout the day enhances and reinforces the benefits of supplemental activity. To fully impact on the quality of living, optimal active living ought to include vigorous physical activity not only of an optimal supplemental dosage but of an increased intensity in daily living as well.

One's reserve energy should be constantly challenged throughout the day. This not only fine tunes the energy capacity but adds the quality dimension to active living.

Decline in energy capacity with age is a normal phenomenon; abstinence from physical activity is not. Unless one aspires to an embraces a vigorous active lifestyle that includes a habitual supplemental dosage of leisure or occupational physical activity, one increases the risk of impairment, frailty, and morbidity along with a shorter life.

Older adults who are sedentary and inactive have a greater risk of injury, disease, and death than those who are physically active. When all the risks of optimal active living are weighed against the benefits, the choice for the older adult is clear. Optimal active living increases the probability of a higher quality of life with a dignified death.

References

Åstrand, P.-O. (1986). Exercise physiology of the mature athlete. In J.R. Sutton & R.M. Brock (Eds.), *Sports medicine for the mature athlete* (pp. 3-13). Indianapolis: Benchmark Press.

Blair, S.N., Kohl, H.W., III, Paffenbarger, R.S., Debra, D.G., Cooper, K.H., & Gibbons, L.W. (1989). Physical fitness and all-cause mortality: A prospective study of healthy men and women. *Journal of the American Medical Association*, **262**, 2395-2401.

Burfoot, R. (1981). 1980: The Olympic year that produced the first non-Olympics. *Runner's World*, pp. 81-95. (Annual issue)

Dearman, J., & Francis, K.T. (1983). Plasma levels of catecholamines, cortisol, and beta-endorphins in male athletes after running 26.2, 6 and 2 miles. *Journal of Sports Medicine and Physical Fitness*, **23**, 30-38.

deVries, H.A., Brodowicz, G.R., Robertson, L.D., Svoboa, M.D., Schendel, J.S., Tichy, A.M., & Tichy, M.W. (1989). Estimating physical working capacity and training changes in the elderly at the fatigue threshold (PWCft). *Ergonomics*, **32**, 967-977.

Emerson, V. (1990). *Next generation rental terminals: Effects of aging design of telephones for the elderly* (TR89-0148). Ottawa, Ontario: Bell–Northern Research.

Fiatarone, M.A., Morely, J.E., Bloom, E.T., Benton, D., Solomon, G.F., & Makinodan, T. (1989). The effect of exercise on natural killer cell activity in young and old subjects. *Journal of Gerontology: Medical Sciences*, **44**, M37-M45.

Fisher, L.R., Cawley, M.I.D., & Holgate, S.T. (1990). Relation between chest expansion, pulmonary function, and exercise tolerance in patients with ankylosing spondylitis. *Annals of the Rheumatic Diseases*, **49**, 921-925.

Goldman, R., & Rockstein, M. (Eds.). (1975). *The physiology and pathology of human aging*. New York: Academic Press.

Harris, R., & Frankel, L.J. (Eds.). (1977). *Guide to fitness after 50*. New York: Plenum Press.

Jette, M., & Landry, F. (in press). Physical activity and cardio-vascular disease. *Revue de Science et Technique des Activites Physique et Sportive*.

Kennelly, A.E. (1906). An approximate law of fatigue in the speeds of racing animals. *Proceedings of the American Academy of Arts and Sciences*, **42**, 275-331.

Lake, F.R., Henderson, K., Briffa, T., Openshaw, J., & Musk, A.W. (1990). Upper-limb and lower-limb exercise training in patients with chronic airflow obstruction. *Chest*, **97**, 1077-1082.

Niinimaa, V., & Shephard, R.J. (1978). Training and oxygen conductance in the elderly: 1. The respiratory system. *Journal of Gerontology*, **33**, 354-361.

Paffenbarger, R.S., Wing, A.L., Hyde, R.T., & Jung, D.L. (1983). Physical activity and incidence of hypertension in college alumni. *American Journal of Epidemiology*, **117**, 245-257.

Rockstein, M. (Ed.). (1974). *Theoretical aspects of aging*. New York: Academic Press.

Shephard, R.J. (1990). The scientific basis of exercise prescribing for the very old. *Journal of the American Geriatrics Society*, **38**, 62-70.

Shephard, R.J. (1991). Fitness and aging. In C. Blais (Ed.), *Aging into the twenty-first century* (pp. 22-35). North York, Ontario: Captus University.

Simonson, E. (1977). Effect of age on work and fatigue-cardiovascular aspects. In R. Harris & L.J. Frankel (Eds.), *Guide to fitness after 50* (pp. 53-65). New York: Plenum Press.

Smith, D.W., & Bierman, E.L. (Eds.). (1973). *The biological ages of man: From conception through old age*. Toronto: Saunders.

Snowdon, D.A., Ostwald, S.K., Kane, R.L., & Keenan, N.L. (1989). Years of life with good and poor mental and physical function in the elderly. *Journal of Clinical Epidemiology*, **42**, 1055-1066.

Stamford, B.A. (1973). Effects of chronic institutionalization on the physical working capacity and trainability of geriatric men. *Journal of Gerontology*, **28**, 441-446.

Strehler, B.L. (1977). *Time, cells, and aging*. New York: Academic Press.

22

Active Living for Persons With Disabilities

22.1
Preparing Children With Mental Disabilities for Active Living
E.J. Watkinson

22.2
From Community Participation in Physical Activity to Olympic Integration
R.D. Steadward

Editor's Note

Because this chapter presents the content of a panel session at the conference, it was integrated into one chapter with two specific perspectives.

22.1

Preparing Children With Mental Disabilities for Active Living

E.J. Watkinson

A major challenge for professionals in the field of physical activity is facilitating the involvement of all Canadians, including those with mental disabilities, in active lifesytles that will enhance their health and happiness. Active living is "a way of life in which physical activity is valued and integrated into daily life" (Active Living Alliance for Canadians with a Disability, 1992, p. 3). Active living may mean quite different things for younger and older individuals, for elite performers and for those who are not so gifted. In childhood active living can take place in many different settings and with many different groups of people (Smith, 1987). In the "mainstream," it includes such things as swimming with family in the summer, taking part in recess on the school playground, or playing soccer in the local community league. It encompasses participation in structured and unstructured activities, in warm and cold weather, indoors and outdoors, alone and with groups of other children and adults.

Active living is viewed today as an almost limitless choice of activities ranging from those that make very few demands on our physiological systems to those that stretch our limits. Even for children the breadth of choice is huge. But for most youngsters with disabilities and for their parents and teachers, the mainstream of children's play is possibly the most desirable setting for active living. Parents want their children to take part in school and community activities as much as possible. But the demands of active living in mainstream physical activity settings are significant: Children play vigorously and they employ complex skills. For adults, active living includes gardening and strolling through the park. For children, however, participation in age-appropriate and culturally appropriate activity means being involved in the activities of the school and the neighborhood. Active living in these settings is physiologically and cognitively demanding.

As children grow older the demands of this active participation increase. Simple skills of running, walking, jumping, climbing, sliding, swinging, and tricycle riding that make up the repertoires of children in preschool are maintained, but as they grow older children acquire reactive and complex skills so they can engage in more cooperative and competitive activity (Wall, 1989). Ball skills, games skills, and more sophisticated swimming, skating, skiing, and riding skills are typically developed by children in the middle-school years. Often, such skills are combined in complex patterns within games and are accompanied by rules and strategies that make their use more meaningful. As children get older, bigger, and stronger, their motor skill repertoires become broader and more complex, requiring quick decisions and reactions to changing perceptual information. The skill demands and setting demands increase as larger and more organized groups of children begin to play together (Lindsay, 1984).

During the early elementary school years, a good deal of active living takes place on the playgrounds of schools at recess, during lunch hour, or at the end of the day. Slides, bars, poles, ladders, swings, and beams are the equipment most often found on elementary school playgrounds, according to Bowers (1988). Playful activity on this equipment and in the open spaces of fields and hard surfaces requires specific motor skills. When a child uses equipment and space in concert with other children, more skillful performance, knowledge of rules and contingencies, and sophisticated social interactions are required.

The slide, for example, is the most common piece of equipment of North American playgrounds (Bowers, 1988). If a child is content to play alone on this apparatus, then the simple skills of climbing up the ladder and going down the slide are sufficient. But if the child wants to engage in vigorous social play with other children the demands are much more. "Alligator House," for example, is played by 5- and 6-year-olds on the spiral slide. The challenge is to go down the slide while avoiding the "alligators" at the bottom. Children must be able to climb up and down the ladder, climb up the slide from the bottom quickly and against opposition, slide down in a mass, pull others up the slide, push some down the slide without hurting them, and get pulled up and bumped in the process. This is a popular kindergarten and first-grade game in at least one Canadian city. Although Alligator House may not be the favored game in all playgrounds, it does represent the activities that take place on most such pieces of equipment. Climbing up the ladder and going down the slide in a sitting position may be the requisite skills for productive solitary play on this particular piece of apparatus (Watkinson & Wall, 1982), but they are clearly not sufficient for vigorous social play of elementary school children. Active living, even in the early elementary years, requires the knowledge of rules and the social competency required for participation, in addition to the motor skills on which the activity is based.

As children grow toward adolescence the demands of their active participation increase tremendously (Wall, 1989). In the preteen years many youngsters join community organizations to participate in sport activities. Although participation in the local softball league is normally guaranteed regardless of skill level, skills, rules, and strategies must be acquired for that participation to be satisfying to the participant and to others. Participants want to know how to bat, how to field grounders, and how to throw the ball to first base. Furthermore, they need to know the basic rules regarding strikes and balls, base running, pitching, and how to throw a player out on a force play. Compared to the rules and understandings of a sliding game these are formidable challenges from both a physical and a cognitive perspective.

What happens when a child lacks these skills and knowledges? Studies indicate that individuals without adequate motor repertoires are unable to participate in the activities of their peers (Evans & Roberts, 1987; Matthews, 1980; Smith & Hurst, 1961). Children may avoid situations in which they do not feel competent (Craft & Hogan, 1985; Crawford & Griffin, 1986; Griffin & Keogh, 1982), or they may be deliberately excluded by their peers. Furthermore, during the school years, children's esteem (especially that of boys) is largely based on their talent in performing motor skills (Evans & Roberts, 1987), and children with higher skill levels are sought as playmates (Cavallaro & Porter, 1980). Children with developmental disabilities may be restricted in their active participation because of a lack of friends (Levinson & Reid, 1991).

It is well documented that the child with a mental disability does not bring an adequate motor repertoire to the recreational or free-play setting (DiRocco, Clark, & Phillips, 1987; Keeran, Grove, & Zachofsky, 1969; Ulrich, 1982). The repertoire should include both age-appropriate and culturally normal skills that are highly valued in the child's own schoolyard or neighborhood. Without such a repertoire the child is forced to watch or sit on the sideline, play alone, or, at the very best, play with children who are younger or less skillful than most of the child's peers. This is not an uncommon sight. On many playgrounds in "mainstreamed" schools children with disabling conditions play in a separate area and employ skills that are immature or different from the culturally normal activities of the rest of the school.

A study of the motor skills of moderately mentally disabled children in Edmonton's public and Catholic schools revealed that none of the 45 children assessed in the study demonstrated independent, "adequate" performance on six critical playground skills without intervention (Watkinson & Muloin, 1988a). This study (Watkinson & Muloin, 1988b) suggested that the students who were low in motor competence on these six skills were also less active in their free play. Perhaps they did not have the motor skills required to enter the normal activities of recess. They tended to spend the majority of their time alone, away from the equipment, in open space. When they were on the equipment the swings were their first choice; they simply sat on the swings, remaining completely inactive. When these children were involved in more advanced forms of social interaction, it was largely with their disabled classmates, not with nondisabled peers.

Literature suggests that social interaction is minimal between disabled and nondisabled children in mainstreamed settings (Cavallaro & Porter, 1980; Gresham, 1982; Ispa, 1981; Kohl & Beckman, 1984; Taylor, Asher, & Williams, 1987). Beckman (1983) found that even in preschool, social exchange occurred more frequently when it involved the most sophisticated and complex behavioral networks such as smiling, laughing, talking, shouting, walking, running, and climbing. Children with mental disabilities exhibit these behavioral chains less frequently and thus may be unable to fully participate in free active play.

Active living in typical childhood settings requires motor skill competency, social interaction skills (including verbal skills), and knowledge of rules and strategies for games and activities. Children who lack these will remain inactive and isolated, so that their opportunities to develop more complex motor and social skills are severely limited (Guralnick, 1986). Inactivity will clearly lead to lack of fitness and further separation of youngsters who are disabled from their skilled peers.

Traditional Strategies for Increasing Participation

In the past 20 years professionals in the field of physical activity have attempted to undo the vicious circle of incompetence and lack of participation through a number of different avenues, some of which are fruitful and others that are not. Recently, we have tried to increase the opportunities for participation through mainstreaming in recreational and educational physical activity settings. We have also tried to modify the environments of the participants to make it easier for youngsters with disabilities to participate. Finally, we have tried to upgrade the skills of youngsters to prepare them for interaction and participation in active lifestyles. The following will look at each of these approaches and attempt to present a model for all three that will increase the physical activity of children with disabilities.

Provide Opportunity

The assumption we make when we try to increase participation simply through providing opportunity is that all individuals will have an equal chance to develop under the circumstances that are typical in physical activity programs and settings. The adoption of integrated programs of physical activity has been encouraged with this assumption in mind. But, as Gresham (1982) found in his review of the literature in the education field, the assumption is faulty because it is based on three predictions, none of which have stood up to scrutiny. The first prediction is that children with disabilities will increase their social interactions with peers in integrated settings. The second predication is that children with disabilities will be socially accepted in such settings. The third prediction is that children with disabilities will learn new social behaviors and other skills through modeling the behaviors of their nondisabled peers. But research has shown clearly that children with disabilities cannot take full advantage of the opportunities that mainstreaming provides in both classroom and free-time activity. In fact children who are moderately mentally disabled are relatively inactive in both segregated and integrated activity settings (Titus & Watkinson, 1987; Watkinson & Muloin, 1988a) in spite of the presence of exciting playground equipment and skilled models. When they participate, it is often with skills that are not culturally normal or age appropriate. When they do interact in a positive social manner it is most often with other classmates who are disabled (Ispa, 1981). They seem to be unable to spontaneously take advantage of the presence of skilled peers to learn new skills or change their behaviors to encourage more involvement. Even when they are provided with instruction in integrated programs, they have difficulty applying their new knowledge appropriately, and their levels of skill maintenance and generalization fall well below those of their peers.

Providing opportunity alone clearly does not encourage active living in children who have mental disabilities. In fact, if parents, teachers, or leaders take pride in the mere presence of these children in integrated settings, they may overlook the children's meager involvement in the activity. It is clear that children react differently to the same environment, and although providing the opportunity for active living may be enough to facilitate vigorous physical activity in most elementary-age children (Kraft, 1989), it does not do the same for children who already lack the skills and knowledge required for participation.

Modify the Environment to Accommodate the Disability

Changing the environment to accommodate the individual disability is a strategy that has been widely adopted in both schools and recreational settings. Instructors and leaders have tried to change the goals of activity to facilitate the inclusion of youngsters with disabilities (e.g., Banks & Aveno, 1986; McGill, 1984); have changed the goals for the individual with a disability to include only partial participation; and have also tried to change the environment by providing supports (e.g., Halle, Gabler-Halle, & Bemben, 1989; Henderson, 1990) and peer tutors (e.g., Donder & Nietupski, 1981; Gold, 1983) or by using additional cues and prompts that help to improve performance (Cuvo et al., 1983; Koh & Watkinson, 1988).

These environmental modifications are a positive part of the solution but they could be viewed as being contrary to the ideals of normalization and equity. Ideally, children who are mentally disabled would be involved in active living in settings that are part of the normal experience of children who are not disabled. Placing children who are disabled in protected, special environments may prevent them from achieving their potential in physical activity. Furthermore, altering instructional and recreational environments may cheat youngsters who are not disabled of their own opportunities to excel. For example, a common environmental modification to integrated programs is to move to a cooperative, rather than a competitive, focus in the activity. Karper, Martinek, and Wilkerson (1985) investigated the differential effects of a competitive and a noncompetitive environment on the acquisition of skills by disabled youngsters in integrated settings and found the less competitive environment to be more supportive of motor development. Although it is likely that cooperative activities will benefit all participants, it is also possible that some youngsters with disabilities will respond very positively to competitive activities and the developmental programs that go with them (e.g., Dahlgren, Boreskie, Dowds, MacTavish, & Watkinson, 1991). Those who are able to should have opportunities to be involved in mainstream competitive activities as well.

Upgrade the Repertoires of the Individual

A third strategy is to upgrade the skills and the fitness of the individual in preparation for participation in the mainstream of physical activity or for active living in segregated settings. There is evidence that movement skills of individuals with severe to mild mental disabilities can be upgraded through programs of instruction in integrated or segregated settings (Beuter, 1983; Fediuk, 1990; Karper & Martinek, 1983, 1985; Rarick & Beuter, 1985; Wehman, 1977). (For a review of studies in skill training with individuals with moderate and severe disabilities see Nietupski, Hamre-Nietupski, & Ayres, 1984.) There is evidence also that individuals with mild to severe mental disabilities can improve their fitness to levels that may be required for active participation (Halle et al., 1989). In fact, data indicate

(Watkinson & Koh, 1988) that moderately mentally disabled children can sustain vigorous activity with heart rates above 150 for periods of 12 min, provided they are verbally prompted and encouraged by teachers who model the activity. This would lead one to believe that children who are moderately mentally disabled are at least physiologically capable of participating in mainstream activity. Children and youths with mental disabilities can gain the skills they require for active living if they are exposed to a systematic instructional program that focuses on specific skills that are lacking in individual repertoires. Individualized instructional programs of short (Watkinson & Muloin, 1988a) or long (Karper & Martinek, 1985) duration can increase the number of skills in children's repertoires. Other studies have demonstrated skill upgrading to the extent that individuals can take part in segregated leisure programs (Banks & Aveno, 1986; Hill, Wehman, & Horst, 1980) and special competitive programs (Dahlgren et al., 1991).

Key aspects of the instruction in these studies include the attention paid to specific skills that suit the equipment or activity available to the child, a focus on only one or two skills until they are performed with some proficiency, the use of task analyses to identify teachable components of the skills, and the application of a systematic prompting continuum that allows the instructor to gradually reduce physical, visual, and verbal prompts (Collier & Reid, 1987; Cuvo et al., 1983; Dunn, 1990; Nietupski et al., 1984; Watkinson & Wall, 1982).

Facilitating Active Living

The three strategies already described may increase the chances of active living for individuals with mental disabilities. Used alone the strategies result in modest effects, but used in concert with each other they may provide the mechanism most likely to improve the lifestyles of people with disabilities. A crucial ingredient of the mix is that each individual's skills and knowledges are upgraded to match the demands of an environment in which he or she is expected to successfully participate. This involves identifying a natural environment in which the child has the opportunity to be active yet one in which the child's predicted level of skill and knowledge will be satisfactory for participation. In such a model, environments are not always modified to accommodate the child, but they are carefully chosen. In addition, the skills and knowledges that the child needs to participate in the environment must be carefully evaluated and upgraded to a level that will put him or her within the bandwidth of what is expected or accepted in such a setting. This strategy clearly involves providing the opportunity, choosing the environment, and changing the child (rather than the environment).

Choosing appropriate activities appears to be a critical aspect of the success of instruction. While acknowledging that children with disabilities can learn motor skills,

professionals also must realize that capacity problems may limit the extent to which some skills can be easily acquired. Skills that are primarily response loaded (Wall, McClements, Bouffard, Findlay, & Taylor, 1985), that is, that do not require quick decisions made under pressure or call for intricate coincidence timing, may be easier to learn. Ball and games skills that require a good deal of timing and planning are much harder to learn and perform than activities such as playground skills, swimming, and bicycle riding. The former skills are applied in stressful situations in which other performers count on the performance of each member of a group, whereas the latter are activities in which the learner participates in parallel with others or even alone. In fact, activities of this nature (walking, swimming, skating, jogging, running, and biking) are identified as the most common activities of Canadian children and youths, including those who have developmental disabilities (Levinson & Reid, 1991).

It is critical, therefore, that instructors know how to identify the age-appropriate and culturally normal games and activities in which their students with disabilities have potential for success. Walking, swimming, skating, and biking activities may be a good starting place for activity prescription. Teachers and leaders must be prepared to make choices in their activity prescriptions, so that children with disabilities are put in the most advantageous position possible when they attempt to take part in active living. Giving a child the motor and social skills he or she needs to enter one neighborhood activity with confidence and competence may be all that can be managed in the school year, but it may profoundly affect the child's happiness. Helping a more severely disabled child to acquire the fitness and skill to walk or ride a tricycle may enable that child to enter the active lifestyles of parents who walk for exercise. Choosing more complex and demanding activity settings will require that the child acquire more complex skills and knowledge. Community softball for 9-year-olds requires the application of complex fielding, throwing, and striking skills under constantly changing conditions. This activity also requires knowledge of highly sophisticated rules regarding strikes and force-outs, fly balls, and base running. In contrast, cycling has fewer strategies and rules and a narrower repertoire of required procedural skills for successful participation. It is important to choose an "optimal challenge" that matches the difficulty of the task to the capability of the child (Weiss, 1991).

Once an activity has been chosen that seems to balance the capabilities of the child with the demands of the environment, instructors have to ask themselves exactly what to teach. Choosing the appropriate skills means knowing how to complete a meaningful task analysis of that activity and having the instructional technology needed to assist the child in acquiring, and maintaining, suitable skills for his or her specific setting

(Reid, 1987b). A knowledge-based model of motor development may help. Different kinds of knowledge contributer to moving well, and these must be identified in the task analysis (Wall et al., 1985). Clearly there is the perceptual-motor or procedural knowledge that allows an individual to execute a movement consistently, with economy, precision, and accuracy (Wall et al., 1985). Knowing how to run, jump, roll, float, wheel, dodge, ride, swing, strike, glide, stop, and catch is important. These skills, which provide the foundation for physical performance, demand instructional attention. Using graded tasks that lead to development of the full procedural skill will help teachers and leaders observe incremental changes in performance.

Teaching procedural skills to children with mental disabilities appears to be most successful if there is a focus on a limited number of specific skills and if the teacher uses a systematic guidance and prompting strategy (Collier & Reid, 1987; Watkinson & Wall, 1982). But it is also essential that the prompts be gradually reduced so that the child performs independently. Gradual removal of the external assistance facilitates the transition to independent and self-initiated performance in a natural setting; it also helps the performer gain the perception of self-efficacy (Craft & Hogan, 1985).

Other kinds of knowledge involved in physical performance should be reflected in the task analysis. Declarative knowledge (Wall et al., 1985) is knowledge about movement. This includes knowing game strategies, knowing about the rules, knowing how to keep fit and healthy, and knowing the principles involved in performance. This knowledge should become part of the content of the child's physical activity program in concert with the knowledge that lets the child perform an action. Activities that rely on excessive amounts of declarative knowledge may be too difficult for some children with disabilities and may prevent their full participation in the activity. Teachers of children with disabilities should choose activities in which the declarative knowledge demands are relatively light and the declarative knowledge required is well learned.

Those who administer the Red Cross swimming program attempt to include the acquisition of declarative knowledge in the program. As children develop performance skill they can increase their knowledge of the strokes, of the principles of buoyancy and propulsion, of the appropriate use of different water entries, and of water safety. Such knowledge may be logically inferred by nondisabled children as they engage in physical activity. But for the child with a disability, the instructor must ensure that this knowledge is learned and used appropriately during activity.

Knowledge of how to monitor one's performance and environment (metacognitive knowledge) is important in the development and performance of skill (Wall et al., 1985). Successful teachers and coaches of children who are mentally disabled often exert a tremendous amount of control over their students during practice and games, leaving little room for self-regulation. Many coaching and instructional materials prescribe carefully designed drills that are monitored and managed by the coach or the teacher. In fact, in many of the applications of these program materials the learner or player is dependent on the coach for every trial that she or he experiences. In contrast, outstanding performers have demonstrated the benefits of self-monitoring during the childhood years. It is time we attempted to incorporate metacognitive skills into our developmental programs. We may be able to teach psychological skills and self-regulating strategies that will help youngsters with disabilities become more independent of their teachers and coaches. These skills and strategies may contribute to sustained involvement in active living (Weiss, 1991). Yet those who need these strategies the most may be the children who are the least likely to encounter them in physical activity programs. More work is clearly needed in this area to determine which strategies can be successfully incorporated into developmental programs.

Finally, some have identified affective knowledge as important to the development and performance of skilled action. As children grow and experience success, failure, happiness, and anxiety, they develop a knowledge base of feelings toward physical activity (for more information see Wall et al., 1985). Early positive feelings can contribute to the development of attitudes that will facilitate the learning of motor skills. But positive feelings do not just happen. They need to be planned and controlled (Weiss, 1991). There is a danger in thinking that development in the affective domain will occur automaticaly and incidentally in integrated programs. This may lead to disproportionate time being devoted to "feeling good" about participating, while attention is diverted from the acquisition of motor skill. Interventions that are designed to enhance positive feelings about the self include both skill instruction and self-efficacy enhancement (Craft & Hogan, 1985).

Low self-concept is characteristic of children who find themselves compared with individuals who appear to have greater ability (Craft & Hogan, 1985). Preparing the child for an activity environment should include an upgrading of skills so that the child perceives that his or her own skill level is within the range of those demonstrated by the social comparison group. Placement of students into mainstream physical activity settings should be based on skill level and ability rather than on a belief in the power of opportunity! Placement in settings where the gap between the youngster with a disability and the peer group is large may only confirm negative self-concepts and self-efficacy.

Theory suggests that skill acquisition can positively affect the development of self-efficacy (Bandura, 1981), particularly if the skills have a significant level of difficulty and are acquired with some effort and without external support (Craft & Hogan, 1985). Craft and Hogan (1985) suggested that teachers should choose skills carefully, use graded success experiences through task analysis, gradually reduce the amount of external assistance provided to the learner, use verbal persuasion, employ similar models, and eliminate competitive experiences for which the child is unprepared. In other words, strategies that can bring about positive increments in procedural skill (Dattilo, 1987; Reid, 1987a; Watkinson, 1987) can also improve self-efficacy in children with disabilities.

Conclusion

We must recognize both the capacity problems and the potential of children with disabilities in preparing them for active living. Having even a small repertoire of culturally normal motor skills may allow the child with mental disabilities to participate confidently in physical activity. For the youngster with severe disabilities these skills may be enough to allow for active participation in family recreation where the social and verbal demands are not excessive. For others these skills may prepare them to take part in active living on the school playground or in the neighborhood. Demonstrable motor competence, based on sound procedural, declarative, and metacognitive knowledge, may affect the acceptance of children who are disabled by those who are not and may affect their own perceptions of competence, influencing their success in environments in which their classmates and peers are participating actively.

References

Active Living Alliance for Canadians with a Disability. (1992). *A blueprint for action.* Ottawa: Author.

Bandura, A. (1981). Self-referent thought: The development of self-efficacy. In J.H. Flavell & L.D. Ross (Eds.), *Development of social cognition: Frontiers and possible futures* (pp. 1-21). New York: Cambridge Press.

Banks, R., & Aveno, A. (1986). Adapted miniature golf: A community leisure program for students with severe physical disabilities. *The Association for Persons with Severe Handicaps,* **11**(3), 209-215.

Beckman, P.J. (1983). The relationship between behavioral characteristics of children and social interaction in an integrated setting. *Journal of the Division of Early Childhood,* **7**, 69-77.

Beuter, A. (1983). Effects of mainstreaming on motor performances of intellectually normal and trainable mentally retarded students. *American Journal of Corrective Therapy,* **37**(2), 48-52.

Bowers, L.E. (1988). Children need playgrounds—but playgrounds need help. *Journal of Physical Education, Recreation and Dance,* **59**(7), 47-51.

Cavallaro, S.A., & Porter, R.H. (1980). Peer preferences of at-risk and normally developing children in a preschool mainstream classroom. *American Journal of Mental Deficiency,* **84**(4), 357-366.

Collier, D., & Reid, G. (1987). A comparison of two models designed to teach autistic children a motor task. *Adapted Physical Activity Quarterly,* **4**, 226-236.

Craft, D.H., & Hogan, P.I. (1985). Development of self-concept and self-efficacy: Considerations for mainstreaming. *Adapted Physical Activity Quarterly,* **2**, 320-327.

Crawford, M.E., & Griffin, N.S. (1986). Testing the validity of the Griffin/Keogh model for movement confidence by analyzing self-report playground involvement decisions of elementary school children. *Research Quarterly for Exercise and Sport,* **57**(1), 8-15.

Cuvo, A.J., Ellis, P.J., Wisotzek, I.E., Davis, P.J., Schilling, D., & Bechtal, R. (1983). Teaching athletic skills to students who are mentally retarded. *TASH Journal,* **8**(1), 72-81.

Dahlgren, W.J., Boreskie, S., Dowds, M., MacTavish, J.B., & Watkinson, E.J. (1991). The Medallion Program: Using the generic sport model to train athletes with mental disabilities. *JOPERD,* (Nov.), 67-73.

Dattilo, J. (1987). Recreation and leisure for individuals with mental retardation: Implications for outdoor recreation. *Therapeutic Recreation Journal,* **21**(1), 9-17.

DiRocco, P.J., Clark, J.E., & Phillips, S.J. (1987). Jumping coordination patterns of mildly mentally retarded children. *Adapted Physical Activity Quarterly,* **4**, 178-191.

Donder, D., & Nietupski, J. (1981). Nonhandicapped adolescents teaching playground skills to their mentally retarded peers: Toward a less restrictive middle school environment. *Education and Training of the Mentally Retarded,* **16**, 270-276.

Dunn, J.M. (1990). Methodological considerations in program development. In C. Doll-Tepper, C. Dahms, B. Doll, & H. Von Selzam (Eds.), *Adapted physical activity* (pp. 201-205). Berlin: Springer-Verlag.

Evans, J., & Roberts, G.C. (1987). Physical competence and the development of children's peer relations. *Quest,* **39**, 23-35.

Fediuk, F. (1990). Effects of an integrated adapted physical education program on psychomotor and cognitive parameters of mentally retarded adolescents. In G. Doll-Tepper, C. Dahms, B. Doll, & H. von Selzam (Eds.), *Adapted physical activity* (pp. 171-175). Berlin: Springer-Verlag.

Gold, D. (1983). One to one support in integrated settings: The leisure buddy program. *Journal of Leisurability,* **10**(4), 14-18.

Gresham, F.M. (1982). Misguided mainstreaming: The case for social skills training with handicapped children. *Exceptional Children,* **48**(5), 422-433.

Griffin, N.S., & Keogh, J.F. (1982). A model for movement confidence. In J. Kelso & J. Clark (Eds.), *The development of movement control and co-ordination* (pp. 213-236). New York:Wiley.

Guralnick, M.J. (1986). The peer relations of young handicapped and nonhandicapped children. In P.S. Strain, M.J. Guralnick, & H.M. Walker (Eds.), *Children's social behavior: Development, assessment, and modification* (pp. 93-140). Orlando: Academic Press, Inc.

Halle, J.W., Gabler-Halle, D., & Bemben, D.A. (1989). Effects of a peer-mediated aerobic conditioning program on fitness measures with children who have moderate and severe disabilities. *The Association for Persons with Severe Handicaps*, **14**(1), 33-47.

Henderson, N. (1990). Moving into mainstreaming—an integrated approach to adapted physical education. In G. Doll-Tepper, C. Dahms, B. Doll, & H. von Selzam (Eds.), *Adapted physical activity* (pp. 167-170). Berlin: Springer-Verlag.

Hill, J., Wehman, P., & Horst, G. (1980). Acquisition and generalization of leisure skills in severely and profoundly retarded youth: Use of an electronic pinball machine. In P. Wehman & J. Hill (Eds.), *Instructional programming for severely handicapped youth* (pp. 43-61). Richmond, VA: Virginia Commonwealth University.

Ispa, J. (1981). Social interactions among teachers, handicapped children, and nonhandicapped children in a mainstreamed preschool. *Journal of Applied Developmental Psychology*, **1**, 231-250.

Karper, W.B., & Martinek, T.J. (1983). The differential influence of instructional factors on motor performance among handicapped and non-handicapped children in mainstreamed physical education classes. *Educational Research Quarterly*, **8**(3), 40-46.

Karper, W.B., & Martinek, T.J. (1985). The integration of handicapped and nonhandicapped children in elementary physical education. *Adapted Physical Activity Quarterly*, **2**, 314-319.

Karper, W.B., Martinek, T.J., & Wilkerson, J.D. (1985). Effects of competitive vs. noncompetitive learning environments on motor skill performance among handicapped and nonhandicapped children in mainstreamed physical education classes. *American Corrective Therapy Journal*, **39**(1), 10-15.

Keeran, C.V., Grove, F.A., & Zachofsky, T. (1969, June). Assessing the playground skills of the severely retarded. *Mental Retardation*, pp. 29-32.

Koh, S.M., & Watkinson, E.J. (1988). Endurance run pacing of moderately mentally handicapped children. *CAHPER Journal*, **54**(6), 12-15.

Kohl, F.L., & Beckman, P.J. (1984). A comparison of handicapped and nonhandicapped preschoolers' interactions across classroom activities. *Journal of the Division for Early Childhood*, **8**, 49-56.

Kraft, R.E. (1989). Behavior of children at recess. *Journal of Physical Education, Recreation and Dance*, **60**(4), 21-24.

Levinson, L.J., & Reid, G. (1991). Patterns of physical activity among youngsters with developmental disabilities. *CAHPER Journal*, **57**(3); 24-28.

Lindsay, P.L. (1984). The physical characteristics of playground games in public elementary schools in Edmonton. *CAHPER Journal*, **50**(6), 8-11.

Matthews, P.R. (1980). Why the mentally retarded do not participate in certain types of recreational activities. *Therapeutic Recreation Journal*, **14**, 44-50.

McGill, J. (1984). Cooperative games as a strategy for integration. *Journal of Leisurability*, **11**(4), 14-18.

Nietupski, J., Hamre-Nietupski, S., & Ayres, B. (1984). Review of task analytic leisure skill training efforts: Practitioner implications and future research needs. *The Association for Persons with Severe Handicaps*. **9**(2), 88-97.

Rarick, G.L., & Beuter, A.C. (1985). The effect of mainstreaming on the motor performance of mentally retarded and nonretarded students. *Adapted Physical Activity Quarterly*. **2**, 227-282.

Reid, G. (1987a). Motor behavior and psychosocial correlates in young handicapped performers. In D. Gould & M.R. Weiss (Eds.), *Advances in pediatric sport sciences: Vol. 2. Behavioral issues* (pp. 235-258). Champaign, IL: Human Kinetics.

Reid, G. (1987b). Skill upgrading programs. *CAHPER Journal*, **53**(5), 6-11.

Smith, M. (1987). Understanding and changing physical activity delivery systems. *CAHPER Journal*, **53**(5), 39-44.

Smith, J.R., & Hurst, J.G. (1961). The relationship of motor abilities and peer acceptance of mentally retarded children. *American Journal of Mental Deficiency*, **66**, 81-85.

Taylor, A.R., Asher, S.R., & Williams, G.A. (1987). The social adaptation of mainstreamed mildly retarded children. *Child Development*, **58**, 1321-1334.

Titus, J., & Watkinson, E.J. (1987). The effects of segregated and integrated programs on the participation and social interaction of mentally handicapped children at play. *Adapted Physical Activity Quarterly*, **4**, 204-219.

Ulrich, D.A. (1982). A comparison of the qualitative motor performance of normal, educable, and trainable mentally retarded students. *IRUC Briefings*, **7**(8), 219-225.

Wall, A.E. (1989, October). *The winds of change in school physical education: Community networking for a lifetime for active living*. Paper presented at the CAHPER convention, Halifax, NS.

Wall, A.E., McClements, J., Bouffard, M., Findlay, H., & Taylor, M.J. (1985). A knowledge-based approach to motor development: Implications for the physically awkward. *Adapted Physical Activity Quarterly*, **2**, 21-42.

Watkinson, E.J. (1987). The development and evaluation of integrated programs. *CAHPER Journal*, **53**(5), 13-20.

Watkinson, E.J., & Koh, M.S. (1988). Heart rate response of moderately mentally handicapped children and youth on the Canada Fitness Award adapted endurance run. *Adapted Physical Activity Quarterly*, **5**, 203-211.

Watkinson, E.J., & Muloin, S.T. (1988a). Playground skills of moderately mentally handicapped youngsters in integrated elementary schools. *The Mental Retardation and Learning Disability Bulletin*, **16**(2), 3-13.

Watkinson, E.J., & Muloin, S.T. (1988b). *The relationship of motor competence and activity participa-tion of mentally handicapped students in integrated physical activity settings*. Final report to the Canadian Fitness and Lifestyle Research Institute, Ottawa.

Watkinson, E.J., & Wall, A.E. (1982). *The PREP play program: Play skill instruction for mentally handicapped children*. Ottawa: CAHPER and Fitness and Amateur Sport Canada.

Wehman, P. (1977). *Helping the mentally retarded acquire play skills: A behavioral approach*. Springfield, IL: Charles C Thomas.

Weiss, M.R. (1991). Psychological skill development in children and adolescents. *The Sport Psychologist*, **5**, 335-354.

22.2

From Community Participation in Physical Activity to Olympic Integration

R.D. Steadward

As people with disabilities strive to become involved in physical activity and sport programs and to obtain the right to integrated involvement in the Olympics, a paradox arises. In 1986, it was estimated that only 28% of disabled individuals were physically active. Furthermore, because existing sport delivery systems primarily were aimed at the "able-bodied" population, there were relatively few opportunities for a person with a disability to take part in physical activity and sport programs regularly (Canadian Summit on Fitness, 1986, cited in).

Ironically, the emergence of the International Paralympic Committee (IPC) in 1989 signaled increased cooperation among sport bodies to gain international and Olympic recognition at the highest level of sport competition for persons with disabilities.

How is it that at one end of the scale, opportunities are limited for integration into sports in schools and communities, while at the international and world level, athletes with disabilities are producing marathon times that so-called able-bodied athletes can only dream about?

The truth is that much work remains to be done at every level if the goal of full integration of people with disabilities into physical activity and sport participation is to be realized.

Toward a Self-Help Philosophy: The Role of Physical Activity for People With Disabilities

It is important that professionals working with persons with disabilities strive for sport excellence as well as physical activity and sport participation for all individuals. However, as Ferguson (1988) has observed, in recent years there has been a shift toward increased personal responsibility for medical care. Furthermore, due to fiscal constraints, there is a movement toward increased self-help not only in medical situations but in recreation as well. For example, The Rainbow Report (1989) underscored the need for increased personal responsibility for health in response to the severe strains on the province of Alberta's health care budget. In fact, a Smart Card was suggested that people and the health care system could use to monitor their own health care expenditures. At the same time, the implication was clear that there is a finite amount of health care funding per person. Although the concept of universality was protected in the Alberta government's response to the Rainbow Report (Partners in Health, 1991), there is little doubt that we all face a changing, and possibly less comprehensive, health care system. It is entirely possible that the disabled population may face declining health care support. Recent cuts in medical benefits to people with disabilities warn us of future trends in health care. Canada may no longer be able to afford to pay for all health needs. Hence, the value of physical activity for health enhancement takes on even greater importance.

The value of physical activity in maintaining health cannot be disputed. This is no less true for persons, young or old, who have disabilities. For example, for those with spinal cord injuries, coronary disease is a leading cause of death. In the past, persons with spinal cord injury were often afflicted with decubital ulcers and infections as a result of weight gain and a progressive cycle of inactivity. Such inactivity was accelerated by a lack of opportunity for physical activity. In addition to health benefits, physical activity also is important to the maintenance of mental health. Quite simply, regular physical activity is essential for the health and well-being of people with disabilities.

The Final Barrier

While the disabled population struggles with the lack of access to physical activity programs in schools and communities, elite athletes with disabilities face problems of full integration and recognition.

The final barrier facing elite sport participants with disabilities is full representation, including medal status, at the Olympic games. The recent formation of the IPC and its Presidential Commission on Integration (International Committee on Integration) represents a move toward the cooperation and cohesion necessary to gain approval of the International Olympic Committee (IOC) and full acceptance into the Olympic games. Many barriers still exist that can be traced to the developmental level of physical activity and sport in schools and communities.

Unfortunately, when elite athletes with disabilities are prevented from participating at the highest realms of competition, this final barrier perpetuates the perception of the general public and the disabled community itself that persons with a disability are less competent than their able-bodied counterparts. As long as this attitude persists, full integration at all levels of physical activity and sport cannot and will not occur.

Physical Activity Delivery System

Several models for evaluating physical activity delivery systems exist. One model, proposed by Smith (1974, 1988) and elaborated on by Fitness Canada, can be used to evaluate physical activity opportunities and sport programs for people with disabilities. The elements of this model are shown in Table 22.1.

Essentially this model has two main features:

1. Opportunity options, which reflect different levels of participation
2. Involvement and development processes that are fundamental to education for initiation and continued involvement in physical activities

The essential questions that arise using this model in relation to people with disabilities are these:

Table 22.1 Physical Activity Delivery System in Canada

Developmental processes	Opportunity options
Inactive population	Unstructured participation
Awareness	Structured participation
Initiation	Recreational competition
Basic skill acquisition	Low-intensity competition
Skill and strategy development	High-intensity competition

Data from Smith (1988).

- Does the model accommodate people with disabilities?
- Can they be categorized under the same participation and opportunity classes as people without disabilities?
- Can they be categorized under the same developmental processes as outlined in the model?
- Is sport excellence for athletes with disabilities synonymous with sport excellence for those without disabilities?
- Do athletes with disabiltiies have the same opportunities for recognition and excellence in competition as their peers without disabilities?

The first three questions are associated with the developmental process and participation aspects of the Smith (1974) Fitness Canada model. The final two questions deal with high-intensity and high-performance sport. The answers to the first three questions depend largely on the education and certification of those who teach people with disabilities. These questions address the level of integration of those with disabilities into physical education and sports.

The final two questions are primarily associated with the historical development of disabled sport organizations, which culminated in the establishment of the IPC. These questions address the final barriers to full Olympic integration.

The questions point to the extremes of the physical activity continuum: the development of skills and attitudes in young children in the schools and the development of sporting excellence. Developmental aspects of sport delivery systems are essential for developing the knowledge and skills young children require for future participation in physical activity programs. A basic assumption of the Smith (1974) Fitness Canada model is that at least some people who begin participating in a sport as children will eventually become elite performers. At the other end of the spectrum, elite athletes are given the opportunity to strive for world-class performance and Olympic medals. Within this continuum, an unusual situation exists for persons with a disability: There are more opportunities for adults than for youths.

In the context of this diverse system of involvement of people with disabilities in physical activity and sport, the degree to which the Fitness Canada model can be applied will now be examined. Each aspect of the model will be addressed, and the particular issues arising with respect to individuals with disabilities will be considered.

The Developmental Processes

The developmental processes are very relevant to integration and education in physical activity. The development of skills and knowledge prepares children for regular participation in physical activity and potential participation in sport at the community, provincial, national, and elite levels. As those with disabilities progress through the developmental process, they learn about their abilities and about opportunities for integration. Also during the developmental years, dreams are born about participating in the Olympics. In addition, at this stage able-bodied youth learn to accept or reject people with disabilities as equals in athletic competition as well as in life. The field of physical activity appears committed to integration. This commitment has been reflected in increased physical education programs for people with disabilities. Goals in those programs have included skill acquisition, physical fitness, and active participation. However, the systematic evaluation of program outcomes has received scant attention (Watkinson, 1988).

The Inactive Population

Inactivity is a particular concern with regard to individuals with disabilities. For example, an adult or child with multiple sclerosis faces a fluctuating health status, but exercise can help to maintain strength and flexibility. In muscular dystrophy patients, regular exercise can reduce the chronic loss of strength and muscle mass. In addition, the psychological benefits of activity for individuals affected by these disorders can be quite impressive. Often overprotective parents, physicians, and teachers exclude children with congenital cardiac problems, spina bifida, and asthma from physical activity when it would in fact benefit them. These adults are overprotective because they do not know the needs, capabilities, interests, and limitations of people with disabilities. In particular, the sedentary lifestyle often associated with post–spinal cord trauma has been linked with increased incidence of coronary artery disease, a leading cause of death for spinal cord patients. It is indeed unfortunate that this aspect of the model is such a good fit for people with disabilities. Given the large percentage of inactive people with disabilities, clearly change is needed in this sector of the model.

Awareness

The awareness component reflects people's need to understand and appreciate the value of physical activity. The major barriers in this component of the model for people with disabilities are the level of integration of children with disabilities into regular physical activity classes and limited access to information about physical activity programs. Although the profession is trying to overcome these barriers, much work remains to be done. Volunteers and professionals need comprehensive education about the needs, interests, capabilities, and exercise limitations of people with disabilities. The quality of leisure counseling activities is of particular importance at this stage (Taylor, 1988).

Many individuals with disabilities need to learn the value of exercise and how to use leisure time if they are to become active. The inadequate professional preparation of teachers and recreation counselors in leisure education of people with disabilities should thus be of great concern.

Initiation

Initiation refers to the processes that introduce people to the value and demands of different physical activities. These processes vary with age and interests and may involve the school, the community, and the family. Until recently, few community programs of physical activity and sport were available for the child or adult with a disability due to a lack of appropriate facilities. In addition, the increasingly litigious nature of society had raised questions about the risks of working with a person with a disability. A lack of knowledge of the capabilities and limitations of people with disabilities and the effects of exercise on them had resulted in reluctance to include them in physical activity programs for fear of injury and negligence suits. Fortunately, many organizations now offer community activities and sports such as track and field, bowling, skiing, basketball, and swimming.

Basic Skill Acquisition, Developmental Skill Acquisition, and Skill and Strategy Development

This aspect of the model deals with the development of basic skills, including simple, reactive, and complex skills, as well as the activity-specific strategies needed for enjoyable involvement in physical activities and recreational sport programs.

A universal theme in physical education literature is the need for a continuum of activity opportunities so children, in particular those with disabilities, can select appropriate levels of integrated or segregated physical activity to optimize their skill development. It is essential that children have the opportunity to master basic skills (running, jumping, catching, throwing, climbing) in a supportive learning environment. This may entail full integration or specialized programming involving one-on-one teaching or specialized group teaching. The offering of such supportive programs is often hampered by a misunderstanding of the terms *integration* and *segregation*. Often, in the name of integration, children with disabilities are put in programs with able-bodied children. In these programs children with disabilities may experience only frustration and failure. These children require success within an integrated setting where individual or small-group help can be given. They need integration with functional specialization, not segregation.

The need for highly trained staff is clear. However, it is disturbing to note that a recent survey by the Canadian Association of Health, Physical Education and Recreation of 1,550 schools and 1,107 teachers indicated some woeful inadequacies in physical education for children with disabilities (cited in Evans, 1988). For example, only 50% of physical educators in adapted physical education reported having a degree. Only 19% had even one course credit in adapted physical education. An additional 19% had taken no physical education courses, and only 11% had participated in workshops or upgrading in the previous 5 years. To improve this aspect of the physical activity delivery system, more attention must be paid to adequate teacher preparation and leadership training and to effective programming. A continuum of physical activity programs is required to allow students to choose appropriate activities for their ability levels (Watkinson, 1988). Furthermore, Goodwin (1988) called for a continuum of programming options in modified or regular programs and for placements based on reliable, valid assessments. In fact, Dickenson (1988) called for a review of the compulsory curriculum, financial assistance for equal access for physical activity opportunities, and a higher profile for staff training and effective leisure counseling. Goodwin has observed specific skills, attitudes, and knowledge unique to adapted physical activity; hence, special training is required to optimize the role of physical activity for people with disabilities in schools and communities.

Thus, in relation to the developmental processes aspect of the Fitness Canada model, three main areas of concern exist:

1. Education of teachers with regard to physical education for students with disabilities
2. The level of integration and, therefore, equality of participation opportunities for skill and knowledge acquisition
3. The need for the present physical activity delivery system to prepare more knowledgeable, skillful young athletes for future elite-level sport participation.

Opportunity Options

Since 1924, when the International Deaf Sports Organization (CISS) was formed, tremendous advances have been made in the development of sport organizations for athletes with disabilities. These developments have created more opportunities for participation and competition in many different sports. At the same time, athletes with disabilities have made impressive improvements in performance due to significant advances in wheelchair design, improved quality and quantity of training methods, better coaching, and a significant increase in research. Yet one barrier still must be overcome: full participation in the Olympic Games with medal recognition. Since its inception in 1989, the IPC has recognized that several barriers remain to this final step in the integration process and that fundamental differences of view exist between the Olympic and Paralympic organizations.

Unstructured Participation

The initial aspect of the opportunity options component of the physical activity delivery system model assumes that individuals must initiate their own activities alone or with the help of others. It is clear from the preceding discussion that people with disabilities have limited access to information about physical activity and rarely have the opportunity to gain such knowledge in quality daily physical education. Discrimination and a lack of accessible facilities have exacerbated this situation. In recent years, disability-specific interest groups have formed in hospitals and other centers. The groups have worked to alleviate these problems, but they continue to seriously limit the participation of people with disabilities in unstructured situations.

Structured Participation and Recreational Competition

Even after the Second World War, people with disabilities had few opportunities, if any, to participate in physical activity. Often they were afraid to participate due to a lack of knowledge. For example, people with spinal cord injuries were not expected to live long, let alone participate in organized sports. Although the CISS began in 1924 and wheelchair basketball appeared in the United States in 1945, interest in physical activity for people with disabilities did not develop until 1948. In that year Sir Ludwig Guttman established the Stoke Mandeville Games, which developed into the International Stoke Mandeville Games Federation (ISMGF), later named the International Stoke Mandeville Wheelchair Sport Federation. Since then many national and international sport organizations have arisen that provide more access to physical activities including nordic skiing, volleyball, shooting, weight lifting, fencing, table tennis, tennis, racquetball, basketball, archery, swimming, downhill skiing, and water skiing. Specialized sports, such as boccia, goal ball, wheelchair rugby, and ice sledging have developed for people with disabilities.

In addition, centers that specialize in sport and fitness programs, as well as health and lifestyle counseling, have arisen out of increased public and government awareness of the needs and rights of people with disabilities. For example, at the Rick Hansen Centre in Edmonton, Alberta, individuals with disabilities can take part in rock climbing, sky diving, canoeing, and sophisticated resistance training. In short, they have access to the same opportunities as able-bodied people. However, few such centers exist, and much remains to be done if they are to be developed nationally and internationally.

In these times of budget cuts, there is a fear that much of the progress toward integration in physical activity and sport programs may be stalled or lost altogether. Neither public apathy nor bureaucratic cost cutting can be allowed to stall the efforts of those who have devoted themselves to securing these opportunities for people with disabilities.

A Paradox. If one questions wheelchair athletes about physical activity and sport participation, many report that they were relatively inactive before their injury. Yet following their injury they often aspire to and achieve the highest levels of athletic performance. In contrast, fewer of those with congenital disabilities and those injured early in life are involved in elite sport. Why do so few of these children become elite athletes?

Children with congenital abnormalities and with traumatic injuries, such as spinal cord injuries, receive limited opportunity for physical activity and are often overprotected in school. Unfortunately, unless they become involved in community sport organizations, they may not receive the information and encouragement they need to make the transition to organized sport participation. Although there is increased awareness of the value of physical activity for youth with disabilities, more people who developed disabilities as adults participate in sports later in life than those who received traumatic injuries as children. There is little doubt that a lack of teacher education and recreation leadership training results in a lack of awareness of the needs, interests, limitations, and capabilities of children with disabilities. This presents an effective developmental barrier to their future participation in physical activity and sport programs.

The Changing Face of Youth Sport: What Effect Will This Have on the Process of Integration? For many years, developmental theorists have argued that it is more appropriate in sports to emphasize age-appropriate skill development than to emphasize competition (Bloom, 1985; Smith, 1988). Unfortunately, until recently sports involvement for children as young as 5 years of age has been based on a competitive sport model. Coaches have only recently seriously questioned the competitive philosophy. It is interesting to note that in Canada the National Coaching Certification Program

(NCCP) has shifted its emphasis to developmental models. The highly respected NCCP program educates coaches from the community to the national level. Certainly, this new developmental model will influence the philosophy and practice of the next generation of volunteer coaches. In recent years, coaches of athletes with disabilities have taken the NCCP program's three theory levels and specific, sport-based programs, either through community or sport-specific organizations. The question thus arises how this will affect the integration of people with disabilities into community physical activity and sport programs. Developmental models, designed to promote skill mastery rather than intense competition, are expected to greatly benefit children with disabilities. No longer left until last to be picked for a game, these children may now develop at their own rates and develop a sense of mastery of important skills.

Low- and High-Intensity Competition and High-Performance Competition

Since 16 athletes participated in the first Stoke Mandeville Games in 1948, the Paralympics have grown to the point where more than 4,000 athletes with disabilities participated in the Barcelona Summer Paralympics in 1992. The competition, no longer limited to spinal cord–injured athletes, has advanced in both size and scope. In Barcelona, amputees, blind athletes, and athletes with spinal cord injuries and cerebral palsy all competed together. The games have grown to include a comprehensive range of activities. As the Paralympic Games have evolved, so too have many other sport organizations.

Since the ISMGF was founded, other organizations have formed, such as the International Sports Organization for the Disabled (ISOD, 1964), the Cerebral Palsy International Sports Association (CP-ISRA, 1978), the International Blind Sports Association (IBSA, 1981), and the International Association of Sports for the Mentally Handicapped (INAS-FMH, 1986), and all have developed mandates of sport excellence. The jealous guarding of territory and the diversity of policies, however, led the International Olympic Committee to request that one organization be formed with which it could interact at the policy level.

An informal organization, the International Coordinating Committee (ICC) was founded in 1983 and later replaced by the International Paralympic Committee (IPC). In 1989, the IPC was formed to serve as the only organization with the right to organize Paralympic games and multidisability world and regional championships and games. The formation of the IPC represented an important step because the organization is sport-specific rather than disability-specific. This organization was able to address the IOC regarding integration at the Olympic games.

Even though there were no Olympic opportunities for athletes with disabilities in 1984, the IOC did sanction a downhill skiing demonstration at the Sarajevo Winter Games. Later that year two demonstration wheelchair races were held at the Los Angeles Summer Olympics. In 1988 further demonstrations were included at the Summer Olympics in Seoul and at the Winter Olympics in Calgary. However, these were not medal events.

It is at this point that development of sport for people with disabilities has stalled. The IPC is now the driving force for the integration of athletes with disabilities into the Olympic games with full medal status. The IPC argues that these athletes fit the excellence mode, are motivated at the highest level, and have the highest possible objectives. The IPC does, however, recognize that all disabilities and levels of disabilities cannot be accommodated and integrated into the games and, as a result, inclusion criteria have been established. The inclusion of athletes with disabilities into the Olympic Games represents one more hurdle for the IOC to accept, just as it has accepted the inclusion of women, developing nations, new sports, and the means to control performance-enhancing drugs. There is no question that if we are to flourish as an organization then we must adapt to the changes demanded of us. Integrating athletes with disabilities into the games would contribute both to the Olympic movement and to the ideals on which the games are based.

Yet many barriers remain to integration, including differences between the Paralympic and Olympic movements.

Barriers

Major Differences Between the Olympic and Paralympic Movements: Impact on Full Integration

Several major differences between the Olympic and Paralympic movements may affect the ease with which full integration into elite competition may be achieved. There are relatively few elite athletes with disabilities compared with the number of able-bodied athletes. This reflects in part a lack of public awareness, funding, and opportunities in some countries. In addition, fewer countries participate in the Paralympics than in the Olympic Games. Perhaps of greatest importance as a potential barrier to full integration into the Olympic games is the classification system of the Paralympics. The number of classifications produces an inordinate number of medal ceremonies and reduced numbers in each event, decreasing competition in favor of absolute equality. Finally, public recognition and acceptance of the Paralympics does not match that of the Olympic Games. Despite the efforts of the Seoul committee (1988) in attracting more than 90,000 spectators to the Opening Ceremonies, the Paralympics still lack public support and interest. Because the competition is not

highly publicized or valued, it is unlikely to attract major sponsors. This in turn will affect IOC rulings with regard to participation. Whether we like it or not, the Olympics, for all its ideals, has become a talent showcase and a business. The Los Angeles Games were a classic example. In such a climate, it is difficult to overcome the barrier of final acceptance.

Public Perception, Education and Support: Prejudices Among Disability Groups

If elite athletes with disabilities are to be accepted, then the public must see a unified front within the disabled community. In 1990 in the Canadian Senate, Matthew Burns suggested that prejudices within the disabled community hinder the removal of public prejudices toward disabled sport. If we accept the comment ''Let he who is without prejudice make the first pitch for integration,'' then political infighting among organizations must cease immediately.

Political Issues

Like the Olympics, the Paralympics have not escaped the effects of politics in sport. For example, the involvement of the South African team in the 1976 games in Toronto resulted in the Canadian government's withdrawing $500,000 in support funds. Although this money was earmarked for sport organizations for people with disabilities, its withdrawal affected the attitude of games organizers regarding apartheid and segregation. An organization fighting for full integration could scarcely afford to appear to endorse segregation, albeit of a different kind.

Developmental Models of Sports Participation: Concerns With Athletic Competition in Youth: A Help or Hindrance to the Disabled Integration Movement

As previously noted, a lack of integration opportunities in schools and a lack of qualified teachers affects the educational and physical activity opportunities of disabled individuals. In addition, early participation acts as a feeder system and motivational environment for later athletic success. However, the Paralympic movement and disabled sport organizations in general must proceed with caution with regard to early selection ideals and involvement of youngsters in competition. As noted, the NCCP has shifted its emphasis to a developmental sport model in which youngsters are encouraged to acquire skills rather than to compete. Such a change portends well for the child with a disability who needs to concentrate on skill development before involvement in games. In addition, organizations like Fun Team Alberta have arisen in response to the increasing alienation of children from organized sport as a function of the "too much too soon" syndrome. The emphasis here is on fun, participation, skill development, and family and community involvement. What better model for integration of children into physical activity programs? Having mastered basic skills in an atmosphere of enjoyment without undue competition, a child may develop the motivation to continue with physical activity and become involved with sport organizations in adulthood.

Perceived Limitations of Disabled People

There is little doubt that people with disabilities see themselves as handicapped in many ways. For example, following spinal cord injury, patients may initially retreat from physical activity and want to eliminate thoughts of further physical activities. This is an understandable reaction to trauma, but such attitudes must change if the individual is to return to physical activity programs. Hence, rehabilitation programs are vital for these individuals. For those with congenital disabilities, the lack of education and knowledge of physical activity can become a self-fulfilling prophecy, particularly where attitudes of teachers and cohorts are less than encouraging.

Organizations: Working for Whom?

Organizations working for integration of people with disabilities at the highest levels of competition must not become bogged down in bureaucracy. They must remember that they are working for their members and strive to develop policies of action, not policies of internal organization (Burns, 1990). Internal struggles, such as those among groups representing people with different disabilities, must be avoided.

Conclusions

Sport and physical activity for people with disabilities only partially fits the physical activity delivery system model proposed by Smith (1984) Fitness Canada. Two key areas need to be addressed. First, more education is needed both for the disabled community in terms of skill and knowledge development and leisure counseling and for the able-bodied community with regard to attitudes toward disability and the athletic potential of people with disabilities. Second, differences between the Paralympic and Olympic movements must be addressed, particularly with regard to philosophy and classification systems, if full medal event participation for elite athletes with disabilities is to become a viable reality.

References

Bloom, B.S. (1985). *Developing talent in young people*. New York: Ballantine.

Burns, M.C. (1990). Integration opportunities in athletics and recreation and other issues of concern to people with physical disabilities. *Senate of Canada Report* Government of Canada.

Dickenson, R. (1988). Some general recommendations for the field of adapted physical activity. In *Jasper Talks Proceedings: Strategies for change in adapted physical activity in Canada* (pp. 36-37). October 9-12, 1986, Jasper, Alberta: CAHPER/ACSEPC.

Evans, J.R. (1988). The role of education in the adapted physical education delivery system: A state of the art review. *Jasper Talks Proceedings: Strategies for change in adapted physical activity in Canada* (pp. 38-39). October 9-12, 1986, Jasper, Alberta: CAHPER/ACSEPC.

Ferguson, T. (1988). Medical megatrends: The consumer as provider of health care. Keynote address. In *Jasper Talks Proceedings: Strategies for change in adapted physical activity in Canada* (pp. 10-12). October 9-12, 1986, Jasper, Alberta: CAHPER/ACSEPC.

Goodwin, D. (1988). The need for specialist training adapted physical activity. *Jasper Talks Proceedings: Strategies for change in adapted physical activity in Canada* (p. 31). October 9-12, 1986, Jasper, Alberta: CAHPER/ACSEPC.

Government of Alberta. (1991, November). *Partners in health: Government of Alberta's response to Premier's commission on future health care for Albertans*. Alberta: Government of Alberta Queen's Printer.

Introduction. (1988). *Jasper Talks Proceedings: Strategies for change in adapted physical activity in Canada*, October 9-12, 1986, p. 4. Jasper, Alberta: CAHPER/ACSEPC.

Smith, M. (1974). A preliminary case for classifying sports environments by participant objectives. *Journal of the Canadian Association of Health, Physical Education and Recreation*.

Smith, M. (1988). Understanding and changing physical activity delivery systems. *Jasper Talks Proceedings: Strategies for change in adapted physical activity in Canada* (pp. 32-35). October 9-12, 1986, Jasper, Alberta: CAHPER/ACSEPC.

Steadward, R. (1988). Issues in adapted physical activity: A knowledge base. *Jasper Talks Proceedings: Strategies for change in adapted physical activity in Canada* (pp. 28-30). October 9-12, 1986, Jasper, Alberta: CAHPER/ACSEPC.

Taylor, J. (1988). Leisure counselling as an integral part of program development. *Jasper Talks Proceedings: Strategies for change in adapted physical activity in Canada* (pp. 17-18). October 9-12, 1986, Jasper, Alberta: CAHPER/ACSEPC.

The Rainbow Report. (1989, December). *Our vision for health*. Alberta: Government of Alberta, Queen's Printer.

Watkinson, J. (1988). Adapted physical activity: The development and evaluation of integrated programs. *Jasper Talks Proceedings: Strategies for change in adapted physical activity in Canada* (pp. 16-17). October 9-12, 1986, Jasper, Alberta: CAHPER/ACSEPC.

23

Workplace Active Living and Total Quality Management: A Paradigm For A New Corporate Culture

Michael H. Cox
Daniel S. Miles

Few would argue that prevention of disease is more cost-effective and humane than treatment. Nevertheless, all societies currently spend far more on disease treatment than prevention. In both humanistic and economic terms, the impact of chronic diseases related to lifestyle, however, has not been controlled through medical treatment. The impact on mortality due to poor lifestyle behaviors in the United States has been estimated at 2.1 million deaths annually (U.S. Department of Health and Human Services, 1990). Similar statistics relating injudicious lifestyles to morbidity and mortality have been steadily accumulating in the scientific and medical literature for the last forty years (Manson et al., 1992; Morris, Heady, Raffle, Roberts, & Parks, 1953). Thus, international health care agendas for the next several years will focus on disease prevention through health promotion. Examples of such efforts are *Healthy People 2000: National Health Promotion and Disease Prevention Objectives* (USDHHS, 1990) in the United States and *Achieving Health for All: A Framework for Health Promotion* (Department of National Health and Welfare, 1986) in Canada. Both documents point to the working environment as an important setting for the delivery of preventive health care.

The workplace has been considered to be an effective venue for primary or even secondary prevention (Cox, 1987). Large numbers of people can be reached in a cost effective and timely manner. Moreover, the opportunity exists to design an environment and create a culture which would allow employees to make prudent health behavior choices. Although it is an attractive hypothesis, the impact of a rather limited number of preventive health programs over the last 20 years remains questionable (Fielding, 1982; Shephard, 1992). In the future, success of such programs will depend on integrating these preventive health programs into the long-term corporate vision, mission, culture, and strategy.

While governmental officials and health professionals challenge industrial leaders to include health promotion programs within the corporate strategy, North American industry is facing many serious challenges. The current challenges to North American industrial leaders are multiple, urgent, and complex and have led them to reassess programs of quality management. Businesses must increase productivity, reduce costs, improve overall efficiency, and deliver a product or provide a service of high quality and lasting value. Furthermore, an emerging global marketplace has intensified competition for goods and services. These challenges have motivated corporations in North America to re-evaluate the way they do business.

Two concepts which are emerging simultaneously in North America and may be compatible within the work setting are *Total Quality Management* (TQM) and *Workplace Active Living* (WAL). This paper describes both and discusses the potential compatibility and integration of the two concepts.

Total Quality Management (TQM): Historical Perspective

Some 40 years ago, an American industrial theorist and expert in statistical quality control, Dr. W. Edwards Deming, presented to the Japanese his concepts of "total quality management." At the time, American industry paid little attention to Deming and his small band of followers. The American approach to industrial problem solving was centered around the worker and his or her work ethic. If a product was defective or a service delivered poorly, it was the workers' fault. The solution to inferior quality was to remove the worker or send him or her to a training course. Some have called this victim blaming. Berwick (1989) calls this "the theory of bad apples" or "quality by inspection."

On the other hand, Deming and his associates maintained that quality begins and ends with management. Quality improvement is a process by which management, through clear consistent communication, creates a corporate culture focused on perfection. Deming calls it a process of "continuous improvement." In organizations driven by quality, imperfection is not tolerated, and defects are considered an opportunity.

Now, American industrialists head for Japan to find the inner secrets of Japanese industrial success. They are finding out that quality is tangible and measurable. Unfortunately, these trips are probably not necessary since most North Americans could tell these industrial leaders that Japanese products conform to rigid standards and perform to specifications. It is accepted that Japanese products do what is expected of them. The marketing slogan for the Lexus automobile captures this philosophy: A Lexus is the result of "the relentless pursuit of perfection."

TQM: Current Approach

Traditionally industry has viewed the concept of quality subjectively. However, TQM advocates maintain, contrary to popular belief, that quality is tangible (Berwick, Godfrey, & Roessner, 1990). A business devoted to quality can produce products and provide services which are error free. The business understands what is required to produce a defect-free product or provide a consumer friendly service. Quality is a process in which things are done right the first time. Problems and errors are prevented.

In the TQM system, performance measurements must be objective, continual, and visible (Schaffer & Thomson,1992). Appropriate measurements help mold the framework for concrete incremental improvements and the establishment of short term goals which align with the long-term corporate vision. The purpose of quality improvement is to institutionalize quality as a process which "becomes more and more an enduring way of life, as it becomes the culture of the company" (Crosby, 1984).

Crosby maintains there are four absolutes in the TQM theory. These absolutes are:

1. *A clear definition of quality.* Each person in the system must work toward doing things right the first time. Management's task is to establish a clear set of requirements and to enable employees to meet those requirements. Quality is defined as conformance to requirements.

2. *A system which denotes quality as prevention.* Implementation of this concept requires complete understanding of all organizational processes to identify where preventive action is needed. Within the prevention process, errors are identified and become opportunities for improvement.

3. *The performance standard must be "zero defects."* Every action within the process must be done as planned.

4. *Quality is measured specifically by evaluating the price of nonconformance.* Quality must be viewed in financial terms. The price of nonconformance is the cost of compensation, and of setting up repair networks. The price of conformance relates to expenditures required to manufacture a product or provide a service correctly.

The process of TQM is in perpetual motion. It is a process whereby knowledge for product improvement and problem prevention is constantly sought (see Figure 23.1). TQM is a systems process. That is, it focuses on the systems from which products and services evolve. Each employee is part of one or more vital corporate systems, not part of a traditional "top-down" management structure. Employee involvement is central to TQM theory. The corporate culture creates an environment of encouragement, support, and facilitation for each worker at all levels of the organization. For a further discussion of the TQM concept, readings are recommended from Shewhart (1925), Deming (1986), Juran (1992), Ishikawa (1986), and Donabedian (1980).

Workplace Active Living (WAL)

Active living is a Canadian concept. Basic to the active living conceptual framework is that physical activity is part of a dynamic life system, which touches the body, mind, and spirit. This philosophy may be a prudent and perhaps more realistic approach to promoting physical activity in a culture than previous efforts. Certainly, traditional approaches attempting to motivate the vast majority of citizens to an active lifestyle have at best shown only marginal success. Moreover, recent scientific data lend further credibility to the active living approach (Blair, Kohl, & Gordon, 1992; Debusk, Stenestrand, Sheehan, & Haskell, 1990).

The long-term vision for the active living concept is for it to become a Canadian cultural trademark. For this to happen, the process of implementation must cross all boundaries of Canadian society and find its way into every community and workplace.

Workplace active living (WAL) is an extension and a part of the active living process (Fitness Canada, 1990). In Canada, a vision toward active living in the workplace has been articulated. This vision is part of a strategic framework largely developed by The Canadian

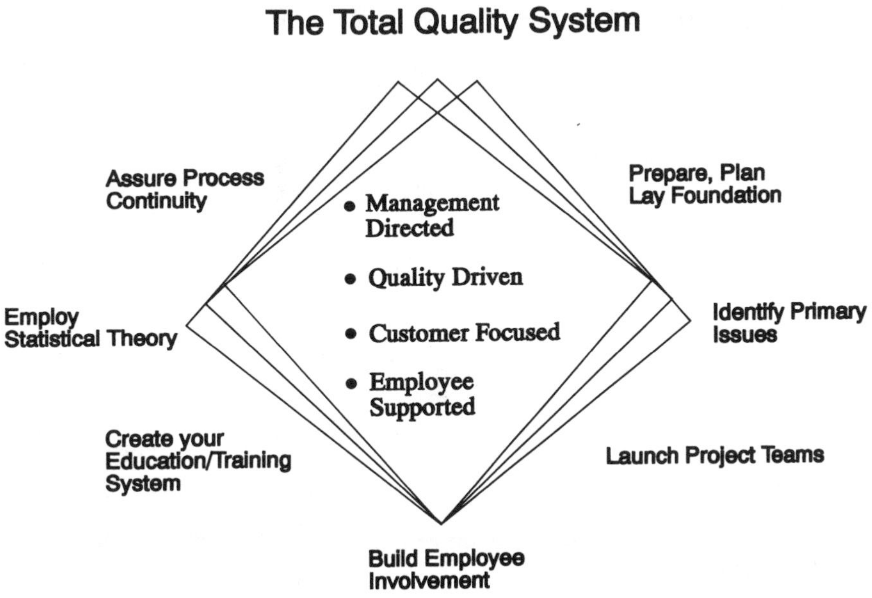

The Total Quality System

Figure 23.1 The seven dynamics of TQM which support a system for continuous improvement (reprinted from Daisey, 1990).

Table 23.1   Guiding Principles for Workplace Active Living (WAL)

- Individual employee interests and needs are important considerations in the planning of programs and services for active living.
- Opportunities and initiatives for active living can improve the level of job satisfaction, enhance the quality of working life, and contribute both to the overall well-being of employees and the organization.
- Supportive workplace environments enhance the success of organizational strategies for active living.
- Committed leadership is an integral component of exemplary workplace initiatives. As such, on-going support, training, and development opportunities are essential.
- Advocacy and educational campaigns directed at decision makers are effective ways to promote the development of active living in the workplace.

Centre for Active Living in the Workplace (CCALW). This strategic framework includes guiding principles, areas of emphasis, and National goal statements developed by the CCALW (see Tables 23.1 and 23.2).

The Development of WAL

Since the 1974 Canadian conference on employee fitness was held (Department of National Health and Welfare, 1975), governments at all levels, both in Canada and the United States, have placed a strong emphasis on development of employee fitness and lifestyle programs. For many years it has been suggested that employee fitness and lifestyle programs could have a significant impact on people involved in risk taking behavior. Factors that have made the employee fitness and lifestyle program approach attractive include

- the ability to reach a large population in a relatively controlled, concentrated, and accessible environment (Cox, 1988; Shephard, 1991);
- reinforcement of positive changes in behavior through industrial or corporate incentives (Stoffelmayr et al., 1992);
- the ability to design integrative models with other work site health promotion programs (Marsh, Vojtecky, & Marsh, 1987); and
- in some cases, corporate willingness to relinquish work time for different aspects of the program.

This is further supported by research which suggests that convenience may be the most universal discriminator as to why people do or do not exercise (Dishman, 1990). In accepting this logic, it is curious that after 20 years of employee fitness and lifestyle programming, these programs are only attracting a minority of employees.

Currently, less than 13% of large Canadian corporations offer such programs, and in the small business sector, employee fitness and lifestyle programs are almost non-existent (Canadian Chamber of Commerce, 1987; Fitness and Lifestyle Research Institute, 1990; Shephard, 1992). Moreover, even in companies considered to have successful programs, long-term adherence rates at best are less than 30% of the total employee population (Brill et al., 1991; Cox, 1984; Fielding, 1984; Stoffelmayr et al., 1992). Furthermore, the most cynical evaluators would suggest that the majority of employees attending these programs were already active and would

Table 23.2 Summary Grid of Strategic Goals and Partnership Categories

Partnership categories Goals	Active living and related organizations	Governments	Management and other decision makers	Program and service providers	Academic and research community	Media
Network development						
Implement blueprint	•	•	•	•	•	•
Develop partnerships	•	•	•	•	•	•
Systems and structures	•	•		•		
Human resource development						
Networks	•		•	•		
Training and development	•			•		
Guidelines	•	•		•	•	
Resource development						
Human and financial assistance	•	•		•		
Products, programs, and services	•	•	•			
Specific target groups	•		•		•	
Collaboration and coordination	•	•	•			•
Promotion						
Spread the message	•	•	•	•		•
Promotion needs	•	•	•			•
Promotion strategies	•	•	•			•
Research and evaluation						
Monitor prevalence and nature		•	•		•	
Develop instruments and tools		•			•	
Link with research	•	•			•	

continue to be active independent of any "in-house" offerings.

Issues such as daily work schedules and the perception of accessibility need to be evaluated. Perhaps most employees perceive such programs as too vigorous or regimented, although to the casual observer these programs may look convenient. Changing into workout clothes, exercising, showering, and giving up a lunch period, however, may not be all that appealing to a large number of workers. For others, particularly those employees who generate a large proportion of the medical and absenteeism costs, the program may be perceived as a health risk. Still others among the workforce may find it embarrassing to change their clothes and exercise with fellow employees, or live up to the media image of the svelte young fashionable executive vigorously exercising without a bead of sweat on their forehead. It follows that concerns about privacy and enjoyment may need to be reviewed.

The perceived barriers to exercise participation typically reported include lack of time, conflicts with work, inconvenience, and no facilities, equipment, or program (Dishman, 1990; Shephard & Cox, 1988). Theoretically, a well-designed employee fitness and lifestyle program should overcome such barriers. Unfortunately, recruitment and retention statistics suggest otherwise (Martin & Dubbert, 1985). Moreover, even complex theoretical behavioral models attempting to characterize both sedentary and active populations have not shown major differences between these two groups in relation to beliefs and behavioral intent (Godin, Desharnais, Jobin, & Cook, 1987; Godin, Shephard, & Colantonio, 1986). Furthermore, there has been some suggestion that even the most sedentary individuals seem to have a latent desire to be active (Godin, Cox, & Shephard, 1983). If this is the case, WAL may provide the catalyst for behavior change given a supportive corporate environment (Wankel, Yardley, & Graham, 1985).

In the United States, the U.S. Department of Health and Human Services (1990) released *Healthy People 2000: National Health Promotion and Disease Prevention Objectives*. Among the specific targets of the 300 objectives are preventive services related to the work site. One objective is to "increase the proportion of worksites offering employer-sponsored physical activity and fitness programs" (p. 103, see Table 23.3). The Healthy People 2000 initiative has provided an exciting destination, but the road map is not well drawn. Similarly, the CCALW has clearly described where they are

Table 23.3 Healthy People 2000 Target Objectives for Implementing Employee Fitness Programs in Companies of Different Sizes

Worksite size	Year 2000 target
50-99 employees	20%
100-249 employees	35%
250-749 employees	50%
≥ 750 employees	80%

and where they want to be, but it has not detailed the path on how to get there. Advocates of WAL must understand corporate cultures and identify those corporations that are ready and willing to make workplace active living part of the way they do business.

Admittedly, WAL is in its infancy, and must draw primarily upon experience from employee fitness and lifestyle programming, as well as research results emanating from such programs over the last 15 years. Although supportive data has been accumulated over this period (Blair, Piserchia, Wilbur, & Crowder, 1986; Cox, Shephard, & Corey, 1981; Sharratt & Cox, 1988; Shephard, 1992), such a heavy focus on traditional employee fitness and lifestyle programs may in itself be limiting. Perhaps, a much broader perspective for the WAL concept may be more prudent as the process develops.

TQM and WAL: Conceptual Compatibility and Integration

TQM requires a defect-free product of lasting quality, while WAL is concerned with disease prevention and the quality of life. Both TQM and WAL aim for incremental improvements and require employee involvement in planning and implementation at all levels of the organization. Another similarity between the two concepts is they create cultures in which quality permeates the corporate environment. This philosophy not only includes products and services, but the very nature of the quality of working life and the company's relationship with employees.

TQM and WAL continually ask and seek answers to three basic questions:

1. Where are we now?
2. Where do we want to be?
3. How can we get there?

For the TQM process to be successful, companies must accept the approach voluntarily. TQM and WAL could be considered jointly to be a natural addition to the intrinsic factors relating to the quality of working life and employee motivation.

In the TQM process, managers spend 100% of their time facilitating the process and workers. A salient feature of the TQM process is that managers and workers continually define the requirements of the parts which make the whole. In the summary grid of strategic goals and partnership categories (review Table 23.2) laid out in *Working Actively Together: Canada's Blueprint Toward Active Living in the Workplace* (Fitness Canada, 1990), management is left out of several key indicators for WAL. In the TQM organization, a successful management relationship with employees is a priority; the WAL process will require the same. The Canadian WAL approach must be more targeted towards a management driven process.

In corporations that have adopted the TQM process, such as Xerox and 3M, the actions and culture of this process are highly visible. Every employee and each function within the corporation is involved and touched by the TQM process. A basic principle of TQM is the concept of involving and empowering employees. Each employee must be a partner in charting the corporate future, defining the corporate culture, and achieving quality goals. Similarly, the concept of WAL helps integrate the corporate environment and individual employee interests and needs. As with TQM, cooperation among employees, employee groups, supervisors, and the entire organization will eventually determine the nature and scope of the WAL process. It is also noteworthy, that a corporate culture and employee population centered in health, safety, and wellness is essential to both processes. It is within these principles that the synergy between WAL and TQM may be found.

For TQM to be successful it is critical that there is total organizational commitment and 100% involvement by the workforce. This is a formidable challenge for the WAL concept and may require rethinking of traditional program approaches which have attempted to create a physically active workforce.

Recent evidence suggests that the health and physical activity paradigm need not be presented as a complex one (Bouchard, Shephard, Stephens, Sutton, & McPherson, 1990). This seems to be particularly true, if the long-term goal is health related, as opposed to performance related, fitness (see Figure 23.2). Moreover, there is data to suggest that individuals do not need to take a "bleed through the eye" approach to exercise or even follow traditional methods of exercise prescription (which may be perceived to be too complex, inconvenient, and time consuming), to reduce disease risk and improve the quality of life (Blair et al., 1989; Debusk et al., 1990).

Future Directions

Lessons from the past 20 years have shown that increasing employee daily physical activity levels remains a

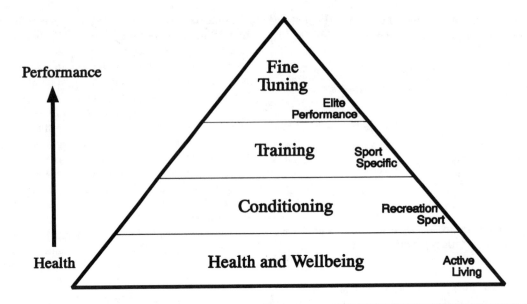

Figure 23.2 The triangle represents the continuum from health related activity for the population at large (base) to performance related training for elite athletes (apex).

challenge. Although increasingly popular, employee fitness and lifestyle programs have limited success in attracting large numbers of participants. Further, the majority of those who do participate may need the program the least. Although employee fitness and lifestyle programs can be part of a corporate culture which stresses positive health norms, a total process is needed to integrate daily physical activity into the lives of all workers.

Opportunity now exists to test the blending of the TQM and WAL processes. Both concepts are relatively new to North American industry and share similar philosophies. An emerging concept of TQM goes well beyond managing technology and is becoming more focused relative to human resources. TQM theory is now addressing a workforce whose demographics are changing. The workforce has become heterogenous; it is older and more inclusive of female, minority, and disabled workers. This is a timely challenge for the WAL concept, since many of these same employee groups now entering the workforce have traditionally been the most resistant to habitual physical activity. Correspondingly, from a public health perspective, these groups may benefit the most from increasing their daily activity levels (Dishman, 1990; Stephens, 1986; Stephens, Craig, & Ferris, 1986; U.S. Department of Health and Human Services, 1990). At the same time it is promising that the level of activity needed to have a profound influence on health and the quality of life may be less than previously envisioned (Blair et al., 1992; Gordon, Kohl, Scott, Gibbons, & Blair, 1992).

"AN AMBULANCE DOWN IN THE VALLEY"

T'was a dangerous cliff as they freely confessed,
Though to walk near its edge was so pleasant.
    But over its edge had slipped a Duke,
And it fooled many a peasant.

The people said something would have to be done,
But their projects did not at all tally.
Some said, "Put a fence around the edge of the cliff,"
Others, "An ambulance down in the valley."

The lament of the crowd was profound and loud,
As their hearts overflowed with pity;
But the ambulance carried the cry of the day,
As it spread to the neighboring cities.
So a collection was made to accumulate aid,
And dwellers in highway and alley,
Gave dollars and cents not to furnish a fence,
But an ambulance down in the valley.

"For the cliff is all right if you're careful," they said,
"And if folks ever slip and are falling;
It's not the slipping and falling that hurts them so much,
As the shock down below when they're stopping."

And so for the years as these mishaps occurred,
Quick forth would the rescuers sally,
To pick up the victims who fell from the cliff,
With the ambulance down in the valley.

(continued)

(Continued)

> Said one in his plea, "It's a marvel to me
> That you'd give so much greater attention,
> To repairing results than to curing the cause;
> Why you'd much better aim at prevention.
> For the mischief, of course, should be stopped at
> the source;
> Come friends and neighbors, let us rally!
> It makes far better sense to rely on a fence,
> Than an ambulance down in the valley.
>
> "He's wrong in his head," the majority said,
> "He would end all our earnest endeavors.
> He's the kind of a man that would shirk his responsi-
> ble work,
> But we will support it forever.
> Aren't we picking up all just as fast as they fall,
> And giving them care liberally?
> Why, a superfluous fence is of no consequence,
> If the ambulance works in the valley."
>
> Now this story seems queer as I've given it here,
> But things oft occur which are stranger.
> More humane we assert to repair the hurt,
> Than the plan of removing the danger.
> The best possible course would be to safeguard
> the source,
> And to attend to things rationally.
> Yes, build up the fence and let us dispense,
> With this ambulance down in the valley.
>
> ANONYMOUS

References

Berwick, D.M. (1989). Sounding board: Continuous improvement as an ideal in health care. *New England Journal of Medicine*, **320**(1): 53-56.

Berwick, D.M., Godfrey, A., & Roessner, J. (1990). *Curing health care: New strategies for quality improvement.* San Francisco: Jossey-Bass.

Blair, S.N., Kohl, H.W. & Gordon, N.F. (1992). Physical activity and health: A lifestyle approach. *Medicine, Exercise, Nutrition and Health*, **1**(1): 54-57.

Blair, S.N., Kohl, H.W., Paffenbarger, R.S., Clark, D.G., Cooper, K.H., & Gibbons, L.W. (1989). Physical fitness and all-cause mortality: A prospective study of healthy men and women. *Journal of the American Medical Association*, **262**, 2395-2401.

Blair, S.N., Piserchia, P.V., Wilbur, C.S., & Crowder, J.H. (1986). A public health intervention model for work-site health promotion. *Journal of the American Medical Association*, **255**, 921-926.

Bouchard, C., Shephard, R.J., Stephens, T., Sutton, J.R., & McPherson, B.D. (Eds.) (1990). *Exercise, fitness and health: A consensus of current knowledge.* Champaign, IL: Human Kinetics.

Brill, P.A., Kohl, H.W., Rogers, T., Collingwood, T.R., Sterling, C.L., & Blair, S.N. (1991). The relationship between sociodemographic characteristics and recruitment, retention, and health improvements in a worksite health promotion program. *American Journal of Health Promotion.* **5**(3): 215-220.

Canadian Chamber of Commerce. (1987). *Fitness and health promotion by Canadian business.* Ottawa: Author.

Cox, M.H. (1984). Fitness and life-style programs for business and industry: Problems in recruitment and retention. *Journal of Cardiovascular Rehabilitation*, **4**, 136-142.

Cox, M.H. (1987). Implementation of fitness and lifestyle programs: Critical issues. In S.H. Klarreich (Ed.), *Health and fitness in the workplace: Health education in business organizations* (pp. 338-354). New York: Praeger.

Cox, M.H. (1988). Costs and benefits. In: M. Collis, M. Cox, R. Gagne, S. Keir, & P. Youldon (Eds.). *Fitness and lifestyle at the workplace* (pp. 13-19). Ottawa: Fitness Canada.

Cox, M.H., Shephard, R.J., & Corey, P. (1981). Influence of an employee fitness programme upon fitness, productivity and absenteeism. *Ergonomics*, **24**, 795-806.

Crosby, P.B. (1984). *Quality without tears: The art of hassle-free management.* New York: New American Library.

Daisey, D.H. (1990). The seven dynamics of implementation. *Total Quality Dynamics*, **1**(2): 4-5.

Debusk, R.F., Stenestrand, U., Sheehan, M., & Haskell, W.L. (1990). Training effects of long versus short bouts of exercise in healthy subjects. *American Journal of Cardiology*, **65**, 1010-1013.

Deming, W.E. (1986). *Out of the crisis.* Cambridge, MA.: Massachusetts Institute of Technology, Center for Advanced Engineering Study.

Department of National Health and Welfare. (1975). *Proceedings of the National Conference on Employee Physical Fitness.* Ottawa: Author.

Department of National Health and Welfare. (1986). *Achieving health for all: A framework for health promotion.* Ottawa: Author.

Dishman, R.K. (1990). Determinants of participation in physical activity. In C. Bouchard, R.J. Shephard, T. Stephens, J.R. Sutton, & B.D. McPherson (Eds.), *Exercise, fitness and health: A consensus of current knowledge* (pp. 75-101). Champaign, IL: Human Kinetics.

Donabedian, A., (1980). *Explorations in quality assessment and monitoring, Volume I: The definition of quality and approaches to its assessment.* Ann Arbor, MI: Health Administration Press.

Fielding, J.E. (1982). Effectiveness of employee health improvement programs. *Journal of Occupational Medicine*, **24**, 907-916.

Fielding, J.E. (1984). Health promotion and disease prevention at the worksite. *Annual Review of Public Health*, **5**, 237-265.

Fitness and Lifestyle Research Institute. (1990). *Campbell's Canada fitness survey. The well-being of Canadians*. Ottawa: Author.

Fitness Canada. (1990). *Working actively together: Canada's blueprint toward active living in the workplace*. Ottawa: Department of National Health and Welfare.

Godin G., Cox, M.H., & Shephard, R.J. (1983). The impact of physical fitness evaluation on behavioural intentions towards regular exercise. *Canadian Journal of Applied Sports Science*, **8**, 240-245.

Godin, G., Desharnais, R., Jobin, J., & Cook, J. (1987). The impact of physical fitness and health-age appraisal upon exercise intentions and behavior. *Journal of Behavioral Medicine*, **10**, 241-250.

Godin, G., Shephard, R.J., & Colantonio, A. (1986). The cognitive profile of those who intend to exercise but do not. *Public Health Report*, **101**, 521-526.

Gordon, N.F., Kohl, H.W., Scott, C.B., Gibbons, L.W., & Blair, S.N. (1992). Reassessment of the guidelines for exercise testing: What alterations to current recommendations are required? *Sports Medicine*, **13**(5): 293-302.

Ishikawa, K. (1986). *Guide to quality control*. White Plains, NY: Kraus International Publications.

Juran, J.M. (1992). *Juran on quality by design*. New York: The Free Press.

Manson, J.E., Tosteson, H., Ridker, P.M., Satterfield, S., Hubert, P., O'Connor, G.T., Buring, J.E., & Hennekens, C.H. (1992). The primary prevention of myocardial infarction. *The New England Journal of Medicine*, **326**(21), pp. 1406-1416.

Marsh, M.J., Vojtecky, M.A., & Marsh, D.D. (1987). Workplace health promotion/protection: Correlates of integrative activities. *Journal of Occupational Medicine*, **29**(4): 353-356.

Martin, J.E., & Dubbert, P.M. (1985). Adherence to exercise. *Exercise and Sports Science Reviews*, **13**, 137-167.

Morris, J.N., Heady, J.A., Raffle, P.A., Roberts, P., & Parks, J.W. (1953). Coronary heart disease and physical activity of work. *Lancet*, **3**, 1111-1120.

Schaffer, R.H., & Thomson, H.A. (1992, January–February). Successful change programs begin with results. *Harvard Business Review*, pp. 80-89.

Sharratt, M.T., & Cox, M.H. (1988). Employee fitness: State of the art. *Canadian Journal of Public Health*, **79**, S40-S43.

Shephard, R. J. (1991). Historical perspectives. A short history of occupational fitness and health promotion. *Preventive Medicine*, **20**, 436-445.

Shephard, R.J. (1992). A critical analysis of work-site fitness programs and their postulated economic benefits. *Medicine and Science in Sports and Exercise*, **24**(3), 354-370.

Shephard, R.J., & Cox, M.H. (1988). Recruitment and retention. In M. Collis, M. Cox, R. Gagne, S. Keir, & P. Youldon (Eds.), *Fitness and lifestyle at the workplace* (pp. 28-32). Ottawa: Fitness Canada.

Shewhart, W.A. (1925). The application of statistics as an aid in maintaining quality of a manufactured product. *Journal of the American Statistics Association*, **20**, 546-548.

Skinner, J.S. (1987). General principles of exercise prescription. In J.S. Skinner (Ed.), *Exercise testing and exercise prescription for special cases* (pp. 21-30). Philadephia: Lea & Febiger.

Stephens, T. (1986). Health practices and health status: Evidence from the Canada Health Survey. *American Journal of Preventive Medicine*, **2**, 209-215.

Stephens, T., Craig, C.L., & Ferris, B.F. (1986). Adult physical activity in Canada: Findings from the Canada Fitness Survey I. *Canadian Journal of Public Health*, **77**, 285-290.

Stoffelmayr, B.E., Mavis, B.E., Stachnik, T., Robison, J., Rogers, M., VanHuss, W., & Carlson, J. (1992). A program model to enhance adherence in worksite based fitness programs. *Journal of Occupational Medicine*, **34**(2), 157-161.

U.S. Department of Health and Human Services. (1990). *Healthy people 2000: National health promotion and disease prevention objectives*. Washington, DC: Author.

Wankel, L.M., Yardley, J.K., & Graham, J. (1985). The effects of motivational interventions upon the exercise adherence of high and low self-motivated adults. *Canadian Journal of Applied Sport Science*, **10**, 147-155.

24

Cost-Benefit Analysis of Workplace Active Living Programs: The Employer Perspective

Jonathan E. Fielding
Kevin K. Knight

The workplace is targeted as the site to motivate and assist the working population to increase their energy expenditure. This initiative is aimed at increasing the physical activity of adults in the United States, Canada, and some other countries (Fielding & Piserchia, 1989).

One rationale for employers to sponsor and subsidize these fitness efforts is that they will directly benefit from the resulting improvements in employee health. Some sponsors express the hope that they will be able to realize a definable dollar return for this investment at a rate commensurate with that received on average from other investments. Physical activity programs may also be considered by some employers as the focal point for a variety of potentially synergistic preventive efforts, such as lipid screening and control, high blood pressure detection and control, and smoking cessation activities. Thus, a fitness program's presence may significantly contribute to the employer's as well as the employee's benefits.

The estimated percentage of U.S. employers with 250 or more employees offering formal exercise programs increased from 2.5% in 1978 to 32.5% in 1985, the last year for which representative national survey data is available. A new study fielded in early 1992 should release results soon.

Employers cite a number of reasons for implementing employee physical activity programs (Boyer & Vaccaro, 1990), including improvement in employee health, moderation in health care cost increases, improvement in employee productivity, reduction of absenteeism, and improvement in the organization's ability to recruit and retain employees.

The increasing prevalence of work site–sponsored fitness programs suggests that more and more employers are convinced of their potential economic benefits. It is

not known to what degree employers believe in making these decisions that the quantifiable evidence supports their conclusion or whether they are prepared to make judgments on the relative magnitude of costs and benefits. Personal experiences of chief executive officers and other senior managers often play a pivotal role in the decision to invest in exercise programs (Boyer & Vaccaro, 1990).

The primary tools for formal evaluation of costs and benefits of workplace exercise programs are cost-benefit analysis (CBA) and cost-effectiveness analysis (CEA). Both techniques attempt to relate monetary input costs to outputs. CBA deals exclusively with outputs that are monetized. In CEA, the outcome variables of interest cannot easily be monetized. For work site health promotion, these variables might be health-related, such as changes in risk factor levels, health status (e.g., quality adjusted life years), or productivity (Fielding 1990a, 1990b, in press; Warner & Luce, 1982). This review will focus on the results of cost benefit analysis.

The types of costs and benefits to be counted depend on the perspective chosen for analysis. In assessing employer-sponsored fitness activities, the costs and benefits to the employee will differ considerably from those to the employer. Employer sponsorship may make the effective cost to the employee zero, especially if participation in fitness activities can be on work time. Any health benefits could accrue in some measure to both employee and employer. The potential benefits and costs to employers of improvements in employee physical activity will be greatly affected by the timing of adverse health consequences and related disability and by possible employee turnover.

This review will primarily focus on the employer perspective because it has been the subject of many published reports and discussions and because, in the United States, employers have shown a willingness to invest in fitness activities, implying a conclusion that the benefits outweigh the costs. An important difference between employer perspectives in Canada and the United States is that in the U.S., a high proportion of costs attributable to poor health habits of employees is borne directly by employers, which is in direct relationship to the health care experience of the group.

Workplace physical activity programs encompass a wide range of interventions, with varying costs and potential benefits. The benefit-to-cost ratio for a particular, well-defined intervention may vary from one employer to another. This is a result of differing degrees of employer responsibility, for example, paying the costs of workers' sedentary lifestyles, the demographic and health risk characteristics of the employed population, impacts of physical fitness on ability to perform specific job tasks, worker readiness to modify activity levels, and success in making these changes as a result of employer-sponsored programs.

In examining the cost-benefit relationship, we are concerned with the effectiveness of employer-sponsored programs in increasing employees' levels of physical activity outside of work requirements. A substantial effect on key fitness variables could be considered a prerequisite to the application of CBA or CEA.

It is important to distinguish between the benefits to an employer of a physically active work force and those resulting from implementation of a work site program. The latter benefits are a function of the ability of a program to increase the physical activity level of employees as well as of the benefits resulting from increased physical activity.

A separate question that some published studies address is whether physically active employees cost employers less. Studies often show differentials in health, health cost, and personal productivity between sedentary and physically active employees. However, causality cannot be assumed becuase of potential bias. Even if we assume that observed gaps could theoretically be removed or eliminated by getting the sedentary population to be more active, gaps cannot be used to assess the cost-benefit or cost-effectiveness of any specific workplace physical activity programs.

From the employer's perspective, there are eight major cost categories for workplace fitness programs:

1. Personnel costs (at prorated individual wage and salary rates) of all work on company time to plan and implement the corporate strategy, including program personnel, others involved in planning, and those participating in the program on company time.
2. Operation and maintenance of on-site facilities. Expenditures for capital equipment should be depreciated based on standard schedules.

3. Off-site activities, such as subsidization of fitness memberships, donations in lieu of direct payment for services, and reimbursement for participation in fitness activities.
4. Materials, supplies, and promotional items associated with fitness activities.
5. Contract services and purchased products other than those included in items 1 through 4.
6. Health care costs, including
   - medical clearance exams and administrative work,
   - care for injuries due to exercise (prorated portion based on incremental physical activity attributable to employer-sponsored efforts),
   - care for exercise-induced illness,
   - incremental employer-paid portion of retiree health benefit costs due to increased longevity, and
   - prorated portion of care for the incremental or decremental share of job injuries that are attributable to the effects of employer-sponsored physical activity programs.

   In the U.S., these costs are experience-rated and paid 100% by employers.
7. Productivity reductions due to absenteeism and other diminutions in product quantity and quality due to exercise-related injuries and illnesses.
8. Incremental retiree pension benefits due to increased longevity associated with enhanced fitness.

Four main types of potential benefits could accrue to an employer who sponsors a physical activity program:

1. Reduction in health costs that may be paid through health benefits, workers compensation, and disability claims. Utilization and related costs may be reduced by generally improved health status, which may lead to a reduced propensity to use health care services. Reductions may also be mediated through lower incidence and intensity of specific health conditions causally related to physical inactivity. These include coronary artery disease mediated through reduction in blood pressure, improvement in lipid profiles, reduction in weight, and an independent effect of physical activity; hypertensive disease; obesity and related disorders; Type II diabetes mellitus; osteoporosis; some cancers, particularly colon cancer; and musculoskeletal disability (Blair, Kohl, Gordon, & Paffenbarger, in press).

2. Improved productivity, of which reduced absenteeism is the most easily and commonly measured element. Effects on both quantity and quality of products and services can potentially be observed in specific occupational settings. Softer measures such as improvements in employee attitudes toward their job and employer, and perceived improvement of personal

productivity can also be observed but are difficult to translate into dollars. Enhanced ability to recruit and retain well-qualified employees can be considered a contribution to improved organizational productivity. Improved image with customers and the general public can translate into improved sales, though this is likely to be specific to the organization, its location, its line of products, its services, and a particular period of time. Potential industrial relations benefits could improve profitability because of reduced grievances or labor contracts that are more favorable to employers. Such benefits are difficult to measure and their extent will differ greatly among organizations.

3. Costs for employer-paid life insurance for active employees may decline to the extent that longevity increases due to increased physical activity.

4. Employer payments for disability, direct or through employer disability insurance, could decrease based on declines in chronic disease incidence and prevalence secondary to increased physical activity.

In the context of this analysis, costs and benefits are measured incrementally. At issue is whether at the margin, employer investment in physical activity programs for employees (and potentially retirees and dependents) will yield an acceptable return on investment.

Using the health file (1975 to January 1992) of the National Library of Medicine's Medlars system, also known as Medline, we searched for employer sponsored physical activity program economic evaluation studies in peer-reviewed publications that attempted to evaluate one or more of the areas of potential benefit. Inclusion of only those studies that evaluated a physical activity program in isolation was not practical, because few studies met this criterion. Studies that did not involve a work site physical activity program and one or more economic outcome variables were not included. Therefore, studies that examined associations between physical activity assessed with a health risk appraisal, and health care costs were excluded because such studies do not assess effects of physical activity programs. Thirteen published reports from nine programs met the inclusion criteria.

Blue Cross and Blue Shield of Indiana: Gibbs, Mulvaney, Henes, and Reed (1985) compared health care costs for 667 participants in a comprehensive health promotion program with those for 892 nonparticipants at the same work site. Participant costs were greater than nonparticipant costs during the first 6 months of the program but averaged 24% less over a 4.75-year period. The authors conclude that savings in health care costs exceeded program costs by a factor of 1.45 over the 4.75 years. Also observed was an average decline of 20% in disability days incurred by participants following program implementation as compared to no change in average disability days for all employees.

Canada Life: Shephard (1992) reported that health care per employee averaged $170 (1990 Canadian dollars) less at the Canada Life Assurance compared as a control company in the first year following implementation of the program. Also noted was a turnover rate in the first program year of 1.8% among frequent participants as compared with an initial company-wide average of 18%. Frequent program participants had an absenteeism rate 22% less than that of others at the program site or employees of the control site 6 months after the program began. A productivity gain of 7% in the program company compared favorably to a 4.3% gain at the control site. Details as to how productivity was limited are reported by Shephard (1986). None of these results were statistically significant at the 0.05 level. The company provided an operating subsidy of $220 per participant, along with equipment valued at $69 per participant and space conservatively valued at $1,125 per participant (all figures in 1990 Canadian dollars). Approximately 25% of eligible employees were paying program dues after 12 years of program implementation. Per-employee costs would thus be one fourth of the per-participant costs cited.

Dupont: Bertera (1990) compared changes in hourly workers' disability days in the 2 years following implementation of a comprehensive health promotion program in 41 program sites with 29,315 employees and 19 control sites with 14,573 employees. In the second year of the program, changes over baseline were a decline of 0.7 days per employee per year at the program sites and 0.3 at the control sites, demonstrating a 0.4 greater decline in program sites (95% confidence interval 0.3, 0.5 days). Among program sites, the change in disability days varied little by level of program intensity in the second year. Cited total program costs averaged $48 (1985 U.S. dollars) per employee in Year 1 and $24 (1986 U.S. dollars) per employee in Year 2. Savings were estimated by applying wage costs to the reduction in disability days, with the result that the program was estimated to have broken even in Year 1 and returned $2.05 for every dollar invested in Year 2.

Johnson & Johnson Live for Life Program: Bly, Jones, and Richardson (1986) compared adjusted changes in health care costs over 5 years (1979 to 1983) in two groups of Johnson & Johnson employees offered a comprehensive health promotion program (N = 5,192, 3,259) and a control group (N = 2,955). Average annual inpatient cost increases were $76 (U.S. dollars) for the control group and $42 and $43 for the two program groups, although the differences were largely confined to the final year of the study. The difference between the program and control groups was statistically significant at the 0.05 level. No difference was noted for outpatient costs. Jones, Bly, and Richardson (1990) compared the absenteeism experience of employees at four program sites (N = 1,406) and five control sites (N = 487) over a 3-year period. After adjusting for potential confounding variables, wage employees at program sites were found to experience an average of 20 fewer sick hours per year than those at control sites in the final year of the study. The difference was statistically significant at the 0.05 level. No meaningful difference was noted for salaried employees at program sites as compared to those at control sites. Holzbach et al. (1990) demonstrated significantly more favorable changes in employee work-related attitudes (organizational commitment, job involvement, growth opportunities, supervision, working conditions, job competence) in program participants as compared to nonparticipants over a 2-year period.

A Large Midwestern Transportation Company: Bell and Blanke (1989) reported that absenteeism did not vary by degree of participation in a work site program among 216 eligible employees in the first 8 months of program operation.

New York State Education Employees: Bjurstrom and Alexiou (1978) tracked changes in absenteeism in a group of 99 New York State Education Department employees who remained in a physical fitness and heart disease intervention program for at least 1 year. Compared to the year prior to joining the program, average sick leave hours were 4.7 hours fewer per employee per year in the first year of program participation.

Prudential: Bowne, Russell, Morgan, Optenberg, and Clarke (1984) tracked major medical costs, disability days, and total disability costs in a group of 184 employees at the Southwestern home office of Prudential Insurance. The employees participated in a work site program for at least 1 year, and at least 1 year of baseline experience was available. Compared to the year prior to program entry, a 45.7% decline in major medical costs, a 20.1% decline in disability days, and a 31.7% decline in disability costs were observed on average in the year following entry into the program, although these results were not statistically significant at the 0.05 level. The average savings was estimated as $353.38 per participant, and the average operational cost was $120.60 per participant (1980 U.S. dollars).

Tenneco: Baun, Bernaki, and Tsai (1986) compared absenteeism and health care costs of participants in a work site program with those of nonparticipants in a random sample of 517 employees during the first year following implementation of the program. Health care costs for exercisers were approximately half those for nonexercisers, but the difference was not statistically significant at the 0.05 level. Male exercisers were absent an average of 9 hours less than nonexercisers, while female exercisers were absent an average of 22 hours less than nonexercisers. The difference was statistically significant for females but not for males. Bernacki and Baun (1984) reported a statistically significant association of job performance ratings and exercise adherence in a group of 3,231 employees of the same corporation.

Travelers Taking Care Program: Lynch, Golaszewski, Clearie, Snow, and Vickery (1990) compared the absenteeism experience of members of a fitness center sponsored by the Travelers corporation (N = 2,232) with nonmembers (N = 5,837). Membership was found to be associated with an annual difference of 1.2 days absent due to illness.

Overall, the studies display considerable heterogeneity in design target population, program components, physical activity programs, and input (e.g., cost) and outcome variables assessed, precluding broad conclusions on the relationship of costs to benefits. The usefulness of existing evaluation of intervention studies in estimating benefits resulting from physical activity programs is limited by the multicomponent nature of the interventions evaluated. However, from an employer perspective, evidence of positive effects is probably more important than being able to identify the responsible program components. In some studies there is evidence that the intervention had a positive impact on one or more categories of benefits, most commonly health care costs and absenteeism. Employers may also assume that the benefits are understated, because some categories are difficult to monetize (productivity) and others may occur beyond the time horizon of the evaluation (e.g., cardiovascular disease reductions secondary to reducing coronary risk factors).

From a scientific perspective, the evidence for a positive ratio of benefits to costs can be considered suggestive but not definitive. Construction of a cost-benefit ratio is difficult, and some assumptions utilized in some of the reported rates of costs to benefits are questionable (Warner, Wickizer, Wolfe, Schildroth, & Samuelson, 1988). A problem common to these studies in varying degrees is potential bias due to lack of random assignment to intervention or control conditions.

The finding that participants score significantly better than nonparticipants on a variety of measures of program benefit suggests that there is a potential gap that could be reduced through effective encouragement of physical activity by sedentary employees. However, such comparisons of self-selected program participants with nonparticipants are likely to be biased because healthier individuals may self-select at a higher rate into fitness programs. Construction of restricted cohorts, where inclusion is conditioned on adherence to a program for some period of time, may also bias results because adverse health events may result in nonadherence. In the absence of a program, individuals who would have participated may choose to exercise on their own. Comparisons of the experience of participants and nonparticipants must be viewed in light of these limitations.

The effects of a work site program depend on the effects of exercise and on the ability of the program to increase exercise adherence. Most programs report overall adherence of less than 25%. The extent to which programs increase exercise adherence is usually not discernible from published studies. An exception is found in Blair, Piserchia, Wilbur, and Crowder (1986), where 20% of women and 30% of men started an exercise program within 2 years of implementation of Johnson & Johnson's Live For Life® program, compared to 7% of women and 19% of men at control sites. Spillover effects of work site programs have been postulated (Shephard, 1990) as a possible mechanism whereby programs might achieve results greater than those expected on the basis of achieved participation levels. The existence of synergies between exercise programs and other health improvement programs might result in important cost savings, although such potential synergies have not been critically evaluated.

Study designs employed to estimate outcomes relevant to a cost-benefit analysis fall into several categories. Studies comparing changes over baselines achieved at sites offering programs with those achieved at sites not offering programs (Bertera, 1990; Bly et al., 1986) have advantages over comparisons of self-selected participants and nonparticipants. However, the nonrandom nature of site selection leaves open questions regarding comparability of sites (Warner, 1992). No published evaluation to date has employed random assignment, at the level of either the individual or the work site.

The costs borne by an employer will depend on national laws, the social environment in which the employer does business, and employer sponsored benefits. From the employer's standpoint, maximizing the ratio of benefits to costs often requires a different strategy than maximizing the overall program benefits in the employed population. To maximize the cost-benefit ratio, an employer might target the group of employees most likely to benefit from the intervention—those with low activity levels, high levels of interest in and commitment to starting and continuing an exercise program, and high levels of risk factors amenable to reduction through exercise. However, to maximize overall program benefit, the employer would target all sedentary employees. It is a reasonable presumption that increases in marginal per capita costs are necessary to induce larger and larger proportions of the work force to adopt and continue a regular exercise program. Therefore, the cost-benefit ratio may be significantly affected by the proportion of employees who are already engaged in regular physical activity when the employer decides to invest in increasing participation.

In conclusion, any cost-benefit analysis of workplace active living programs must be based on many assumptions because of the inadequate characterization of the effects of workplace programs. In spite of this uncertainty, many employers have been willing to invest substantial sums in such programs, a decision encouraged by the well-documented benefits of exercise on health and by the ability of well-structured programs to persuade a substantial minority of employees to engage in higher levels of physical activity. The decision to implement programs is ultimately subjective, and in that

sense not unlike the decisions faced by employers in a variety of other areas.

References

Baun, W.B., Bernacki, E.J., & Tsai, S.P. (1986). A preliminary investigation: Effect of a corporate fitness program on absenteeism and health care cost. *Journal of Occupational Medicine*, **28**, 18-22.

Bell, B.C., & Blanke, D. (1989). The effects of a work-site fitness program on employee absenteeism. *Health Values*, **13**(6), 3-11.

Bernacki, E.J., & Baun, W.B. (1984). The relationship of job performance to exercise adherence in a corporate fitness program. *Journal of Occupational Medicine*, **26**, 529-531.

Bertera, R.L. (1990). The effects of workplace health promotion on absenteeism and employment costs in a large industrial population. *American Journal of Public Health*, **80**, 1101-1105.

Bjurstrom, L.A., & Alexiou, N.G. (1978). A program of heart disease intervention for public employees: 2. A five year report. *Journal of Occupational Medicine*, **20**, 521-531.

Blair, S.N., Kohl, H.W., Gordon, N.F., & Paffenbarger, R.S., Jr. (in press). How much physical activity is good for health? *Annual Review of Public Health*.

Blair, S.N., Piserchia, P.V., Wilbur, C.S., & Crowder, J.H. (1986). A public health intervention model for work-site health promotion: 2. Impact on exercise and physical fitness in a health promotion plan after 24 months. *Journal of the American Medical Association*, **255**, 921-926.

Bly, J.L., Jones, R.C., & Richardson, J.E. (1986). Impact of worksite health promotion on health care costs and utilization: 2. Evaluation of Johnson & Johnson's Live for Life Program. *Journal of the American Medical Association*, **256**, 3235-3240.

Bowne, D.W., Russell, M.L., Morgan, J.L., Optenberg, S.A., & Clarke, A.E. (1984). Reduced disability and health care costs in an industrial fitness program. *Journal of Occupational Medicine*, **26**, 809-816.

Boyer, M.L., & Vaccaro, V.A. (1990). The benefits of a physically active workforce: An organizational perspective. *Occupational Medicine: State of the Art Reviews*, **5**, 691-706.

Fielding, J.E. (1990a). The challenges of work-place health promotion. In S.M. Weiss, J.E. Fielding, & A. Baum (Eds.), *Health at work* (pp. 13-28). Hillsdale, NJ: Erlbaum.

Fielding, J.E. (1990b). Cost-benefit and cost-effectiveness analysis in work-place health promotion programs. In S.M. Weiss, J.E. Fielding, & A. Baum (Eds.), *Health at work* (pp. 170-177). Hillsdale, NJ: Erlbaum.

Fielding, J.E. (in press). The role of cost-benefit and cost-effectiveness analysis in corporate decision making for worksite health promotion programs. In D.M. DeJoy & M.G. Wilson (Eds.), *Critical issues in worksite health promotion*. New York: Macmillan.

Fielding, J.E., & Piserchia, P.V. (1989). Frequency of worksite health promotion activities. *American Journal of Public Health*, **79**, 16-20.

Gibbs, J.O., Mulvaney, D., Henes, C., & Reed, R.W. (1985). Worksite health promotion: 2. Five-year trend in employee health care costs. *Journal of Occupational Medicine*, **27**, 826-830.

Holzbach, R.L., Piserchia, P.V., McFadden, D.W., Hartwell, T.D., Herrmann, A., & Fielding, J.E. (1990). Effect of a comprehensive health promotion program on employee attitudes. *Journal of Occupational Medicine*, **32**, 973-978.

Jones, R.C., Bly, J.L., & Richardson, J.E. (1990). A study of a work site health promotion program and absenteeism. *Journal of Occupational Medicine*, **32**, 95-99.

Lynch, W.D., Golaszewski, T.J., Clearie, A.F., Snow, D., & Vickery, D.M. (1990). Impact of a facility-based corporate fitness program on the number of absences from work due to illness. *Journal of Occupational Medicine*, **32**, 9-12.

Shephard, R.J. (1986). *Economic benefits of enhanced fitness*. Champaign, IL: Human Kinetics.

Shephard, R.J. (1990). Costs and benefits of an exercising versus a nonexercising society. In C. Bouchard, R.J. Shephard, T. Stephens, J.R. Sutton, & B.D. McPherson (Eds.), *Exercise, fitness, and health: A consensus of current knowledge* (pp. 49-60). Champaign, IL: Human Kinetics.

Shephard, R.J. (1992). Twelve years experience of a fitness program for the salaried employees of a Toronto life assurance company. *American Journal of Health Promotion*, **6**, 292-301.

Shipley, R.H., Orleans, C.T., Wilbur, C.S., Piserchia, P.V., & McFadden, D.W. (1988). Effect of the Johnson & Johnson LIVE FOR LIFE Program on employee smoking. *Preventive Medicine*, **17**, 25-34.

Warner, K.E. (1992). Effects of workplace health promotion not demonstrated [Letter to the editor]. *American Journal of Public Health*, **82**, 126.

Warner, K.E., & Luce, B.R. (1982). *Cost-benefit and cost-effectiveness analysis in health care: Principles, practice and potential*. Ann Arbor, MI: Health Administration Press.

Warner, K.E., Wickizer, T.M., Wolfe, R.A., Schildroth, J.E., & Samuelson, M.H. (1988). Economic implications of workplace health promotion programs: Review of the literature. *Journal of Occupational Medicine*, **30**, 106-112.

Part IV

Community Determinants of Active Living

Although in many instances the promotion of active living is individual and personalized, consideration should also be given to the impact of community determinants and interventions. In Part IV, practitioners and researchers provide information on how to promote active living from a community perspective.

First, Carron addresses the importance of conducting needs assessment and program evaluation in the promotion of physical activity and fitness. Carron suggests a wealth of means and strategies to achieve these ends. Hunter broadens the concept of active living to deal with the concept of an active living community. Hunter then offers a series of strategies designed to transform communities into active living communities. Burton describes the development of the active living movement and relates it to a similar movement that is emerging around the concept of sustainable living. Burton compares and contrasts the two movements and suggests ways to enhance their development.

Lord examines the concept of empowerment from the perspective of theory, process, and practice. Lord introduces different sources of personal empowerment and makes a strong case for implementing them in professional interventions. Labonté examines the concept of community empowerment through consideration of health as well-being, differing approaches to health, empowering goals, and a continuum of strategies. Labonté concludes that we can create a "fitter" society if we continue to ask hard questions and take actions we deem appropriate toward achieving this end. Gottlieb describes the omnipresent concept of social support by examining relevant literature and presenting cogent examples and illustrations. Gottlieb suggests that physical activity should be viewed as not only inherently rewarding but also socially rewarding.

In further elaborating on the issue of social support, Horne presents data on the effectiveness of an active living program specifically designed to provide social support, namely the Stay-at-Home Parents Network. Through a description of the development of the program, Horne aptly illustrates the challenges and intricacies involved in developing programs that include a social support component. Crocker discusses social support with special reference to persons with disabilities. Through his review of pertinent literature, Crocker suggests that social support can serve two separate stress-reducing functions—problem solving and emotional gratification.

O'Brien Cousins examines the issue of social support in older persons. Through an examination of the relevant literature, O'Brien Cousins offers a wealth of suggestions on promoting physical activity in older persons. In the final chapter, Keating and Etkin separately address the difficulties encountered in extending active living programs to populations labeled as "hard to reach." Keating and Etkin identify several myths that permeate practice and thinking in this area and offer suggestions for improving professional interventions.

25

Needs Assessment and Program Evaluation for Fitness, Health, Wellness, and Lifestyle

Albert V. Carron

When you cannot measure it, when you cannot express it in numbers, your knowledge is of a meager and unsatisfactory kind.

Lord Kelvin

It is Facts that are needed: Facts, Facts, Facts. When facts have been supplied, each of us can try to reason from them.

James Bryce

These two quotes by Lord Kelvin and James Bryce highlight a fundamental human issue, namely, that it is impossible for us to know how to initiate an enterprise, to understand how we are progressing with it, or, ultimately, to determine how successful we have been in its execution without some form of measurement and evaluation. Evaluation is a fundamental human activity, the cornerstone of our daily lives, taking many different forms.

On a personal level, each of us continually acts as a scientist engaging in a form of evaluation that Fritz Heider (1944, 1958) referred to as *common sense*, or *naive psychology*. We constantly assess, evaluate, and then develop theories to understand, explain, and predict our personal behavior as well as the behavior of others. These commonsense theories form the basis for our subsequent behavior—they assist us in imposing stability and predictability on our interpersonal and physical environments.

Although we do not want to eliminate the use of common sense (in fact, we cannot), it does have its limitations as an evaluation process—limitations that make it a poor substitute for more rigorous scientific evaluations (Kerlinger, 1973). Our commonsense theories are usually generated on the basis of a limited number of observations made in only a few, select situations. Scientific theories, on the other hand, are the product of numerous observations obtained in a wide cross-section of situations. For example, numerous research studies have highlighted the incredible complexity of anorexia nervosa and helped to identify the various attitudinal and psychological patterns associated with its development (cf. Garner & Olmstead, 1984). However, there is a tendency for the layperson to view anorexia in simple cause-effect terms. It is doubtful that common sense could help us completely understand the etiology of anorexia.

Another limitation of common sense is that although scientists constantly search for alternative explanations that might disprove a theory, the layperson typically seeks out verifications for his or her theories. Our current understanding of the benefits of weight training illustrates how research has worked to dispel the once popular theory that weight training detracts from flexibility and speed. Almost every modern elite athlete engages in a systematic program of weight training; a dramatic evolution from a time when using weights was frowned upon because it produced a muscle-bound condition.

The concept of control, that is, the use of baseline or comparison groups or conditions to serve as a reference, also distinguishes the scientific process from common sense. Many early reports on the benefits of work site health promotion programs were of minimal scientific value because they lacked baseline measures or control groups against which to compare program effects (Katz & Showstack, 1990).

And, finally, human behavior is complex. Therefore, the scientist, unlike the layperson, is more prone to search for the complex interrelationship among variables. For example, simply counting heads might show increased participation in a work site health promotion program (using common sense). However, more in-depth analyses (using scientific processes) might also show that most participants are already relatively healthy or are in white collar positions (e.g., Baun, Bernacki, & Tsai, 1986).

Common sense does have its place in our daily lives, but it is not a substitute for evaluation research. At an institutional level (in clubs, schools, organizations, associations, businesses, or government) *evaluation research*, a systematic, scientific approach, must be used. Rossi and Freeman (1982) have defined evaluation research as "a robust area of activity devoted to collecting, analyzing, and interpreting information on the need for, implementation of, and impact of intervention efforts to better the lot of humankind by improving social conditions and community life" (p. 15).

One purpose of this report is to outline the general processes associated with needs assessment and program evaluation. Evaluations may be undertaken at three stages: prior to the initiation of a program (preplanning stage), during its progress (ongoing monitoring), and following its completion (output stage). In this paper, the nature of the important issues and questions in each stage are discussed. The paper also presents an overview of the protocols necessary to evaluate the impact of intervention programs that are often used to effect change in some attitude, cognition, or behavior. In order to reliably assess whether an intervention program has been successful, specific protocols associated with sound scientific research are necessary.

A Framework for Intervention Programs

It is convenient to present the processes involved in the development and evaluation of intervention programs as a three-stage, linear model consisting of input, through, and output phases (see Figure 25.1). The *input phase*, which occurs prior to the introduction of an intervention program, is concerned with needs assessment and preplanning. The *through phase*, which occurs after the intervention program is underway, is concerned with ongoing monitoring. And finally, the *output phase*, which occurs at the completion of the program, is concerned with evaluating program effectiveness or impact.

Preplanning Stage

In the preplanning (input) stage, the principle concerns are related to establishing the focus of the fitness, health, wellness, or lifestyle program. Seven types of general issues are pertinent (Rossi & Freeman, 1982) prior to the introduction of any intervention program and spark the need for answers to certain questions:

- Identifying the target problem. What is the focus of concern, that is, the outcomes, behaviors, attitudes, and cognitions that must be changed?

- Identifying the target population. What group or set of individuals is the general focus for the potential intervention?
- Identifying the population at risk. Does the target problem have a greater probability of detrimentally affecting one subgroup more than others?
- Determining the mechanisms for recruiting or obtaining the cooperation of targets. What protocol or inducements will secure the involvement of the target population?
- Assessing the feasibility of specific types of programs that must be established. What intervention programs would be effective with the target problems?
- Determining the population interests. What intervention programs would be effective with the target population?
- Evaluating the cost-effectiveness of alternative approaches. Can more than one program effectively solve the problem? Which is more cost-effective?

A health education planning framework called PRECEDE was developed by Green, Kreuter, Deeds, and Partridge (1980) to provide a systematic protocol for answering these seven fundamental issues in the needs assessment process. With the PRECEDE framework, the initial concern is with desired outcomes. When the desired outcomes are identified, it becomes necessary to determine their predisposing factors, their enabling factors, and their reinforcing factors. Predisposing factors are the rationale or motivations underlying a health problem—the reasons why adherence has been problematic. Enabling factors represent the individual and insitutional resources and skills necessary to produce the desired outcome, for example, the financial resources present. Reinforcing factors are the positive or negative contingencies associated with involvement in the program. In combination, these elements help identify the components of the intervention program.

According to Bertera (1990), the PRECEDE health education planning framework was used extensively by the DuPont Company to plan its health promotion and wellness education program. Initially, priority health problems were identified by examining company morbidity, mortality, and disability statistics. The employees' present health behaviors and their intentions to engage in lifestyle-related activities (e.g., weight loss or exercise) within the subsequent 6-month period were then assessed. Employee attitudes and health knowledge were measured to help understand predisposing factors. The enabling factors requirement—the necessity of having sufficient skills and resources available to implement the intervention—was satisfied through general corporate support, the involvement of company medical and employee relations personnel, the use of departmental coordinators, the on-site training of those coordinators, the development of informational materials, and

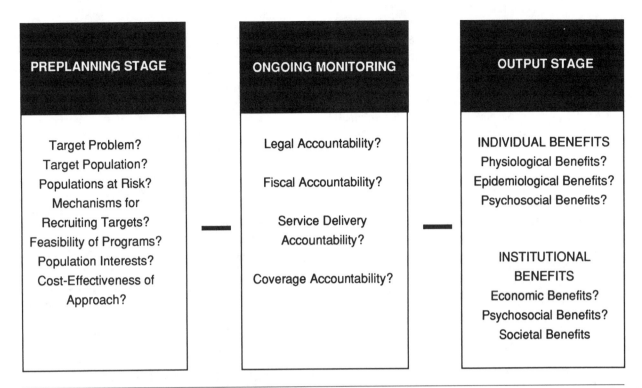

PREPLANNING STAGE	ONGOING MONITORING	OUTPUT STAGE
Target Problem? Target Population? Populations at Risk? Mechanisms for Recruiting Targets? Feasibility of Programs? Population Interests? Cost-Effectiveness of Approach?	Legal Accountability? Fiscal Accountability? Service Delivery Accountability? Coverage Accountability?	INDIVIDUAL BENEFITS Physiological Benefits? Epidemiological Benefits? Psychosocial Benefits? INSTITUTIONAL BENEFITS Economic Benefits? Psychosocial Benefits? Societal Benefits

Figure 25.1 A conceptual framework to examine the process of needs assessment and program evaluation in fitness, health, lifestyle, and wellness programs (reprinted from Rossi & Freeman, 1982).

ultimately the corporate budget. The reinforcing factors requirement was satisfied by publicizing and acknowledging the work of coordinators in the workplace and the accomplishments of participants in the program through special plaques and certificates. When the intervention program was introduced, it was directed toward smoking cessation, blood pressure control, lipid control, weight control, stress management, fitness, substance abuse prevention, and other topics of interest suggested by employees.

Ongoing Monitoring

In the ongoing monitoring (throughput) phase of any intervention program, the critical issues are associated with accountability. Thus, assessment in this phase focuses on the manner in which the service is being delivered, and four important accountability questions become pertinent (Rossi & Freeman, 1982).

One of these questions is related to legal accountability: Does the intervention program intrude on personal rights or expose the participant to serious injuries? In a discussion of legal accountability, Herbert and Herbert (1990) pointed out six potential areas of emphasis in employee health promotion programs: education (e.g., work site safety), screening (e.g., blood pressure), smoking cessation, drug and/or alcohol, exercise and activity, and recreational activities. Each of these has legal implications associated with contract law or tort law.

A contractual problem might arise from employer legal obligations that are part of the employee benefits package. For example, a company may have a contractual agreement to introduce an exercise program or provide annual physical examinations. Or a contractual agreement may forbid the company from instituting drug testing or a smoking cessation program.

Tort law, on the other hand, includes personal injuries and other wrongs resulting from actions in the workplace. A company with a stress testing program, for example, has a responsibility to adhere to professional guidelines relating to the use of properly trained personnel. If nonqualified or unlicensed personnel are used and a fatality occurs, the company could be found negligent. As a result, one important element in the ongoing monitoring of that stress-testing program would be to ensure that the personnel running the program possessed the required qualifications (and were maintaining or upgrading those qualifications through continuing education when necessary). Accountability from a legal viewpoint means that the program is in accordance with contractual agreements and is conducted in such a manner as to reduce the likelihood of civil actions.

A second accountability question in the ongoing monitoring stage is associated with fiscal accountability. A program initiator should ask, Are the financial resources set aside for the intervention program being used appropriately (i.e., within the guidelines established by the budget)?

A third question concerns service delivery accountability. Is the intervention program in operation the one that was originally planned? Intervention programs can undergo gradual changes in focus over time because of the changing expertise of administrators or the changing interests of clients. If proper procedures were followed during the preplanning phase to develop the original intervention program, it becomes necessary to determine whether the revised program is accomplishing the original goals.

A fourth question is associated with coverage accountability. Are the beneficiaries of the program the original target population? Are there constituents or subgroups of the target population not being served by the intervention program? Coverage accountability is probably the fundamental issue in ongoing assessment. If both a problem (e.g., coronary heart disease) and a target population (e.g., blue collar workers) have been identified and a program developed (e.g., aerobics fitness classes), it is important to determine whether the target population is participating in the program. For example, considerable research evidence shows that the percentage of white collar workers who participate in employee fitness programs varies from 15% to 30%; for blue collar workers, the participation rate varies from 3% to 5%. There is also evidence that initially healthier individuals participate more in health promotion programs than individuals who are at "greater risk." In short, those who might benefit most tend not to take advantage of employee health programs (cf. Gebhardt & Crump, 1990).

Coverage accountability is illustrated in an analysis of an employee fitness program carried out by Shephard and Cox (1980). After the program was introduced, an assessment was made to determine what groups were participating in the program and to what extent. It was observed that the percentages of males and females

- who never attended any fitness classes were 23.6% and 10.0%,
- who attended initially but then dropped out were 11.8% and 19.6%,
- who exhibited low adherence were 27.3% and 27.9%, and
- who maintained high adherence throughout the course of the program were 37.3% and 42.5%.

Assessment of Outputs

In the output phase of any intervention program (review Figure 25.1), the critical issues revolve around the assessment of program effectiveness in terms of changes in people's states or behaviors, the costs of the program versus its benefits, success rates, and so on. Hill, Glassford, Burgess, and Rudnicki (1988) pointed out that the two principal areas in which the effectiveness of fitness, health, wellness, and lifestyle programs are

judged pertain to individual benefits and institutional benefits. Individual benefits are related to assessing whether an intervention program has a positive impact on individual participants; institutional benefits are related to assessing whether the intervention program benefited the agency that sponsored it.

Hill et al. (1988) also suggested that the issue of positive individual benefits can be evaluated from three aspects. The first aspect, physiological benefits, is assessed by such parameters as maximum oxygen uptake, body weight, percent body fat, resting heart rate, blood pressure, incidence of orthopedic spinal problems, and stress-related indicators (e.g., cholesterol levels). The second, epidemiological benefits, is assessed through measures of morbidity, disability, and disease. The third aspect, psychosocial benefits, is assessed by measuring such factors as individual morale, satisfaction, interpersonal relations, feelings of self-worth, mental health, anxiety, and self-image.

Hill et al. (1988) also pointed out that institutional benefits can be evaluated from three perspectives as well: economic, psychosocial, and societal. Economic benefits refer to factors such as health care costs, absenteeism, productivity, decreased turnover, and premature death. The psychosocial benefits that might accrue to an institution are similar to those that benefit the individual: management-labor relations, work atmosphere and morale, recruitment, and employee stability. The potential societal benefits include decreased health care costs and increased health and vitality of the population.

The program's goals determine the importance that is attached to each of these benefits. In employee fitness, health, wellness, and lifestyle programs, for example, the most fundamental benefits at the instituional level are usually economic ones. Does the program decrease absenteeism, increase productivity, reduce health costs, or reduce training costs (i.e., by reducing illness, death, or employee turnover)? Most studies that focus on a program's economic benefits appear to be anecdotal accounts of analyses with significant limitations in underlying assumptions, data, or research methodologies (Warner, Wickizer, Wolfe, Schildroth, & Samuelson, 1988). One significant exception to this criticism is the research carried out at the Johnson and Johnson Company (Breslow, Fielding, Herrman, & Wilbur, 1990).

In 1978, Johnson and Johnson introduced a comprehensive health promotion program called Live For Life, which targeted the entire work site and all employees. A preliminary health and lifestyle screening measure, the Health Profile, was used to obtain behavioral, attitudinal, and biometric information (blood pressure, blood lipids, body fat, height and weight). The methods of intervention consisted of behavioral programs focusing on nutrition, exercise, weight control, smoking cessation, stress management, blood pressure control, and others. Educational seminars were also provided to outline the program and the benefits associated with a healthy lifestyle. Six outcomes were desired from the intervention program:

1. An increase in health relevant knowledge, attitudes, and behavior (i.e., relating to tobacco, alcohol, exercise, and seat belts)
2. A reduction in body risk factors (e.g., blood pressure, cholesterol, and fitness levels)
3. An improvement in health status (e.g., reduced disability and disease occurrence)
4. A reduction in the mortality rate
5. Economic benefits (e.g., reduced health care costs, absenteeism, worker's compensation, or disability)
6. An improvement in indirect measures of productivity (e.g., morale, job attitudes)

To assess the economic effectiveness of the program, a quasiexperimental design was used. Group 1, the control group which consisted of 5,192 employees, had not been exposed to the Live For Life program at the time of the analysis. Group 2, consisting of 3,259 employees, had a program in place from 18 to 30 months. And Group 3, consisting of 2,995 employees, had been involved in the Live For Life program for over 30 months. Inpatient costs increased at a significantly slower rate for Groups 2 and 3 ($43 and $42, respectively) than for the control group ($76). The differences in total costs to the company for the control versus intervention groups over the 5-year period examined was approximately $1.22 million.

The Process of Evaluation Research

Fitness, health, wellness, and lifestyle intervention programs are introduced to produce desired outcomes. Consequently, a fundamental question to evaluate any intervention program is, has that program been successful? The only way this question can be answered reliably is by comparing the intervention group with some baseline measure that is either provided by individuals or groups not exposed to the program or is provided through the use of preprogram values from the intervention group. *Comparative* or *single group* research designs are the basic protocols to help practitioners and researchers determine whether a program has been successful (Rossi & Freeman, 1982).

Comparative Designs

The most fundamental protocol used to assess intervention effects is to compare individuals (or, depending on the focus of analysis, groups, clubs, companies, or schools) who have participated in a program with those who have not. The program participants typically are referred to as the experimental (intervention or treatment) condition and the nonparticipants represent the control condition. The intervention program carried out by Shephard and Cox (1980) used this design. Two comparable insurance companies were interested in introducing an employee fitness program; one company agreed to postpone implementation for a year and served as the control condition. Consequently, the differences in physiological, psychological, and strength indices between employees in the treatment condition and the control condition could be compared.

Comparability between subjects in the treatment and control conditions is mandatory to ensure that any changes observed (or not observed) can be attributed to the intervention condition and not to some other extraneous factor on which the subjects differed. Rossi and Freeman (1982) listed three areas in which comparability between intervention and control conditions is important: composition, experiences, and predispositions. In terms of composition, the comparability of the subjects could be questioned if, for example, an intervention site was a white collar business whereas the control site was a blue collar plant. Comparability could also differ because of the experiences of the subjects in the treatment and control conditions. Experiences that occur over time, or as a result of maturation, are different for subjects of different ages. Thus, if the subjects in the treatment and control conditions have different average ages, the impact of any fitness or health intervention could be muted or exaggerated. Another area in which subjects in the treatment and control conditions could differ is their predispositions. For example, there is no doubt that individuals who are initially healthier will more readily volunteer and participate in fitness, health, wellness, and lifestyle programs (Baun, Bernacki, & Tsai, 1986). Thus, unless subjects in the treatment and control conditions are initially comparable in their predispositions toward exercise and health, conclusions about the efficacy of the treatment can be problematic.

Two protocols that can be used to obtain comparability across conditions are *randomization* and *unbiased selection* (Rossi & Freeman, 1982). Randomization occurs when the assignment of subjects to control and treatment conditions is a function of chance. Any subject has an equal opportunity to be in either the control or treatment condition, and any differences in composition, experiences, and predispositions are due to chance. Unbiased selection occurs when subjects are systematically assigned to the various conditions in a study according to some order of rotation.

In those instances where randomization and unbiased selection are not possible, a *constructed control* approach could be used. Typically, constructed control designs match subjects in the treatment and control conditions by selecting subjects with characteristics considered to be potentially important to the outcome of the intervention. Some of the demographic variables frequently used for matching individuals include age, sex, education, socioeconomic status, marital status, occupation, ethnicity, and labor force participation (Rossi & Freeman, 1982).

Single Group Designs

In some instances, the use of a control condition for comparison purposes is not possible. For example, in an industrial setting, a new contractual agreement between management and labor might require the immediate implementation of a health program for all employees. If there is no company sufficiently similar to the target company to provide a valid comparison, then it would be necessary to use a single-group protocol to assess the impact of the health program (Rossi & Freeman, 1982).

One such approach uses *reflexive controls*; the target group serves as its own control. Outcome measures obtained before the intervention or treatment is introduced are compared with outcome measures obtained after the implementation of the program. This approach was used by Porter, Morrell, and Moriarty (1986) to test the impact of what they referred to as an inoculation prevention strategy, a method used to lessen three factors known to be highly related to the development of anorexia nervosa: perfectionism, a drive for thinness, and interpersonal distrust. The early and preadolescent children involved in the study completed a self-report questionnaire, called the Eating Disorder Inventory (Garner & Olmstead, 1984), prior to and following a half-day prevention program. The children's scores before and after the prevention programs were then compared.

A second approach is to use *generic controls*, that is, normative or standardized values reported for the population. Generic controls were used by Tiidus, Shephard, and Montelpare (1989) to analyze the 7-day dietary intake of middle-aged and older middle-class adults. Their subjects participated in a 2-hour training session in which detailed instructions were provided on recording amount and type of food intake. At the completion of the recording period, the reported portions of food ingested were converted into a summary of nutrient intake using the Canadian nutrient file developed by Health and Welfare Canada (1977). The sample's intake of key nutrients was then compared with the normative standards established for Canada, the United Kingdom, and the United States.

In cases where generic controls (i.e., norms or standardized values) are not available, it might be necessary to use what Rossi and Freeman (1982) have referred to as *shadow controls*, that is, the judgments of experts, program administrators, or the subjects themselves. This was the approach used by Haslam (1990) to determine whether the educational objectives set out in Canada's National Coaching Certification Program (NCCP) adequately reflected the skills necessary to be an effective coach. To assess the validity of the program's educational objectives the Delphi technique was used. The technique is one where experts are consulted independently, provide feedback on the group's opinions, and support those opinions with reasons. The process is repeated until a consensus is achieved. Opinions of master course conductors and provincial coaching coordinators for the NCCP were obtained in Haslam's (1990) study.

Epilogue

The interest in fitness, health, wellness, and positive lifestyles is steadily increasing in society—in business and industry, educational institutions, the private sector, special populations, and across the age spectrum. Not surprisingly, these different areas of society are increasingly providing programs involving fitness development, educational enhancement (e.g., worksite safety), wellness appraisal (e.g., blood pressure), smoking cessation, drug and alcohol reduction, and general recreation involvement. But given limitations in resources—personnel, finances, or facilities—questions pertaining to need, accountability, and impact will inevitably arise. Does the program meet the needs of the target population? Does it have a significant impact on the target problem? The answer to these and other questions relating to needs assessment and program evaluation can only be answered through well-conducted evaluation research.

Acknowledgment

I would like to thank Steve Bray, who assisted me with the literature search for this paper, and Larry Brawley, Kevin Spink, and Neil Widmeyer, who reacted to an earlier draft.

References

Baun, W.B., Bernacki, E.J., & Tsai, S.P. (1986). Effect of a corporate fitness program on absenteeism and health care costs. *Journal of Occupational Medicine*, **28**, 18-22.

Bertera, R.L. (1990). Planning and implementing health promotion in the workplace: A case study of the Du Pont Company experience. *Health Education Quarterly*, **17**, 307-327.

Breslow, L., Fielding, J., Herrman, A.A., & Wilbur, C.S. (1990). Worksite health promotion: Its evolution and the Johnson & Johnson experience. *Preventive Medicine*, **19**, 13-21.

Garner, D., & Olmstead, M. (1984). *Eating disorder inventory manual*. Odessa, FL: Psychological Assessment Resources.

Gebhardt, D.L., & Crump, C.E. (1990). Employee fitness and wellness programs in the workplace. *American Psychologist*, **45**, 262-272.

Green, L.W., Kreuter, M.W., Deeds, S.G., & Partridge, K.B. (1980). *Health education planning: A diagnostic approach*. Palo Alto, CA: Mayfield.

Haslam, I.R. (1990). Expert assessment of the National Coaching Certification Program (NCCP) theory component. *Canadian Journal of Sport Sciences*, **15**, 201-212.

Health and Welfare Canada. (1977). Adaptation of *Nutritive value of foods* (House and Garden Bulletin No. 72). Washington, DC: U.S. Dept. of Agriculture.

Heider, F. (1944). Social perception and phenomenal causality. *Psychological Review*, **51**, 358-374.

Heider, F. (1958). *The psychology of interpersonal relations*. New York: Wiley.

Herbert, D.L., & Herbert, W.G. (1990). Legal issues in the delivery of worksite health promotion. *Occupational Medicine: State of the Art Reviews*, **5**, 851-861.

Hill, R., Glassford, G., Burgess, A., & Rudnicki, J. (1988). Employee fitness and lifestyle programs, part one: Introduction, rationale, and benefits. *Journal of the Canadian Association for Health, Physical Education and Recreation*, **54**, 10-14.

Katz, P.P., & Showstack, J.A. (1990). Is it worth it: Evaluating the economic impact of worksite health promotion. *Occupational Medicine: State of the Art Reviews*, **No. 5**, pp. 837-851.

Kerlinger, F.E. (1973). *Foundations of behavioral research* (2nd ed.). New York: Holt, Rinehart, & Winston.

Porter, J.E., Morrell, T.L., & Moriarty, D. (1986). Evaluation of a pilot project for early and pre-adolescents. *Journal of the Canadian Association for Health, Physical Education and Recreation*, **52**, 21-26.

Rossi, P.H., Freeman, H.E. (1982). *Evaluation: A systematic approach* (2nd ed.). Beverly Hills, CA: Sage.

Shephard, R.J., & Cox, M. (1980). Some characteristics of participants in an industrial fitness programme. *Canadian Journal of Applied Sport Science*, **5** 69-76.

Tiidus, P., Shephard, R.J., & Montelpare, W. (1989). Overall intake of energy and key nutrients: Data for middle-aged and older middle-class adults. *Canadian Journal of Sport Sciences*, **14**, 173-177.

Warner, K.E., Wickizer, T.M., Wolfe, R.A., Schildroth, J.E., & Samuelson, M.H. (1988). Economic implications of workplace health promotion programs: Review of the literature. *Journal of Occupational Medicine*, **30**, 106-112.

26

Community Determinants and Benefits of Active Living

Don Hunter

The official genesis of active living was the 1986 Canadian Summit on Fitness; an event that brought together national leaders from a variety of settings to examine the current state of the fitness movement and to map out future directions. It was evident that the field did have a great deal to celebrate. Significant strides had been made to encourage Canadians to become physically active. At the same time, there was clearly a need for a change in focus if the movement was to progress even further.

Participants at the 1986 summit, particularly those who worked at the implementation level in communities, called for a more holistic view of physical activity; one that saw it as part of total well-being. An overemphasis on physiological fitness helped to create an image of fitness that was irrelevant to many individuals while appearing to exclude others, including people with disabilities. There was also a concern that Fitness Canada had too narrow a view of their mandate and needed to go beyond the "sweating vigorously at least three times a week" definition of fitness in relation to the initiatives they would support.

The development of active living by Fitness Canada was an attempt to find a concept that was more holistic, inclusive, and relevant to Canadians. More importantly, Fitness Canada sought an effective vehicle to encourage more Canadians to value physical activity and make it part of their everyday life.

At the same time the active living concept was emerging, a growing number of studies concluded that moderate levels of physical activity did provide health benefits if done on a regular basis. Walking, gardening, and other activities could also be more easily incorporated into the everyday routines and environments of many individuals.

The first substantive attempt to define active living took place in January, 1990 when Fitness Canada hosted a symposium of 50 individuals to examine the term and its potential meaning. This group included practitioners

from education, health, social and community services, and other allied fields. Although there was an attempt to achieve a common definition of active living, the discussions focused on the potential of the concept to influence lifestyles in various community settings. Despite the improbability of reaching a consensus when 50 people tried to include their point of view, the Ottawa symposium eventually led to the development of the definitions and conceptual overviews now used by Fitness Canada (1991a) to describe active living. It also became evident that active living would ultimately be developed, defined, or disappear, by means of its implementation and evolution in communities, schools, and workplaces.

The Nature of an Active Living Community

An active living community is one that fosters healthy and active lifestyles. Although the central focus is on self-empowerment, active living communities ensure that a supportive base of opportunities and resources are available within sustainable environments. An active living community is characterized by its efforts to cultivate

- an increase in numbers of residents who adopt active lifestyle patterns,
- positive health practices,
- a supportive base of opportunities,
- a strong sense of community identity,
- an integrated community network that supports collaborative actions, and
- a strong commitment to the environment.

Efforts to develop these characteristics are not new to most communities, and the concepts surrounding active living are certainly not foreign to many organizations involved in leisure services. The essence of becoming an active living community, however, is to make additional efforts that transcend traditional services.

Creating an Active Living Community

The critical issue is how communities can more effectively encourage healthy and active lifestyles. There are six primary areas where efforts should occur in developing an active living community. All are important, and all are inter-related. These areas are as follows:

1. Forging partnerships
2. Creating awareness and community identity
3. Fostering individual commitment
4. Providing a supportive resource base
5. Initiating public policy
6. Ensuring environmentally sensitive approaches

Many of the examples used in this paper reflect the active living community project in Saanich, British Columbia as described in a special Active Living publication by the Canadian Parks and Recreation Association (1992). The municipality of Saanich is the largest of the communities that collectively make up Greater Victoria and has a population of 96,000. Saanich is one of a number of Canadian communities that is making special efforts to encourage residents to adopt healthy and active lifestyles.

Partnerships

The shift to a more holistic approach to fitness is consistent with a trend toward integrated planning and collaborative action within communities. These holistic approaches, whether through a Healthy Communities committee or an ad-hoc interagency effort, are influencing community decision making in areas such as health, transportation, education, community planning, and social services.

The creation of an active living committee, with representation from a broad spectrum of community organizations, is viewed as a prerequisite to developing an active living community. If communities have an existing network, such as a Healthy Communities committee, it is important to link active living to that network. Municipal parks and recreation departments are generally best positioned to bring organizations together and to provide the administrative support that an active living committee requires.

The typical community partners include: school districts, community health services, social and family serving agencies, mental health services, YM/YWCAs, persons with disabilities, universities or colleges, environmental groups, youth, municipal parks and recreation

departments, and related government departments. Most communities that have attempted to form a committee have found that these agencies think the term active living is both understandable and supportable because its holistic approach easily encompasses their mandates.

An effective active living committee is one that goes beyond information sharing and extends into collaborative planning. In fact, the key role of the committee is to develop a strategic plan for active living, to encourage further community partnerships, and to actually implement the priority initiatives.

Awareness and Community Identity

If active living is going to have an impact, people need to be aware of the term and its potential value to them. There are a number of ways that this may be accomplished:

• *Visibility and meaning*: The terms "active living" and "active living community" can be used on logos, brochures, community signage, and program materials. Use of the terms needs to be complemented by materials that describe their meaning. Publications by Stewart (1991) and Fitness Canada (1991a) serve as excellent resources.

• *Awareness of opportunities*: Instilling the desire to make physical activity a regular part of one's lifestyle is aided by making people aware of community resources, especially resources that can be used at convenient times. A specific guide to active living resources including references to trail networks, safe cycle paths and routes, access to facilities and programs, and special experiences (e.g., scenic views, historical and heritage points of interest), can help link people with active lifestyle opportunities.

• *Community events*: Major community events can help to foster an active living community identity. For example, Saanich ran an Active Living Fair and integrated active living into other local events. In addition, there are a number of national events such as Fitweek, National Access Awareness Week, and heart, lung, and substance abuse related theme weeks that can be excellent vehicles for the promotion of active living concepts while also enhancing the identity of the community as a healthy and active place to live.

• *Leader awareness*: In creating a broad community awareness of active living, it is essential that the staff and volunteers of the partner organizations not be forgotten. In Saanich, special seminars are held with leaders to create enthusiasm and foster commitment for the active living project.

Many of these efforts to create greater awareness of active living and to enhance its identity in the community can be supplemented through involvement of the media and corporations. Their efforts should focus on fostering individual awareness and commitment to an active lifestyle, and on promoting active living opportunities.

Individual Commitment

All active living initiatives must focus on encouraging individuals to do two things: make a personal commitment to an active lifestyle, and actually incorporate physical activities of their choice into their life. Although awareness and attitude change are important, they don't necessarily lead to changes in actual behavior.

An overemphasis on physiological fitness often creates an image that many consider to be personally irrelevant or unobtainable. Striving to achieve a level of exercise intensity that optimizes health benefits is commendable and valid for many individuals; however, it has inhibited too many others, including those people who once were active but now feel guilty about losing their former level of fitness. Active living encourages people to participate in activities of their own choice, at their own pace, and that are in harmony with other aspects of their lives. This new approach is reflected in the various *Blueprints for Action* articles developed by Fitness Canada and written with the input of advisory committees representing the concerned fields. The *Blueprints* focus on target groups such as older adults (1990), people with disabilities (1991b), and children and youth (1991c).

Individual commitment can be fostered in a number of ways:

- *From dependence to independence*: In an attempt to capture and maintain market share, many leisure and fitness agencies often create client dependence, rather than encourage people to become more independent. The physical activity field needs to refocus on helping people make their own choices, use their own personal and neighborhood resources, and then use leisure and fitness agencies as an additional resource to lifestyle choices. Independence was emphasized in a catalogue of comprehensive benefits of parks and recreation departments developed by the Parks and Recreation Federation of Ontario (1991).

- *Integration of positive health practices*: The concept of active living has received support from many involved in health promotion. They believe that physical activity needs to be seen in relationship to nutrition, weight control, smoking cessation, and substance abuse prevention. As a result, physical activity related programs in schools, communities, and workplaces should be integrated with health promotion information so individuals are best equipped to make positive lifestyle choices.

The health promotion field is steadily emphasizing prevention, and it views an active lifestyle as an essential ingredient.

- *Active living education*: To reach certain target groups, more specific active living education will be needed in schools, workplaces, and communities. Recent changes in school curriculum development suggest that more holistic approaches will be applied to lifestyle education and that community involvement will be crucial to its success. Traditional community programs need to be complemented by lifestyle assessment and counseling. The various *Blueprints for Action* (Fitness Canada, 1990, 1991b, 1991c) are excellent resources in planning and developing active living initiatives for a variety of target groups including youth, older adults, and people with disabilities.

Community Resource Base

An active living community provides its residents with a supportive base of programs, facilities, and outdoor areas. These include:

- facility spaces that support participation, including fitness studios, aerobic rooms, and running tracks;
- facility schedules that cater to individualized activities, for example, swim lanes that are available at all times for lap swimming;
- trail networks for pedestrians including neighborhood linkage systems and major community trails;
- bicycle networks that serve recreational users and act as an alternative transportation system for the commuter;
- trails to access natural areas; and
- programs that provide the required information, planning, and skill base to educate people to become independent.

Public Policy

There is a need for public policy that supports active living. For example, policies that prohibit smoking in public buildings can reduce the impact of secondary smoke inhalation. Policies can also ensure access and equity for people with disabilities and the economically disadvantaged. Public policy can also create formal agreements that support resource sharing and collaborative initiatives between organizations. Joint facility use agreements between municipalities and school districts are an example, but should be broadened beyond simple joint facility use to include lifestyle programming. Finally, public policies that help the positive use of the environment, open spaces, and pedestrian and bicycle transportation systems can influence the development of an active living community.

Environmental Commitment

The active living community should be committed to sustainable environments. Municipal parks and recreation departments are the stewards of a significant portion of open spaces in the community. As such, they play a major role in preserving natural open spaces and developing resources, programs, and land management practices that are environmentally sensitive in terms of energy and materials consumption. The outdoor environment obviously has great potential for active living and also is an important part of a community's identity. Active living is fostered through pedestrian and bicycle trail networks, playfields and informal open spaces, and natural areas that invite exploration and provide escape from built environments. Interpretive programs can bring people closer to nature in their own community. Finally, active living group activities such as stream cleaning or tree planting programs can enhance community involvement and identity.

Summary

Although active living is a term that describes what currently occurs in many communities, the concept of becoming an active living community means taking a holistic approach to physical activity as well as the environment. An active living community should strive to go beyond its traditional services and encourage healthier and more active lifestyles.

Responding effectively to the emerging needs of our communities requires an integrated approach; one where people in the physical activity field balance traditional services with involvement in broader lifestyle and social issues in the community. The critical first step is forging partnerships with community agencies and organizations that are also committed to enhancing the quality of life in the community.

References

Canadian Parks and Recreation Association. (1992). Saanich: An Active Living community in action. *Active Living Insert: Recreation Canada*, **50**(1), 6-10.

Fitness Canada. (1990). *Move through the years: A blueprint for action*. Ottawa: Government of Canada.

Fitness Canada. (1991a). *Active living: A conceptual overview*. Ottawa: Government of Canada.

Fitness Canada. (1991b). *Active living for Canadians with a disability: A blueprint for action*. Ottawa: Government of Canada.

Fitness Canada. (1991c). *Because they're young: A blueprint for action*. Ottawa: Government of Canada.

Parks and Recreation Federation of Ontario. (1991). *A catalogue of the benefits of parks and recreation*. Toronto: Government of Ontario.

Stewart, G.S. (1991). *Active living*. Vancouver, BC: Alliance for Health and Fitness.

27

Issues in Policy Development for Active Living and Sustainable Living in Canada

Thomas L. Burton

Two important public policy themes have recurred in Canada during the 20th century. The first has to do with the significance of fitness and exercise to the well-being of the nation and its citizens. The second relates to the condition of the natural environment and the ways in which this affects everyday living. As these two themes have waxed and waned in the political arena, they have been perceived by the public as separate domains. There is growing evidence, however, that the two are not only related but, in fact, are closely interwoven. This interweaving has occurred, principally, because of the way in which public policies for each have evolved.

A Historical Perspective on Active Living

The beginnings of federal government involvement in fitness in Canada can be traced to the PRO–REC programs in British Columbia during the Great Depression. On November 9, 1934, the minister of education for the province announced the establishment of recreation and physical education classes to protect the youth of British Columbia from the degenerating effects of enforced idleness caused by unemployment and to develop morale and character (McFarland, 1970). The success of these classes attracted the attention of the federal Purvis Commission, which had been established in 1936 to investigate the needs of unemployed youth. Following the Purvis Commision's report in 1937, the government of Canada began a program of assistance to the provinces for physical training and recreation projects, through the Unemployment and Agricultural Assistance Act. Thus began the national interest in physical fitness.

Over the next half century, federal government interest in physical fitness ebbed and flowed with the politics of the day. The passage of the National Physical Fitness Act in 1943 signaled the first direct federal involvement in the physical development of Canadians through sports, athletics, and fitness activities. A National Council on Physical Fitness was created, which interpreted its mandate broadly to include physical, recreational, and cultural activities. The repeal of the National Physical Fitness Act in 1954 signaled a federal withdrawal from the field, ostensibly because the perceived need for fitness as part of the daily regimen was now met adequately through the expanding provincial and municipal programs and through the schools.

It wasn't long, however, before the federal government reentered the field, through the Fitness and Amateur Sport Act of 1961. The principal impetus for this new initiative was the poor showing of Canadian athletes in international competition in the preceding years. Paradoxically, although the new act excluded the word *physical* from its title, the interpretation of *fitness* was not nearly as broad as had been the case earlier. Instead, there was a growing emphasis upon the development of elite sport, made most evident in the creation of the carded athlete system. It was only in the early 1970s that much attention was again given to the fitness of the population at large, through the ParticipACTION program. But, although the establishment of ParticipACTION signaled a greater disquiet about general fitness levels in Canada, the bulk of federal activity was still directed at the elite sport system.

It was not until the mid-1980s that a new initiative was launched to address the question of physical fitness in the Canadian population as a whole. The 1986 Canadian Summit on Fitness set out to reexamine the concept of fitness. Delegates acknowledged the need to widen the meaning of the word *fitness* from a narrowly defined physical condition to one that reflected personal well-being in an overarching sense. The concept of active living was developed to describe a situation in which physical activity is integrated into everyday life. Active living broadens the notion of traditional fitness to include nontraditional, unstructured, and unregulated activities, such as gardening and flying a kite. It extends traditional fitness to connect fitness to other aspects of lifestyle such as healthy eating and stress management. And it reaches beyond fitness to emphasize physical activity as part of the social domain of life, through the family, workplace, school, and other social institutions.

A Historical Perspective on Environmental Concern

Concern for the natural environment in Canada has gone through three distinct phases during the 20th century. The principles of the 19th-century conservation movement first took tangible form in the activities of the federal Commission of Conservation, which existed from 1909 to 1921. The commission's philosophy was unashamedly utilitarian, with emphasis given to the complementarity of development and conservation. The principal concern was not that natural resources were being exploited, but that in many cases they were being exploited wastefully. The conservation movement was a crusade against waste and mismanagement in development, not against development itself (Burton, 1972). As such, the movement was dominated by resource management professionals: foresters, land surveyors, and engineers.

Environmental concern waned in Canada following the demise of the Commission of Conservation in 1921. During the 1960s, however, there was a reawakening. The principles of the conservation movement were resurrected in a wider context and took shape in the form of a new environmental movement. The concern was still with waste and mismanagement, but where the conservationists of the 1910s had battled with the quantitative dimensions of waste, the enviornmentalists of the 1960s voiced alarm over the deteriorating quality of the environment. As a result, the debate spilled over from the professional and political domains to the wider public arena. But because the focus remained on large-scale developments, public involvement was limited principally to organized pressure groups. Although the new movement gave priority to ecological considerations over economic ones, emphasized aesthetics over science, and adopted a policy of worldwide population control, its influence was seen most clearly in the passage of federal and provincial environmental impact assessment legislation. The movement did not succeed in generating a broadly based environmental ethic in the population at large.

Since the end of the 1980s, a third phase of concern has emerged and is gaining strength. Its thrust is the adoption of environmental principles in everyday living: Sound environmental practices are considered to be central to everyday living. The concept of sustainable living broadens the notion of conservation to include the practices of individuals as well as those of businesses and governments. It extends conservation to connect environmental quality to other aspects of life, including health and wellness. And it reaches beyond conservation to emphasize sound environmental practices as part of the wider societal domain—in the home, at school, in business, and elsewhere.

Attitudes and Behavior

Both active living and sustainable living are by no means universally espoused. Results of the 1988 Survey on Well-Being in Canada showed that only one third (33%) of Canadians were physically active in their leisure time, and only about one quarter (24%) were moderately active. Only one half (50%) had positive attitudes toward vigorous activity, and only about two fifths (42%) intended to participate in vigorous physical activity at least three times weekly in the year following the study, with an additional 30% intending to do so one to two times per week (Stephens & Craig, 1990). This fragmentation within the general population was even more evident when particular population groups were examined. In every age group, males were significantly more physically active in their leisure time than females. Persons with university degrees were almost twice as active as persons without high school diplomas. And, with the exception of students and retired persons (people who have extremely flexible leisure time patterns), blue-collar workers were the most physically active occupational group in leisure, followed closely by those in managerial and professional occupations.

There has been no comparable national survey of environmental behavior and attitudes, but national public opinion polls suggest that commitment to sustainable living is equally fragmented. The level of popular concern has clearly risen during the past half dozen years. In June 1986, about three fifths (62%) of Canadians described the quality of the environment in their own communities as either excellent or good. Three years later, the figure had dropped to about one half (53%), and almost as many (47%) described their environmental quality as fair or poor (Gregg & Posner, 1990). In the popular mind, the environment was second only to the economy as the most important problem facing the nation in 1989. Perhaps the most significant national statistic, however, has to do with perceptions of environmental responsibility. About one third (35%) of the respondents in the 1989 poll indicated that individuals rather than governments are primarily responsible for protecting the environment (Gregg & Posner, 1990). Three years earlier the proportion had been about half this figure (18%). Moreover, many of these people acted on their beliefs—buying recycled goods, boycotting products made by polluting industries, recycling cans and bottles, and so on. And, like those most involved in active living, these "green activists" came disproportionately from particular segments of the population. They were most numerous among middle-aged persons with a university education in higher paid professional and managerial occupations.

Beyond the domain of personal action, however, Canadians are ambivalent about what to do to protect the environment. Although, for example, three quarters (75%) of the respondents to the 1989 survey thought that Canada should build a toxic waste disposal facility somewhere in the country, more than half (56%) insisted that it could not be located anywhere near their communities (Gregg & Posner, 1990). Similarly, although about two thirds (67%) acknowledged that existing garbage disposal systems were inadequate, almost three quarters (73%) were opposed to new landfill sites within their own communities. In short, although large majorities favor drastic action on some matters, there is much greater division on other matters.

Challenges for Public Policy

From its inception in the 1960s, Canada's social policy has been founded on the principle of universality. Economic prosperity through the 1960s and 1970s meant that social policies were generally designed without reference to such considerations as efficiency, work incentives, initiative, and personal economic means. Policy was driven by considerations of universality and security rather than inequality and adjustment. Social programs were aimed less at the development of a social safety net to help disadvantaged individuals adjust to economic dislocations and more at the provision of a social security blanket available to all. Fiscal, economic, and sociodemographic changes during the 1980s, however, raised significant questions about the viability of such a philosophy and approach and presented major new challenges for both social and environmental policy.

In the past several years, social programs have been seriously constrained by the fiscal burden carried by Canadians. Annual budget deficits of the federal and provincial governments and debt servicing are increasingly constricting policymaking. In 1988, expenditures by all levels of government on the principal social services (health care, education, housing, social security, and culture and recreation) accounted for one half (50.4%) of total government spending (Horry & Walker, 1991). Interest charges on government debt amounted to almost one fifth (18.2%) of the total. The three levels of Canadian government collectively spent almost as much on debt servicing as they did on social security: 18.2% compared to 22.4%, respectively. Moreover, the ratio of debt servicing to social services expenditure is rising. In 1970, social services spending accounted for 54.8% of the total, and interest charges amounted to 8.5%. Even in 1980, debt servicing took only one tenth (10.9%) of the total, whereas social services accounted for more than one half (52%). Put simply, social policy—and, to a lesser extent, policy in other domains—is

increasingly subject to fiscal restraint. The policy challenge, then, is to reorient social programs to conform with fiscal constraint, while maintaining an appropriate social safety net for those affected adversely by the economic and sociodemographic changes presently occurring. Environmental policies, too, must be fashioned in this context of fiscal restraint.

The economic challenge to social and environmental policies derives from Canada's need to adjust to the realities of the new world economic order. Economic prosperity will be enjoyed by those countries that can most readily reorient their allocation of resources toward the "sunrise industries": biomedical technology, tourism, computer hardware and software, recreation and sport equipment, personal services, and so on. The challenge to policy is to ensure that social and environmental programs encourage this economic adjustment rather than constrain it and, at the same time, meet individual and social needs that emerge from this new economic order.

The final challenge is the sociodemographic one. Courchene (1990) has observed that the needs of those who rely on social services are not well met by the entitlements currently provided through social policy. The structure of the Canadian population has changed markedly during the past 2 decades and will continue to do so in the foreseeable future. The traditional nuclear family with one parent employed outside the home is no longer the dominant domestic arrangement in Canada. Single-parent families, blended families, single-person households, families in which both parents are employed outside the home, and other models are evident in great numbers. These arrangements, and such issues as population aging, increased industrial obsolescence, and the growing premium that economic activity places on knowledge and information, are increasingly demanding a major reorientation of social and related environmental policy goals.

Policy Choices

These fiscal, economic, and sociodemographic challenges have drawn attention to a series of fundamental policy choices, or trade-offs, that Canadians will increasingly be required to make. The most important of these are universality versus targeting, public provision versus privatization, democratization versus professionalization, centralization versus decentralization, and rationalism versus incrementalism.

There can be no social safety net in an economy that fails to adjust to major structural change. Nor can such security be found for very long in a society that insists on funding social programs through continuing budget deficits. Thus, Canada's social policies must increasingly be tailored to fit within economic and fiscal policies. Social programs must emphasize not the same treatment for all, but differential treatment among groups, with the purpose of providing more equitable opportunities. Paradoxically, equity requires unequal provision of services. There is a recognition of the need for programs that direct social support to those most in need, but in such a way as to provide incentives for people to work their way out of this need for support. The principle of universality must increasingly give way to the notion of targeting.

There is a popular misconception that social programs must invariably be provided by public sector agencies. Yet, in reality, there has always been a distinction between payment for social services and the provision of them. In some cases, such as education, the service is both paid for and provided by public agencies—in this case school boards. In other instances, such as health care, the state pays for a service that is provided by private practitioners. In yet other areas, such as culture and recreation, a mix of public and private provision, with and without user fees, has been the consistent pattern. Privatization of services that were formerly provided by public sector agencies has accelerated in Canada in recent years. This trend has received added impetus from the fiscal, economic, and sociodemographic challenges that Canadians face. Indeed, Lindbeck (1986) has argued that as the state breaks new ground in the development of social policy, established public services have a greater likelihood of being privatized. As the state becomes more involved, for example, in the provision of day care or maternity benefits, it may choose to privatize its public swimming programs and campgrounds. There seems little doubt that the privatization of public services will continue, especially in the sport, fitness, culture, and recreation sector, although the rate of change will likely vary over time and across jurisdictions.

As the level of state involvement in the provision of social, economic, and environmental programs has risen, so has the state's dependence on professionals and experts for the delivery of these programs. Many new professions and ''semiprofessions'' have been developed to service emerging public sector programs. In the domain of active living, the past 2 decades have seen the development of professional sports administrators, certified coaches, recreation therapists, certified fitness appraisers, and more. In the realm of sustainable living, there are now specialist environmental scientists and planners. All of these groups derive their identification from the attainment of particular (often new) forms of knowledge and are associated, in varying degrees, with the possession of specified credentials. This trend to greater professionalization must, however, contend with an opposite trend toward increased democratization. The public participation movement that blossomed in the 1960s appears to be experiencing a new resurgence. There are growing demands for direct public involvement in both the development and implementation of social and environmental policy.

The history of social policy in Canada has been one of increasing centralization—at both the federal and provincial levels. Responsibilities for health care, education, welfare, housing, and culture and recreation were systematically centralized during the 1960s and 1970s. Sport and fitness were very much a part of this, exemplified by the establishment of various federal and provincial centers to house national and provincial recreation and sport governing bodies. The pace of centralization slowed during the early 1980s, but only since the late 1980s has there been a shift toward decentralization. It is no longer assumed that greater efficiency and more effective services are natural outcomes of greater centralization of decision making, especially at the policy level. And even when centralization can be shown to lead to greater efficiency, it can be argued that the price, in the form of increased discordance, segmentation, and alienation, may not be worth the benefits.

The story of public policymaking has also been one of heightened efforts at rationalization, defined by MacIntosh and Whitson (1990) as a process by which human institutions are increasingly subjected to scientific analysis and redesign in the pursuit of greater technical and bureaucratic efficiency and productivity. Slack and Hinings (1987) have shown how this rationalization has been increasingly sought in sport and recreation organizations. Rationalization promotes planning, coordination, and tight administrative structures, and it emphasizes control. The rationalist model emanates from a preoccupation with the needs to identify causality, to establish facts, and to distinguish facts from values (Burton, 1989). Yet, in reality, most public policies simply are not developed rationally—at least, not comprehensively. It is also doubtful that there really are any social facts that are entirely divorced from values. The ways in which we view the social and environmental worlds shape the facts that we produce about them. The definition of poverty, for example, is not abstract and immutable but rather specific to time and place. In the real world, policymaking is a subjective, diffuse, and political exercise in muddling through to an acceptable state of affairs, not a logical, scientific, and deductive reasoning process for arriving at an optimum human condition.

Quality of Life

Active living and sustainable living are both part of a much larger entity called ''quality of life.'' It is abundantly clear that many Canadians want to improve the quality of their lives, even at the expense of some of its quantitative dimensions. Over four fifths (83%) of respondents to a national opinion poll in 1989 indicated that they would support enforced recycling, over three quarters (76%) would ban plastic and foam products, and over two thirds (67%) would even support severe restrictions on automobile use—if these actions would likely lead to significant protection of the environment (Gregg & Posner, 1990).

These types of actions clearly fall within the purview of governments. It is increasingly evident, however, that Canadians perceive the primary responsibility for pursuing and obtaining an improved quality of life falling upon individuals rather than upon governments. The concepts of active living and sustainable living are both embedded in the notion of personal responsibility. Both are wedded to daily life. Both, of necessity, must focus upon the individual and the family. And public policies for both must also be directed principally at individuals and groups.

We know, however, that those who practice active living and sustainable living are a minority of Canadians—albeit a sizable one. The 1988 National Survey on Well-Being in Canada showed that more than two fifths (43%) of the population are physically inactive, with a further one quarter (24%) only moderately active (Stephens & Craig, 1990). Similarly, a national opinion poll in 1989 showed that only slightly more than one half of the population actually engage in various kinds of sustainable living activities: about half (56%) recycle bottles and cans, and about two fifths (41%) have stopped buying products from identified polluters (Gregg & Posner, 1990). There are still large numbers of Canadians who do not practice active living and sustainable living at all, or who do so in only an incidental and limited way. When this differential pattern of involvement is placed alongside the fiscal, economic, and sociodemographic challenges that currently face Canadian governments, it seems fairly clear that policies for both active living and sustainable living will change. We will likely see a greater emphasis in the future upon targeting, privatization, democratization, decentralization, and incrementalism.

With respect to targeting, policies for active living will need to focus not upon the Canadian population at large but upon target groups within the population, such as women, persons with disabilities, and sales and clerical workers, all of whom are underrepresented among the physically active. In like manner, policies for sustainable living will need to focus upon groups that are underrepresented among the environmentally active, such as high school dropouts, blue-collar workers, low-income people, and so on. The intent will be to focus on the "unconverted," not those who are already involved.

In regard to public provision and privatization, it is worth noting that policies for recreation and culture and for the environment already emphasize a greater role for the private sector in both funding and service provision. The Alberta Ministry of Recreation and Parks, for example, envisages an expanded role for the private sector in its recreation, parks, and sports programs and facilities in the 1990s (Alberta Recreation and Parks, 1988), while the Federal Green Plan for Canada's environment will rely heavily on the development of partnerships with the private sector (Government of Canada, 1990).

In the case of democratization and professionalization, there is an apparent contradiction in present policies. On the one hand, policies for fitness and sport emphasize the need for greater professionalization through the development of a wide array of certification schemes. At the same time, these policies stress the importance of volunteers to the development and implementation of programs. There is also an awareness of the need for people to take greater responsibility for their own health and well-being. There is, in fact, an inherent tension in policymaking between professionalization and democratization.

There is evidence, too, that policies will increasingly foster decentralization of service delivery. A case in point is the 1990 Canadian Museum Policy, which proposes greater decentralization of services and control to the regional level in Canada (Communications Canada, 1990). We will likely see this trend emerging in other domains of active living and sustainable living in the 1990s.

Finally, there is the question of rationalization in public policy. It is doubtful that policy formulation will ever actively encourage spontaneity or intelligent muddling through. It is in the nature of our social and governmental institutions to seek to be (and to appear) rational. However, there is likely to be a retreat from comprehensive rationalism, with its emphasis upon the comprehensive and rational treatment of variables that are themselves comprehensive and rational (Burton, 1989), toward a more incremental approach that emphasizes change through trade-offs between variables. Whereas rational policies are typically conceived as being total, holistic, comprehensive, and optimal, incremental policies are characteristically remedial, serial, exploratory, and fragmented. As Hall (1980) remarked, "Muddling through is no bad prescription for the ordering of public affairs, if it is done with intelligence and forethought" (p. xxvii).

Conclusion

The most important point concerning policy development for active living and sustainable living is that they are not separate and discrete areas but are part of something much larger: quality of life. Canada's Green Plan argues that human health and the environment are inextricably linked and suggests, further, that this relationship is not limited solely to physical health. In words that echo those of the 1988 Canadian Summit on Fitness, Canada's Green Plan maintains that the "spiritual, psychological, social, and emotional health of individuals is affected by the health of the environment as well" (Government of Canada, 1990, p. 27). What is being said, in effect, is that active living and sustainable living are parts of the same policy puzzle. It is imperative, then, that policies for the two should be developed in tandem. Proposed policies for active living must be evaluated in terms of their implications for sustainable living, and vice versa, because human health and well-being are important considerations in every environmental issue.

References

Alberta Recreation and Parks. (1988). *Foundations for action: Corporate aims for the ministry of recreation and parks*. Edmonton: Government of Alberta.

Burton, T.L. (1972). *Natural resource policy in Canada*. Toronto: McClelland & Stewart.

Burton, T.L. (1989). Leisure forecasting, policymaking, and planning. In E.L. Jackson & T.L. Burton (Eds.), *Understanding leisure and recreation: Mapping the past, charting the future* (pp. 211-244). State College, PA: Venture.

Communications Canada. (1990). *Canadian museum policy*. Ottawa: Supply & Services Canada.

Courchene, T. (1990). Social policy. In T.E. Kierans (Ed.), *Getting it right* (pp. 65-88). Toronto: C.D. Howe Institue.

Government of Canada. (1990). *Canada's green plan*. Ottawa: Supply & Services Canada.

Gregg, A., & Posner, M. (1990). *The big picture*. Toronto: MacFarlane, Walter & Ross.

Hall, P. (1980). *Great planning disasters*. Berkeley, CA: University of California Press.

Horry, I.D., & Walker, M.A. (1991). *Government spending facts*. Vancouver: Fraser Institute.

Lindbeck, A. (1986, January-February). Limits to the welfare state. *Challenge*, pp. 31-36.

MacIntosh, D., & Whitson, D. (1990). *The game planners: Transforming Canada's sport system*. Montreal, Kingston, ON: McGill–Queen's University Press.

McFarland, E.M. (1970). *The development of public recreation in Canada*. Ottawa: Canadian Parks/Recreation Association.

Slack, T., & Hinings, B. (1987). Planning and organizational change: A conceptual framework for the analysis of amateur sport organizations. *Canadian Journal of Sport Sciences*, **12**, 185-193.

Stephens, T., & Craig, C.L. (1990). *The well-being of Canadians*. Ottawa: Canadian Fitness and Lifestyle Research Institute.

28

Personal Empowerment and Active Living

John Lord

Active living has been defined as a way of life in which activity is valued and integrated into daily life. Focusing on the whole person (physical, social, mental, and spiritual), the concept of active living emphasizes individual well-being. In this sense, active living is intricately linked to health. However, the concept of active living is unlikely to have wide relevance unless it is also understood in terms of a critical health determinant: empowerment. Citizens who are disempowered, lack valued resources, or are isolated from community life will be unlikely to be able to optimize their health or active living. Rappaport (1987) argues that empowerment as a paradigm can help us understand how to promote health and enable power sharing in communities and programs.

In this paper I will explore empowerment as a concept, process, and practice. In particular, I will relate research on personal empowerment to active living and participation.

Empowerment as a Concept

Several fields of endeavor have begun to incorporate the language of empowerment. Health promotion, for example, is defined by the World Health Organization as "the process of enabling people to increase control over, and to improve, their health" (World Health Organization, 1987, p. 1). In social work, empowerment is seen by some critics as an alternative to the professional control exercised by social workers and the systems within which they work. In the area of family support, a growing network of researchers and practitioners is interested in the concept of empowerment (Cochran & Wolfer, 1983; Dunst, Trivette, & Deal, 1988).

We can begin to understand empowerment by examining the concepts of power and powerlessness. Power is defined by the Cornell Empowerment Group as the "capacity of some persons and organizations to produce intended, foreseen, and unforeseen effects on others" (Cornell Empowerment Group, 1989, p. 1). At the indi-

vidual level, powerlessness can be seen as the expectation of a person that his or her own actions will be ineffective in influencing the outcome of life events (Keiffer, 1984). Lerner (1986) makes a distinction between real and surplus powerlessness. Real powerlessness results from economic inequities and oppressive control exercised by systems and other people. Surplus powerlessness, on the other hand, is an internalized belief that change cannot occur, a belief that results in apathy and an unwillingness of the person to struggle for more control and influence. In our work, many of our research participants experienced both real and surplus powerlessness.

Most of the literature also associates empowerment with personal control. Julian Rappaport (1981) says, "By empowerment I mean our aim should be to enhance the possibilities for people to control their own lives" (p. 7). Furthermore, he notes that "there is built into the term (empowerment) a quality of the relationship between a person and his or her community, environment and something outside one's self" (p. 125).

The concept of empowerment is complex and ecological. Individuals are situated in families and communities and live their lives within a social context. At the Centre for Research and Education, we study personal empowerment by looking at the "person in the environment" and by trying to understand the life experience of each person in relation to family, groups, and other aspects of community life. That the individual is the focus of our concern does not mean we ignore the social context within which people live (Germain & Gitterman, 1980; Rappaport, 1987).

Rappaport (1987) notes that empowerment "conveys both a psychological sense of personal control or influence and a concern with actual social influence, political power, and legal rights" (p. 121). In this sense, empowerment can exist at three levels: at the personal level, where empowerment is the experience of gaining increasing control, influence, and participation in daily life; at the small group level, where empowerment involves the shared experience, analysis, and increasing influence of small groups on their own efforts and their community; and at the community level, where empowerment revolves around the utilization of resources and strategies to enhance community control.

Empowerment as a Process

The concept of active living is rich with qualitative notions of participation, involvement, interaction, meaning, and personal experience. Surprisingly to a qualitative researcher, most of the people conducting research in this field do so from conventional, quantitative paradigms. In using a qualitative, phenomenological approach to these questions, we have gained new and important insights into the process of empowerment, community participation, and active living.

In our research at the Centre for Research and Education, we seek to understand empowerment and participation from the perspective of the citizen. The research has focused on how people have experienced powerlessness, personal control, and participation. We have explored the meanings that people attach to these experiences and how they construct their lives in relation to their social context. Our research used participants' experiences, stories, and insights as a way of building our understanding of the process of empowerment. The frameworks of qualitative research and biographical analysis were used to guide the research process. We have utilized in-depth individual interviews and small, focused groups to help us understand the process that people go through as they gain more control in their lives. To date, we have conducted in-depth biographical interviews with developmentally and physically disabled citizens, low-income women, and citizens who have had extensive involvement in the mental health system.

It is worth highlighting the depth of feeling with which people described their experiences. In one sense, many people were almost desperate to tell their story. Several participants noted that it was the first time they had tried to tell their own story. As researchers, we saw ourselves as part of an intricate process, honoring people's experiences and probing carefully to draw out insights. As we listened, we sensed the vulnerability, the struggles, and the hopes of people's lives in transition (Lord, 1991; Lord & Farlow, 1990).

In this paper, we shall not report on those individual research projects but rather present a brief summary of research themes that can inform us about the role of empowerment and participation in active living.

Powerlessness

Powerlessness for our research participants was both a *global* and a *situational* experience.

- Some people experienced a sense of total powerlessness and became, for a period, unable to see themselves as capable of having control or influencing others.
- Other people experienced powerlessness in some areas of their life but were able to maintain control and self-esteem in other areas. Some individuals who were institutionalized, for example, never lost hope that their life could be better. This sense of self-efficacy became paramount for many of them later in the empowerment process.

The conditions of powerlessness experienced by our participants are similar to Goldenberg's conditions of oppression, which include containment, expendability, and compartmentalization (Goldenberg, 1978). Examining our findings on people with disabilities can explain the lived experience of these conditions. Growing up with a disability in our culture is to feel diminished and maneuvered by myths (Freire, 1985). One of the cruelest myths experienced by people with disabilities is that their difference is somehow not socially acceptable. One woman noted that "people just don't include me as I am." Many participants recalled the profound sense of devaluation and social isolation they felt as young people. One person's experience was typical: "I sat at home a lot of the time. I could go out for walks but I didn't really get involved. There wasn't too much to do then. That's not really living."

The consequences for individuals of prolonged dependency on service systems included low self-esteem and limited options and experience in decision making. For some, resignation or helplessness accompanied prolonged dependency. Most participants also had very small, uninvolved social networks, which contributed to social isolation. For individuals with a disability since birth, imposed segregation meant there were few opportunities to develop natural networks. The combination of social isolation and low expectations limited people's capacity to dream. It also affected their ability to believe in themselves and to take control of their lives. Many participants led very passive lives.

Gaining Awareness: Impetus to Empowerment

The transition toward personal empowerment is a uniquely individual and ongoing process. The impetus toward personal empowerment began for our participants with increased awareness. For some, gaining awareness was a gradual process but for others it appeared to be more dramatic. In either case, the increased awareness was precipitated by one or more of the following scenarios:

- being involved in a crisis or "life transition,"
- acting on anger or frustration,
- responding to new information, or
- responding to a change in context.

These situations acted as catalysts for the empowerment process and led to two vital changes in each participant:

1) becoming aware of their own capacities and of alternatives to the experience of powerlessness, and
2) developing new directions for themselves.

As we shall see, these are critical elements of personal empowerment.

As individuals began to gain a voice and become aware of their own capacities, they realized there were alternatives to passivity. People often realized they could increase their area of influence. For most people, these were tentative beginnings and important first steps in the transition to empowerment. However, for most of the people with whom we worked, the process of personal empowerment was a constant struggle.

Support From People: A Critical Element in Expanding Personal Empowerment

As participants talked about their lives, time and time again they mentioned other people who had been important and who had made a difference to their gaining control and increased self-efficacy. Of all the factors that were identified as being helpful, *people's support* was mentioned most often. For some participants, support from other people was the catalyst that enabled them to begin the journey toward personal empowerment. For most people, however, the support provided by others was more critical to expanding their empowerment once they had begun the journey. People's support appeared to be most useful when the person had already started to become aware of alternatives. While the meaning of personal support and its perceived importance varied from person to person, certain types of support have a significant effect on the process of empowerment.

Social support is often mentioned as a significant contributor to health and well-being (Gottlieb, 1985; Saulnier, 1982). Interestingly, many of the relationships that participants described as empowering resulted from the effect of a single person on their lives. As people outlined their experiences, it became apparent that positive, one-to-one support was seen as the most important contributor to individual empowerment. When that support was interactive, it enabled the person to be involved in decision making, and provided an opportunity for the person to gain clarity of vision in his or her life.

One kind of support is of particular value to active living. Many participants mentioned the support of a mentor, a person who acted as a significant role model, enabling the individual to take more initiative and control and to begin to develop more confidence in participation. Primarily, mentors were individuals who believed in the other person. One man said of his friend,

"He was a person who had a belief in my ability that I hadn't even anticipated." This belief seemed critical for some of our participants to expand their vision and self-confidence.

Sometimes the mentor role was limited to an individual providing appropriate information at the right time. Many people who became disabled later in life, for example, recalled how important it was to meet for the first time someone with a similar disability. One man noted,

One of my doctors had introduced me to someone else in a wheelchair and asked him to come in and speak with me. And I bombarded him with questions because I was really keen to know what I might be able to do for myself and what lay ahead. I was thankful for the doctor for arranging that and for having this person come in to see me. And thanks to this experience, later on in another hospital, I asked that we institute this peer support for other people and we began to have organized sessions.

Mentors enabled people who were struggling to expand their dreams and awareness and to think differently. Several participants who had experienced this process explained how a mentor helped them envision possibilities and options, a critical part of empowerment. Sometimes the mentor provided the impetus by directly challenging the person to change. Most often the mentor was a role model or presented the issues and alternatives in a new way. Jean, for example, had been afraid to speak out in public, but as she watched her friend Carol deal with the welfare office and the school system, she wondered if she could learn to be more assertive. The first time she decided to speak out, Jean rehearsed her speech with Carol. The two women then went to the meeting together. Jean recalled "the surge in confidence" she felt as a result of that initial success with Carol's support.

While people supports were extremely valuable, it is interesting that the people who became the most empowered attributed some of their change to themselves. This sense of self-efficacy is an important piece in the empowerment puzzle (Bandura, 1986). It involves both responsibility and a belief that you can have control over your surroundings and influence decisions that affect your life. As people expand their participation and empowerment, they increase their sense of self-efficacy.

The Role of Resources and Services

Resources and services that contributed to empowerment were those that expanded choice and options. Participants never mentioned congregated, bureaucratic, or institutional services as being helpful or as contributing in any way to their sense of personal empowerment.

Participants identified common characteristics of services that provided support in a way that contributed to empowerment. These same attributes were mentioned by all groups and included supports that were personalized, responsive, interactive, and encouraging of consumer control. Perhaps what is most significant about these findings is that individualized resources and services facilitate participation, which is the most potent of the factors facilitating empowerment. Because active living involves personal choice, facilitators and service providers need to be cognizant of the importance of individualizing approaches to fitness, leisure, and community participation.

Participation and Personal Empowerment

Participation significantly advanced the process of personal empowerment for all of the men and women who have been part of our research studies. Our participants have helped us understand participation as both the process of becoming engaged in activities and social groups, and the sense of being acknowledged and accepted as active, contributing community members.

We found that the process of participation was itself empowering. The process appears to be two-fold. On the one hand, as people gained self-confidence by utilizing the people and resources in their lives, they sought more avenues for participation. On the other hand, participation in a community activity enhanced self-confidence, which in turn expanded personal control. Usually participation was a conscious engagement that altered people's relationship with their social world and increased their sense of control and self-efficacy.

The experiences of our participants demonstrate that participation contributes to personal empowerment by

- enhancing contact and thereby reducing social isolation,
- expanding competence and confidence, and
- creating contexts for meaningful contributions and involvements.

These findings provide important insights for the active living movement. For most of our participants, personal empowerment was expanded through participation in community activities that were based on common cultural, political, or recreational interests. The value of participation in activities of common interest reiterates the community nature of participation for active living. It is in community that people come together around common interests. People who join fitness clubs, running groups, sport clubs, service groups, recreational groups, or women's groups all come together around a common interest.

Regardless of the type of participation, participants in our research often noted that "contributing" helped advance their self-esteem and empowerment. This finding is significant. People with disabilities and other marginalized groups have typically had few opportunities to contribute to community life (Lusthaus, 1986; Redkop & Bender, 1988). More often people have been treated as clients and have been recipients, not contributors. In the initial part of their empowerment process, people generally had too little energy and too few options to even consider how to contribute. As their lives unfolded, opportunities for participating and contributing became more possible; as examples, people felt more confidence in themselves, had more valued resources, or experienced more helpful people in their lives.

While all our participants became more active as they experienced greater empowerment, the range and depth of the involvement varied widely. Some individuals, including all participants with developmental disabilities, required invitations and support from others to become involved. The struggle to remain active was very real for several people and their lives seemed to still be quite vulnerable. Others seemed to have blossomed once they increased their involvement; they had broader social networks, valued resources, and a belief in themselves that contrasted sharply with earlier periods of powerlessness.

Table 28.1 illustrates the elements of the personal empowerment process. What is fascinating for active living is that people become more active as they increase their control and involvement in decisions that affected their lives.

Implications for Practice

The research presented here in many ways reflects a substantial criticism of many common practices. Our participants' experiences show that the process of becoming more empowered involves continual struggle against systems that label, reject, and segregate. It is clear that "more of the same" will seldom contribute to personal empowerment.

Five implications for practice can be identified. First, building on our research approach, people responsible for community resources and services will learn a great deal by listening to the people they support. By truly listening, we can deepen our understanding of the context of people's lives and provide the strong sense of value that many of our participants noted was missing early in their transition from powerlessness to power.

Second, empowering practices build on the strengths and capacities of each person. Programs that are exclusive or restrictive do not allow individual preferences to flourish. Recreation workers in particular need to identify people's gifts and strengths. As some of our research participants noted, part of the professional's role may be to enable people to fit those strengths with community activities of common interest.

Third, practices that are empowering enable people to have more control over the resources and services

Table 28.1 Elements of the Personal Empowerment Process

Experiencing powerlessness	Gaining awareness	Learning new roles	Initiating/ participating	Contributing
• Social isolation	• Acting on anger	• Connecting with others	• Joining groups	• Being a role model
• Service dependency	• Responding to information	• Linking with resources	• Involvement in community activities	• Having influence
• Limited choices	• Responding to new contexts	• Expanding choices/ opportunities	• Expanding participatory competence	• Increasing self-efficacy

Passive - Active

Note. Reprinted from Lord, 1991.

designated for them. In designing community programs, we need to recognize that for a power transfer to occur and equality to be established, the program participants must be the ones to identify the problems and the solutions. Or, as one writer has put it in terms of empowerment, the program must become a "vehicle designed, constructed, and piloted by those being served" (Fried, 1980, p. 3). Our research has shown that resources and services that were most helpful for empowerment were those in which personal control was a requirement for effective participation.

Fourth, professionals conscious of empowerment will find ways to reach out to people who have traditionally not been included in community activities. It is critical to remember that escape from systems that have contributed to dependency and powerlessness is an equally important part of the process of empowerment. In this research, for example, access to community activities and to expanded social networks enabled people to increase their choices and opportunities. Community health, fitness, and recreation workers could consider how their interventions maintain people in dependent situations or how they enable people to access other community resources and opportunities. To what extent, for example, is there support for people to participate in self-help groups or to become connected to a mentor? To build upon people's strengths, are there mechanisms whereby people with disabilities, older citizens, or recent immigrants can be linked with community organizations that are based on common interest rather than devaluing labels?

Fifth, understanding empowerment means we need to pay attention to power relationships. Citizens with whom we have conducted our research note that professionals often have power over them. As professionals, we need to consider how our language, mannerisms, and organizational structures maintain power over people. Moving toward partnership with a variety of communities and citizens requires sharing power with people

in ways that can be empowering to professionals and citizens alike.

We have much to learn about empowerment as a concept, process, and practice and particularly about its relationship to health and quality of life. Understanding the lived experience of people who have gone through a process of change has begun to shed light on critical issues for professional practice.

References

Bandura, A. (1986). *Social foundations of thought and action: A social cognitive theory.* Englewood Cliffs, NJ: Prentice Hall.

Cochran, M., & Wolfer, M. (1983). Beyond the deficit model: Empowerment of parents with information and informal supports. In I. Siegel & L. Laosa (Eds.), *Changing families* (pp. 225-246). New York: Plenum.

Cornell Empowerment Group. (1989). Empowerment and family support. *Networking Bulletin,* **1**(1).

Dunst, C., Trivette, C., & Deal, A. (1988). *Enabling and empowering families: Principles and guidelines for practice.* Cambridge, MA: Bookline Books.

Freire, R. (1985). *The politics of education: Culture, power, & liberation.* South Hadley, MA: Bergin and Garvey.

Fried, R. (1980). *Empowerment versus delivery of services.* NH: New Hampshire Department of Education.

Germain, C.B., & Gitterman, A. (1980). *The life model of social work practice.* New York: Columbia University Press.

Goldenberg, I. (1978). *Oppression and social intervention.* Chicago: Nelson.

Gottlieb, B. (1985). Social networks and social support: An overview of research, practice, & policy implications, *Health Education Quarterly,* **12**(1), pp. 5-22.

Keiffer, C. (1984). Citizen empowerment: A developmental perspective. *Prevention in Human Services*, **3**, 16.

Lerner, M. (1986). *Surplus powerlessness*. Oakland, CA: The Institute for Labor and Mental Health.

Lord, J. (1991). *Lives in transition: The process of personal empowerment*. Kitchener, ON: Centre for Research & Education in Human Services.

Lord, J., & Farlow, D. (1990). A study of personal empowerment. *Health Promotion*, **29**(2), 2-8.

Lusthaus, E. (1986). Making a contribution: An emerging social role for persons with a mental handicap. *Entourage*, **1**(2), 24.

Rappaport, J. (1981). In praise of paradox: A social policy of empowerment over prevention. *American Journal of Community Psychology*, **9**(1), 15-26.

Rappaport, J. (1987). Terms of empowerment/exemplars of prevention: Toward a theory for community psychology. *American Journal of Community Psychology*, **15**(2), 121-148.

Redkop, C., & Bender, U. (1988). *Who am I? What am I?* Grand Rapids, MI: Academic Books.

Saulnier, K. (1982). Network, change, and crisis: The web of support. *Canadian Journal of Community Mental Health*, **1**(1), 5-23.

Weiss, H.B. (1990). The challenges of empowerment in the family supports movement. *Networking Bulletin*, **1**(2), 3-8.

World Health Organization. (1987). Ottawa charter for health promotion. *Canadian Journal of Public Health*, **77**(6), 1.

29

Community Empowerment and Fitness

Ronald Labonté

We know that physical fitness correlates with emotional "fitness"—a state of feeling well about oneself and one's capacities. We also know that good physical fitness is associated with a reduced risk of cardiovascular disease, which makes it a concern of many people in public health.

But there is a physiological bias about most professional definitions of fitness, active living, and exercise. Fitness is "the ability to perform work satisfactorily" (World Health Organization, as cited in Quinney, Wall, & Gauvin, 1992). Active living is "a way of life in which physical activity is valued and integrated into daily life." Exercise is a goal-directed "form of leisure physical activity" conforming to "mode intensity, frequency, and duration of activity." Notably absent from these definitions is any notion of *meaning*. Is artistic expression work? Who judges satisfactory work performance? Is the goal of fitness functional only in terms of employment, or should it embody more explicit spiritual and psychological values? Could active living not also imply those core sociospiritual values of generosity, caring for others, and commitment to community well-being (Ornstein & Sobel, 1987)? Does exercise apply only to the body, or should we not also speak of the need to "exercise" critical, social, and moral behavior?

Health as Well-Being

Although public health has long held to the first half of the World Health Organization's definition ("a complete state of physical, mental, and social well-being"), health services remain focused on the second half ("the absence of disease or infirmity"). Much of our health promotion, wellness, and fitness work becomes defined in relation to disease, specifically disease prevention. Yet people's experiences of health are more about their experiences of capacity and connectives than about their experiences of disease or disability; Jean Miller eloquently defines health as "the increased becoming of what we are most deeply" (cited in Hill, 1990, p. 65).

The few health surveys that have asked open-ended questions about people's experience of health validate this idea (e.g., Blaxter, 1990).

People's experiences of health usually relate to such phenomena as

- feeling vital, and full of energy,
- having good social relationships,
- experiencing a sense of control over one's life and one's living conditions,
- being able to do things one enjoys,
- having a sense of purpose in life, and
- experiencing a connectedness to "community" (Blaxter, 1990; Registered Nurses Association of British Columbia, 1990).

Having a disease, especially a seriously disabling disease, makes it more difficult to experience these phenomena, but it does not make it impossible. People who have physical disabilities, who are near death, or who have unhealthy lifestyles or diagnosed diseases often report themselves as "healthy" precisely because they feel vital, loved, in control, joyful, with purpose, and connected.

At the same time, people who lack the social and personal resources to achieve these feelings tend to experience more disease. Disease is still a useful endpoint for understanding "health determinants," it is simply no longer the only endpoint. It is joined now by people's more socially defined experiences of well-being.

The social dimension of our health experiences is supported empirically. Without caring, respectful relationships, our health withers and our risk of morbidity and mortality increases. People who are relatively isolated (who lack adequate social networks or supportive relationships) suffer 2 to 4 times the risk of mortality, independent of all other known health risk factors (House, Landis, & Umberson, 1988).

From this vantage, the greatest disease reduction and health enhancement fitness programs engender may relate more to the socializing they create than the cardiopulmonary functioning they increase and endorphins they release. This is particularly so for isolated persons who may be drawn into fitness and leisure programs. To what extent should, and can, fitness programs more deliberately structure ongoing socialization for these persons? Does an intimate, in-the-basement home-visit fitness program make more sense for isolated mothers than the mega-chic step-program classes of 100 anonymous faces?

Differing Approaches to Health

Three broad clusterings of health problems have been identified, each of which embeds assumptions about how activities should be planned, implemented, and evaluated (Table 29.1) (Labonté, 1989). These three approaches represent *organizational biases*: Hospitals tend to work from a medical approach, state agencies from a behavioral approach, and community workers from a socioenvironmental approach. These organizational tendencies may constrain the ability of workers employed within these organizations to act effectively or legitimately within a different approach.

Allowing individuals and groups greater power to define health for themselves (wellness instead of just disease) and to define their health problems (which may be quite different from how health agencies or professionals view health problems) is one of the most important principles of a health promotion practice. Yet most health agencies work from a community-based perspective, where the problem is already named (i.e., a disease or behavior) rather than from a community development perspective, where the problem is named by the groups with which the agency works.

Community development programming embodies several collaborative principles:

- Community groups have the right to define their own health problems.
- At the same time, agencies and professionals, with their particular information or knowledge, have a responsibility to identify health problems for communities.
- Health agencies and community groups have reciprocal moral duties to negotiate with each other about how the health problems important to each of them can be acted upon and supported by both. This may involve a *convergence* of the named problem (a consensus) or agreement on how to manage the *divergence* (a mutually supporting dissension).
- Community groups hold responsibility for their own actions on their health problems, including the responsibility to manage these actions.
- Agency staff work to support community groups in their actions; that is, they are resources to actions on community group-defined health problems.
- Agencies cannot be all things to all groups and so must give priority to some groups over others. Priority should be given to those individuals and groups whose health is compromised by unfair living conditions.

There is no simple way of defining "unfair" conditions or of tracing their impacts on health and disease. Figure 29.1 nevertheless attempts to summarize the major interconnections between what are now called the "determinants of health."

People in lower socioeconomic status groups (usually measured by income level, educational attainment, or occupational status) are more likely to experience disease and premature death; to work in dangerous, stressful jobs; and to live in polluted neighborhoods (Gustavesen, 1988; Harding, 1987; Marmot & McDowall, 1986; Wilkins & Adams, 1983; Wilkinson, 1986; World Health Organization, 1984). They are more likely to experience less social support and report fewer social networks (Auslander, 1988; Berkman, 1986), to have low self-esteem, be unhappy, and experience anxieties, depression, self-blame, and low perceived power (Harding, 1987; Lerner, 1986). These psychosocial risk factors increase physiological risk factors associated with increased disease risk, that is, high blood pressure and

Table 29.1 Leading Health Problems by Three Approaches

Medical approach	Behavioral approach	Socioenvironmental approach
Cardiovascular disease	Smoking	Poverty
Cancer	Poor eating habits	Unemployment
AIDS	Lack of fitness	Powerlessness
Diabetes	Drug abuse	Isolation
Obesity	Alcohol abuse	Pollution
Mental disease	Poor stress coping	Stressors
Hypertension	Lack of lifeskills	Hazardous living and Working conditions

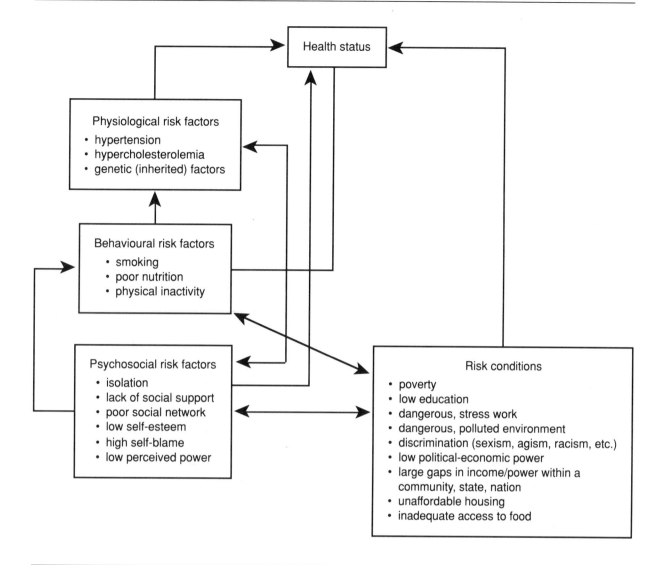

Figure 29.1 The socioenvironmental approach to health.

cholesterol levels and release of stress hormones (Berkman, 1986; Brindley, 1981; House, Landis, & Umberson, 1988).

People experiencing psychosocial risk factors and socioenvironmental risk conditions are more likely to engage in health-damaging behaviors. This reflects, in part, a "stress-buffering, stress coping" strategy in the relative absence of social support or social networks (Hibbard, 1988). Because they experience less social support and greater isolation, these people are also less likely to be active in community groups concerned with improving living, working, economic, political, or environmental conditions (Auslander, 1988; Minkler, 1985). This reinforces isolation and self-blame.

This web of health determinants creates and reinforces a pervasive sense of relative powerlessness, a feeling of not being able to control one's life or living conditions. This lack of control, both real and perceived, is one of the fundamental dynamics underlying poverty–

disease correlations (Haan, Kaplan, & Kamacho-Dickey, 1984; Syme, 1986).

In any hierarchical social structure, persons at the bottom of the hierarchy suffer more disease and death. The size of the gap between top and bottom may be the most important underpinning health determinant (Wilkinson, 1986). Among Organization for Economic Cooperation and Development nations, those countries having the greatest after-tax income equality also have the lowest infant mortality rates and longest life expectancies, independent of the absolute level of income in the country (Wilkinson, 1986). The reasons for this are not clear, but they probably relate to psychological feelings of fairness, control, shared purpose, and collective self-esteem (Ornstein & Sobel, 1987; Sullivan, 1991).

How much wealth a nation creates is only part of a fundamental health question. A nation needs sufficient national income to prevent physiologically compromising poverty. But once that is achieved (which is arguably the case in wealthy countries such as Canada), a more basic health concern is how equitably that wealth and the decision-making power it provides is shared within the nation.

An empowering health promotion or fitness practice, then, becomes one of enabling meaningful participation by professionals, agencies, and their communities of interest in intersectoral actions directed toward the larger issues of socioeconomic and political equity. Because injustice creates illness and disease does not render creating justice the singular task of health, fitness, and leisure professionals; it does require the active participation of those professionals in what might loosely be called social justice movements.

Empowering Goals

In our role as health or fitness promoters, we must deal explicitly with issues of power. *Power*, at its simplest, means the capacity to do or to act. People in our society do not have similar capacities, partly because of various inequalities in

- access to resources (money, goods),
- status (based on occupation, gender, ethnicity, age, ableness, sexual preference), and
- authority (the right to decide for others, in effect limiting others' capacities to act).

These external or "objective" inequalities often become internalized, experienced more as personal than as social problems.

Empowerment is the term used to describe processes through which these internal feelings of powerlessness are transformed and group actions initiated to change the physical and social living conditions that create or reinforce inequalities in power (Labonté, 1990; Rappaport, 1987). Empowerment is not something that occurs purely from within ("only I can empower myself"); nor is it something that can be done for others ("we need to empower this or that group to be healthier"). Rather, empowerment describes our intentional efforts to create more equitable relationships with one another, relationships in which there is greater equality in resources, status, and authority. This requires that those with more resources, status, and authority "give up" some of their power, so that others might "take" it.

A Continuum of Strategies

Attaining the goals listed in Table 29.2 requires a broad range of professional and organizational strategies. One model of these strategies is described in Figure 29.2, the Continuum of Empowering Strategies. This model implies that actions along the entire continuum should be planned and supported. These strategies represent an organizational responsibility; that is, no one staff person

necessarily possesses the skills (or time) to work at each of the five nodes. Rather, the Continuum of Empowering Strategies is the responsibility of the agency (or network of agencies) as a totality. Part of this responsibility is ensuring that the empowering actions of professionals within a given agency or interagency network are linked.

Personal Empowerment

- **Developmental case work**
- **Enhancing personal perceptions of control and power**

This node on the continuum is that of direct service. Poorer groups and communities often first organize around the need for services or for more democratic and useful forms of service delivery. The two pillars that allow services to be empowering are that they are offered in a supportive, noncontrolling way and that they are not the limit of the services and resources offered by the agency. People suffering physical or emotional distresses "have the right, here and now, to support in the face of difficulties" (Jackson, Mitchell, & Wright, 1988, p. 4). This support should be offered in ways that

- respect the autonomy of the individual,
- are culturally sensitive,
- seek to understand the psychosocial and socio-environmental contexts of the problems, and
- move constantly toward a greater capacity by the individual to act upon both the symptoms and the roots of his or her distresses.

At the same time, if health or social service agencies limit their services to individual care or to crisis management, they may facilitate personal empowerment but still reinforce a structural powerlessness.

Recreational services often function as clearinghouses for other community services. Professionals in

Table 29.2 Empowerment Goals

Improvements in:

- personal sense of power
- group identity
- ability to reflect critically and to solve problems
- power equity in social relationships
- self-discipline and ability to work with others

For less powerful groups, increases in:

- access to resources
- collective bargaining power
- political legitimation of demands

Data from Kindervattner, cited in Quinney, Wall, & Gauvin (1992).

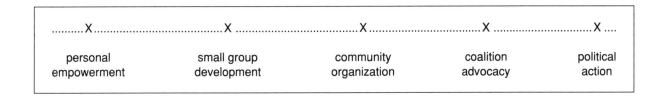

| personal empowerment | small group development | community organization | coalition advocacy | political action |

Figure 29.2 The Continuum of empowering strategies.

these centers may come to know reasonably well the concerns, issues, and interests of those residents who use the facilities. Fitness and leisure professionals are well placed to ask more difficult questions about the socioenvironmental health of their facilities' users and of the localities in which they exist. Although it may be rare for such facilities to offer personal counseling and case-work services, it would be regrettable if they failed to market such services or invite other agencies to consider creative ways of reaching and supporting the hard to reach through the venue and the metaphor of "re-creation."

Small Group Development

- **Improving social support**
- **Promoting personal behavior change**
- **Providing support for lifestyle choices**

Personal empowerment requires opportunities for individuals to overcome their isolation and the "learned helplessness" it can create (Seligman, 1975). This is usually accomplished through group work, when individuals together begin to normalize their experiences of distress, disease, or powerlessness by discovering that they are not alone in their problems and that, therefore, their problems are not uniquely about themselves. Despite their healthful potential, small groups, like personal services, are still insufficient empowering strategies. Current government promotion of self-help groups may mask more political solutions to longstanding health inequalities. Self-help groups often choose specifically to remain separate from more political forms of group action or organizing, yet such forms of action and organizing are required if socioenvironmental risk conditions are to be significantly improved.

One facet of a fitness-specific small group was described earlier: the basement home-visit 60-minute workout. Myriad leisure activities could similarly be offered in people's homes, creating multiple intersecting potentials:

- shaping the leisure or fitness activities themselves;
- creating supportive small groups, which may begin to identify personal and socioenvironmental health concerns (at which point the fitness or leisure animator appraises her or his ability to match the demands

of the group and seeks other help as needed; "empowerment," recall, is an organizational practice, not a lone ranger mission);
- overcoming isolation and improving the organizational capacity of participants; and
- laying the groundwork for people who choose to begin working politically on more broadly defined socioenvironmental health issues.

Community Organization

- **Developing local actions on community-defined health issues**
- **Critical community–professional dialogue**
- **Raising conflict to the conscious level**

Small-group development organizes people around issues or problems that are unique to group members. Community organization as a continuum node describes the process of organizing people around problems or issues that are larger than group members' own immediate concerns.

Community organization involves the decision by professionals and their agencies of which communities to work with. There is growing acceptance within the health sector of an "advocacy" framework of action. This framework recognizes that priority communities for organizing support are those whose income, educational, occupational, and general social class positioning places them low in the hierarchy of political and economic power (Watt & Rodmell, 1988).

There are a wide range of community organizing techniques. I will not review these techniques but will identify two important aspects of community organizing as an empowering strategy.

First, community organizing often involves conflict. Relatively powerless communities usually seek to correct power imbalances by limiting the power of other "communities" (politicians, business interests, bureaucracies) over them. Many powerless groups create their identity as a community only in opposition to those groups that are more powerful than themselves (Roberts, 1979; Ward, 1987). Conflict, in these instances, is a basic ingredient of participatory democracy. Provided that conflict is a prelude to meaningful negotiations around power issues between groups, it is a sign of social health, not of social sickness.

Second, although *community* has many different meanings, most of them include the notion of local groups working on local problems.

This notion of community, with its fully decentralized decision making, may allow for programs unique to community groups and their perceived needs. But it can also deny the reality that most economic and social policy is national and transnational in nature. Local decision making exists only within narrow limits and is unlikely to include substantial control over economic resources. As Alan Durning of the Worldwatch Institute (1989, p. 168) recently commented, "Small may be beautiful, but it may also be insignificant." Thus, community organizing, like personal services and small groups, is a necessary but insufficient empowering strategy.

How might fitness and leisure professionals engage in community organizing? The Parks and Recreation Department of the City of Toronto has struggled with this question for many years. It hires several community workers who talk with other agencies and with locality groups. Out of these conversations, new ways to develop and provide traditional recreational programs are created. More importantly, projects that seem to have little to do with traditional fitness and recreational activities are supported through financial grants and human resources. One parks and recreation program, cosponsored by several local community agencies, hired a community outreach worker to spend time with unemployed youth in a low-income neighborhood. Several youth developed and participated in employment creation projects, in which they were paid to attend leadership training courses and to work in such local social services as day cares, community centers, and recreation facilities, where they organized program activities for other youths.

A recreation program in Vancouver hired a community worker to organize neighborhood meetings to talk about health and safety concerns. These meetings stimulated the other agencies in the neighborhood—churches, schools, service clubs—to create new activities that residents identified as important and committed themselves to implementing. These activities give residents a better sense of their own ability to control their lives (important to their well-being), as well as opportunities to socialize and recreate.

Coalition Advocacy

- **Lobbying for healthier public policies**
- **Achieving strategic consensus**
- **Collaboration and conflict resolution**

Local actions are conditioned and constrained by larger structures of power. Coalition advocacy is a necessary tonic to the limitations of community organizing. Advocacy means taking a position on an issue, initiating actions in a deliberate attempt to influence private and public policy choices. Advocacy actions usually are directed at more senior government or private sector levels. It is described as "coalition advocacy" because often the lobbying is done by a number of groups who temporarily come together to advocate a particular policy change or reform.

Health, fitness, and leisure professionals and their agencies can support coalition advocacy in at least three ways.

First, and in keeping with the community development notion of being a resource to a process, professionals and their agencies can aid community groups in their own advocacy by offering knowledge, analytical skills, information on how the political and bureaucratic structures function, and so on. Their support for advocacy is an extension of their support for community organizing.

Second, agencies can support the advocacy efforts of these external groups by legitimizing their health concerns. This doesn't mean the agency takes the same position on the issue as the local advocacy group. But when the agency acknowledges in its policy statements that poverty and pollution are important health issues, it makes it easier for local groups to get on the agenda of public and private sector decision-making forums.

Third, health, fitness, and leisure professionals can increase the strength of their own political voices. Through local or provincial associations, professionals can take positions on such broad "healthy public policy" issues as social welfare reform, housing needs or affordability, employment policies, environmental standards, or any other concerns that may be expressed by their clients. (Healthy public policy is one of the conceptual axioms of the new health promotion. It means that the health of the public is directly affected by policies in nonhealth sectors; therefore health professionals should begin to hold these sectors accountable for the health effects of their policy decisions.) An organized political voice of caring professionals may be crucial in moving us toward more just and sustainable forms of social organization.

Coalition advocacy may represent the easiest starting point for fitness and leisure professionals to join with their public health colleagues in the hugely defined empowerment process. Many public health agencies are now turning greater attention toward the determinants of health (Figure 29.1); to the extent that their voices are joined and enriched by other professional groups, their work in advocating for healthier public policies will be easier and more successful.

Political Action

- **Support for broad-based social movements**
- **Creating a vision of a sustainable, preferred future**
- **Enhancing participatory democracy**

Political action represents an intensification of actions initiated under the rubric of coalition advocacy. The line between coalition advocacy and political action is somewhat blurry. One important difference, however, lies in the role played by social movements and in the creation of new forms of intersectoral policy planning.

There is no single definition of a social movement, but many such movements exist, including the women's movement, the environmental movement, the labor movement, the peace movement, various ethnocultural rights and antiracist movements, the gay and lesbian rights movement, and the antipsychiatry (mental patients' rights) movement. A social movement differs from a coalition of individual groups. A coalition forms around a particular issue that cuts across and unifies the differing values of member groups. A social movement, while comprising different groups, holds to certain key values and brings these values to many different issues. Social movements challenge the conventional ways in which society is viewed by its members, particularly by its more powerful members (Laclau, 1990; Melucci, 1989). Although social movements usually lack direct political or economic decision-making power, they are often influential in shaping opinions and attitudes.

Political action as a continuum node requires that health, fitness, and leisure professionals and their agencies seek to learn more from the different values and viewpoints advocated by social movements.

Conclusion: Can We Create a "Fitter" Society?

The continuum description derives from a public health and social welfare practice. Can it fit a fitness practice? I believe so. The continuum essentially asks us to continue asking hard questions about the totality of the experience of human health, not so much to embalm it or to systematically plan for some "total health generation" by the year 2018 but rather to prod: What kind of society do we think we deserve? What contribution toward creation of that society can we make in our daily lives, our daily works? How can our organizations embody more the qualities of fitness, community, and caring that we cherish in our holistic visions of wellness?

What vision of a healthy community, a healthy country, do we hold? What actions can we, and our organizations, take to advance that vision a little closer to being real? The answers to these questions do not lie simply in more training, skills development, or scientific research. The answers also involve values and faith.

Faith, in the words of philosopher, literary critic, and theologian Northrop Frye, "starts with a vision of reality that is something other than history or logic, which accepts the world as it is, and on the basis of that vision it can begin to remake the world" (1991, p. 19).

References

Auslander, G. (1988). Social networks and the functional health status of the poor: A secondary analysis of data from the National Survey of Personal Health Practices and Consequences. *Journal of Community Health*, **13**, 4.

Berkman, L. (1986). Social networks, support, and health: Taking the next step forward. *American Journal of Epidemiology*, **123**, 559-561.

Blaxter, M. (1990). *Health and lifestyles*. New York: Routledge.

Brindley, D.N. (1981). Regulations of hepatic triacyglycerol synthesis and liprotein metabolism by glucocorticoids. *Clinical Science*, **61** 129-133.

Durning, A. (1989). Mobilizing at the grassroots. In L. Brown, C. Flavin, L. Heise, et al. (Eds.) *State of the world 1989*. New York: Norton.

City of Toronto. (1991). *Health inequalities in the City of Toronto*. Toronto: Department of Public Health.

Frye, N. (1991). *The double vision*. Toronto: University of Toronto Press.

Gustavesen, B. (1988). Democratizing occupational health: The Scandinavian experience. *International Journal of Health Services*, **18**(4), 675-689.

Haan, M., Kaplan, G., & Kamacho-Dickey, P. (1984). *Poverty and health: A prospective study of Alameda County residents*. Paper presented at the annual meeting of the Society for Epidemiologic Research, Houston, TX.

Harding, M. (1987). *The relationship between economic status and health status: A synthesis*. A background report prepared for the Ontario Social Assistance Review Committee, Toronto.

Hibbard, J.H. (1988). Age, social ties, and health behaviours: An exploratory study. *Health Education Review*, **3**, 131-139.

Hill, M. (1990). On creating a theory of feminist therapy. In L.S. Brown & M.P. Root (Eds.), *Diversity and complexity in feminist psychotherapy* (pp. 53-65). New York: Haworth.

House, J.S., Landis, K.R., & Umberson, D. (1988). Social relationships and health. *Science*, **241**, 540-545.

Jackson, T., Mitchell, S., & Wright, M. (1988). *The community development continuum*. Melbourne: Community Development in Health.

Killian, A. (1988). Conscientization: An empowering, nonformal educational approach. *Community Development Journal*, **23**(2), 118.

Labonté, R. (1989). Community health promotion strategies. In C.J. Martin & D.V. McQueen (Eds.), *Readings for a new public health* (pp. 235-249). Edinburgh: Edinburgh University Press.

Labonté, R. (1990). Empowerment: Notes on community and professional dimensions. *Canadian Research on Social Policy*, **26**, 64-75.

Lalonde, M. (1974). *A new perspective on the health of Canadians*. Ottawa: Health and Welfare Canada.

Lerner, M. (1986). *Surplus powerlessness*. Oakland, CA: Institute for Labour and Mental Health.

Marmot, M.G., & McDowall, M.E. (1986, August). Mortality and widening social inequities. *Lancet*, **2**, 393-415.

McIntyre, S. (1986). The patterning of health by social position in contemporary Britain: Directions for sociological research. *Social Science and Medicine*, **23**(4), 393-415.

Melucci, A. (1989). *Nomads of the present*. Auckland, New Zealand: Radius Books.

Millar, W., & Wigle, D. (1986). Socioeconomic disparities in risk factors for cardiovascular disease. *Canadian Medical Association Journal*, **134**, 127-132.

Minkler, M. (1985). Social support and the elderly. In S. Cohen & S.L. Syme (Eds.), *Social support and health*. Toronto: Academic Press.

Ornstein, R., & Sobel, D. (1987). *The healing brain*. Toronto: Simon & Schuster.

Premier's Council on Health Strategy. (1991). *Nurturing health: A framework on the determinants of health*. Toronto: Author.

Quinney, H.A., Wall, A.E., & Gauvin, L. (1992). *Physical activity, fitness, and health: Policy and practice*. Unpublished manuscript.

Rappaport, J. (1987). Terms of empowerment/examplars of prevention: Toward a theory for community psychology. *American Journal of Community Psychology*, **15**(2), 121-148.

Registered Nurses Association of British Columbia. (1990). *Little Mountain Riley Park Health Project Report*. Vancouver: Author.

Roberts, H. (1979). *Community development: Learning and action*. Toronto: University of Toronto Press.

Seligman, M. (1975). *Helplessness: On depression, development, and death*. San Francisco: W.H. Freeman.

Sullivan, T. (1991). Strategic planning for health. *Health Promotion*, **30**(1), 2-8, 13.

Syme, L.S. (1986). *Strategies for health promotion*. Unpublished manuscript, University of California, Berkeley.

Ward, J. (1987). Community development with marginal people: The role of conflict. *Community Development Journal*, **22**(1), 18-21.

Watt, A., & Rodmell, S. (1988). Community involvement in health promotion: Progress or panacea? *Health Promotion*, **2**(4), 359-368.

Wilkins, R., & Adams, O. (1983). *Healthfulness of life*. Montreal: Institute for Research on Public Policy.

Wilkinson, R. (1986). Income and mortality. In R. Wilkinson (Ed.), *Class and health: Research and longitudinal data*. London: Tavistock.

World Health Organization. (1984). *The health burden of social inequities*. Copenhagen: WHO Regional Office for Europe.

World Health Organization. (1986). *Ottawa charter for health promotion*. Ottawa: Canadian Public Health Association.

30

The Meaning and Importance of Social Support

Benjamin H. Gottlieb

The primary purpose of this chapter is to elucidate the meaning of the concept of social support, approaches to its measurement, and its bearing on health behavior and health status. In addition, I describe some of the processes through which social support confers beneficial effects and outline interventions that involve the mobilization and augmentation of support. Although I review mainly mental health literature, I spotlight examples of the application of the concept of social support to the topics of physical activity, fitness, and active living.

Origins of the Concept of Social Support

The concept of social support was first introduced into the literature by social psychiatrist Gerald Caplan (1974) and by epidemiologist John Cassel (1974). Both were interested in the role that ordinary citizens played in helping one another cope with stressful life events, and both suggested that a promising approach to the prevention of mental disorder and the promotion of mental health could be based on strategies of structuring social ties in ways that strengthened their ability to meet people's psychosocial needs, particularly under stressful conditions.

As a practitioner, Caplan was particularly interested in the ways professionals could optimize the supportive functions and extend the reach of naturally occurring social networks. He exhorted professionals to learn from and further develop certain kinds of neighborhood-based, natural systems of service delivery, and he discussed the importance of developing mutual aid and support groups, linking neighbors with similar needs and complementary resources, and generally identifying ways of delivering human services that capitalized on informal helping resources. Based on his observations, Caplan (1974) concluded that natural support systems

offer three kinds of supportive provisions to their members:

(a) The significant others help the individual mobilize his psychological resources and master his emotional burdens; (b) they share his tasks; and (c) they provide him with extra supplies of money, material tools, skills, and cognitive guidance to improve his handling of his situation. (p. 20)

Although Caplan's formulations brought shape and meaning to our understanding of the forms of support that people give and receive, they left the mistaken impression with many readers that there were such entities as "support systems" in the community waiting to be mobilized when crises and stressful transitions called for their deployment. To this day, many human services professionals refer to client support systems in a kind of romantic way, implicitly ignoring the fact that even the closest of human relationships can have an adverse impact on mental health. It follows that the task for social programs is to optimize the expression of support and to increase the frequency and relevance of supportive exchanges between people, not to try to engineer relationships that are exclusively supportive in character.

Cassel's legacy has been to stimulate more basic research devoted to exploring the nature of social support and the strength and mechanisms of its effects on health. Two kinds of studies were instigated: a series of epidemiological investigations that related social support to morbidity and mortality, and studies examining the sources and types of support that are capable of moderating or cushioning the impact of a variety of stressful life events and transitions on health. Before reviewing the design and general findings of these two complementary lines of research, I will describe the ways in which social support has been conceived and gauged by the studies' investigators.

Concepts and Measures of Social Support

Several definitions of the social support construct have been offered since Caplan and Cassel wrote their groundbreaking papers, and they have been used to guide the development of empirical measures. Perhaps the most influential has been Cobb's (1976), which is strictly cognitive-perceptual in nature, emphasizing that social support is in the ''eye of the beholder'' and predicated upon the recipient's perceptions and interpretations of the communications of others. He writes that

> social support is conceived to be information belonging to one or more of the following three classes: 1. Information leading the subject to believe he is cared for and loved. 2. Information leading the subject to believe that he is esteemed and valued. 3. Information leading the subject to believe that he belongs to a network of communication and mutual obligation. (p. 301)

The definition offered by Heller, Swindle, and Dusenbury (1986) centers largely on the functions of support. It suggests that social support can be conveyed through social activities as much as through help-related interactions as long as they either enhance esteem or offer coping assistance.

> A social activity is said to involve social support if it is perceived by the recipient of that activity as esteem enhancing or if it involves the provision of stress-related personal aid (emotional support, cognitive restructuring, or instrumental aid). (p. 467)

Finally, in my own definition of social support I try to take into account both its functions and the process through which they are communicated: Social support refers to processes of interaction in relationships and social institutions that shore up coping, esteem, belonging, and competence through actual or predictable exchanges of tangible or psychosocial resources.

Several features of this definition bear explication. My emphasis on the notion of exchange calls attention to the reciprocal or mutual nature of interactions that involve social support; the participants both receive and extend support. Support is expressed not only through relationships, but also through social institutions. Schools, places of worship, hospitals, and community centers are settings for gaining support because they can serve a socially integrative function and because they can adopt policies, design roles for their staff, and create settings that shore up coping, esteem, belonging, and competence.

The benefits of support stem as much from the knowledge that one can rely on others as they do from the actual exchange of resources. The inclusion of predictable exchanges in my definition captures the psychological sense of support that sustains people during adversity or periods of chronic hardship. The definition spotlights the fact that social support is conveyed through relationships. It arises from the process of interaction and relationship development, and its meaning is typically colored by the character of the relationship between the two parties. Indeed, the protective effect of social support lies in this process, not in the variable itself.

Empirical measures of social support selectively incorporate various elements of these three definitions. Tardy (1985), Barrera (1986), and most recently, Heitzmann and Kaplan (1988) have reviewed the attributes and psychometric properties of the legion of measures that have appeared in the past 15 years. Tardy's (1985) review is particularly useful because he provides a comprehensive framework for making decisions about the features of support that researchers and program planners may wish to emphasize. I will briefly review each of these features before returning to my discussion of the effects of social support on health.

The first dimension for potential assessment refers to what Tardy (1985) calls the *direction* of support. Because it has been suggested that the benefits of support stem from the opportunity to render support to others, not just to receive it, the extent of symmetry in supportive exchanges can be tapped. If the maintenance of social ties is predicated on equitable social exchanges, then benefits may accrue from both the receipt and donation of aid.

Disposition is the second dimension Tardy (1985) enumerates. It spotlights the distinction between the support that is actually delivered or mobilized and the psychological sense of support. It is noteworthy that the most popular measures of support chiefly concentrate on the latter, namely perceptions of available support. They include Sarason, Levine, Basham, and Sarason's (1983) Social Support Questionnaire, Procidano and Heller's (1983) measure of perceived social support from family and friends, Cohen, Mermelstein, Karmarck, and Hoberman's (1985) Interpersonal Support Evaluation List, and Cutrona and Russell's (1987) Social Provisions Scale. The most widely used measure of enacted or received support is Barrera, Sandler, and Ramsay's (1981) Inventory of Socially Supportive Behaviors (ISSB) which gauges the actual exchange, utilization, or delivery of different types of support within a defined period of time.

Tardy (1985) labels the third dimension *description–evaluation*. He observes that in some inquiries respondents are requested to describe the support they have obtained or could receive, while in others they are asked to evaluate the quality or quantity of this support, thereby tapping support satisfaction. This distinction spotlights yet another aspect of the objective versus subjective issue, but here it pertains to the respondent's judgments about the adequacy of the support tendered to them.

The last two dimensions Tardy (1985) cites are *content* and *network*. Content refers to the different types of social support that have been identified by researchers and theorists, including

- socializing and companionship;
- cognitive guidance or advice;
- support that builds or reinforces self-esteem or valued social identities, sometimes called appraisal or esteem support;
- tangible support, including material goods, services, and money; and
- emotional support, consisting of love, affection, moral support, empathy, and attachment.

What is important to reiterate here is that different stressors arouse different needs for support, and that even at different stages of coping with a given stressor, the supportive requirements to be met will differ.

Just as people's supportive needs are matched with the type and stage of the stressor they face, so too is the match between the source and the type of support. Tardy's (1985) fifth dimension of support, namely the *network* dimension, addresses the information that is gained about the actors with whom individuals exchange support. Typically they include such categories of associates as friends, family members, co-workers, neighbors, and co-participants in leisure and voluntary activities. There are also certain structural properties of networks that may be important to gauge because there is evidence that they bear on people's adaptation to role transitions and their utilization of health and human services. For example, it has been shown that people who participate in dense or close-knit networks that are composed of demographically homogeneous associates can obtain rapid aid during times of crisis because of the speed of internal communication. At the same time, because of the uniform and solitary nature of these networks, they seem to constrain behavior and to block access to novel information about services in the larger community (Wilcox & Birkel, 1983).

A final dimension of support should be added to Tardy's (1985) list. It involves an assessment of the extent to which network members create conflict, stress, or tension in addition to providing support. This dimension forces recognition of the fact that people are not exclusively supportive, that negative interactions with others may cancel out their supportive functions, and that it may be possible to strengthen relationships by removing conflict or managing it better rather than by enhancing support.

Social Support and Health: Epidemiological and Life Event Studies

The epidemiological studies linking social support to health have examined mortality and morbidity among large samples over a relatively long time. They adopt the most macroscopic approach to the measurement of social support, gauging the quantity of social relationships and the frequency of interaction with others. For example, Berkman and Syme (1979) measured the extent of four types of social ties—marriage, contacts with extended family and friends, church membership, and other formal and informal group affiliations. From these data, they derived a "social network index" which, 8 years later, proved to be a significant predictor of mortality even after controlling for biomedical risk factors such as smoking, diet, exercise, and initial health status. The same approach was taken in several subsequent studies, with very similar findings; the greatest increase in mortality risk occurred among the most socially isolated proportion of the sample (see House, Landis, and Umberson [1988] for a review of these epidemiological studies). The implication of these findings is that health protection is afforded by social integration and that prospective health status is compromised by social isolation. Why and how this is so are not addressed by these studies.

Studies examining particular life events have been far more numerous than these epidemiological inquiries. They inquire whether people who receive or perceive that they have access to particular types of support from particular sources are at lower risk of developing negative outcomes, such as psychiatric symptomatology or poor health, compared to those experiencing the same adversity who lack such actual or perceived support. Examples include investigations of the mental health of women undergoing the transition to parenthood (Gottlieb & Pancer, 1988), the adjustment of various samples of bereaved people, the adaptation of new immigrants, the adjustment of adults and children in the wake of marital separation, and the stress resulting from job loss.

In some studies, attention is narrowed to a very small number of associates or even to a single network member whose support or lack of support is seen as critical to the well-being of the respondent. For example, Brown and Harris (1978) found that the presence of a confidant afforded protection against depression among working class women who were full-time mothers of preschool children and who were exposed to stress-provoking events. More generally, a confidant may be more capable of moderating feelings of emotional isolation than may more casual community contacts, who may be more important in moderating feelings of social isolation.

How Does Support Arise and Work?

There are abundant ideas but a paucity of empirical evidence about the mechanisms or processes whereby social support protects and promotes health, and about the individual and environmental determinants of social support. The former topic concerns the reasons why and the ways in which social support improves coping or fosters positive health behaviors by influencing human thought, emotion, and actions. For example, the epidemiological data linking social ties to decreased risk of mortality and morbidity have been explained in terms of the role that the social network plays in facilitating health promoting behaviors such as proper sleep, diet, and exercise, and placing pressure on people to abandon health injurious behaviors such as smoking and drug abuse.

People's associates may also indirectly influence health by functioning as an informal diagnostic and referral system (Gottlieb, 1982), detecting signs and symptoms of ill health or emotional disequilibrium, and speeding consultation with professional practitioners early on. For example, an individual may observe that his frequent squash partner is having difficulty catching his breath and that he requires longer breaks between games. His partner may also disclose the fact that he occasionally experiences chest pain in the locker room after a match. If, rather than ignoring or minimizing the symptoms, the observer suggests that his partner seek medical consultation, his referral may be of significant value in preventing more serious injury or disease.

A different set of more psychological hypotheses about social support's mechanisms of action have been proposed by those studying self-help and support groups. In this context, it has been suggested that the support of peers in similar stressful circumstances or life contexts can reduce the uncertainty people experience in novel circumstances, add to their sense of control and personal efficacy, instill a sense of hope—partly through exposure to veteran sufferers who have adjusted well to the same affliction or personal problem, offer new ideas about coping strategies, and normalize feelings. Peer support can also validate and affirm new roles and identities following life transitions (Gottlieb, 1988). Other hypotheses about the supportive processes that promote coping and foster adjustment among self-help group members include their active participation in the role of helper, the ability of the group to help its members make meaning of their adversity, and the tendency for group members to form ongoing relationships with one another, thereby recruiting new, supportive figures into their natural networks. Over time, the boundary between the self-help group and the personal network of the participants becomes more fluid.

This last point concerning the blending of support group members with the membership of the natural network is only one example of a more general process that applies to the formation of personal relationships. The social fabric is woven in part of cross-cutting strands of relationships developed on the basis of activities pursued with others in multiple settings. They arise from certain organizational and institutional affiliations, such as those based on work, religion, and schooling, and from leisure activities such as volunteering, camping, and the pursuit of sports and exercise. Repeated and pleasurable contact with co-participants in these activity settings, combined with their shared interest in the activity, create hospitable conditions for the formation of personal relationships. Naturally, individual differences and the strength of the motive to affiliate will determine whether and which particular relationships are initiated, but situational factors are otherwise quite favorable for social ties to be formed.

This phenomenon is abundantly illustrated in the sport and physical fitness realms. Fitness centers and aerobics classes have proved to be excellent places to make new friends, especially when the social mix of co-participants stays constant over a prolonged period of time. Golf and racquet clubs, especially those attached to a housing complex, promote abundant socializing both on and off the course and court. Fitness trails and bicycle paths offer much the same kinds of opportunities for repeated casual social contact. Moreover, outdoor forms of exercise and court sports appear to be immune from the industry that is eliminating the potential for developing new relationships by marketing equipment for home exercise.

Even if relationships are not spawned in settings where exercise takes place in large or small group contexts, and even if there is no verbal interaction between the parties, the sheer presence of co-participants makes them agents of certain indirect forms of social influence. Their behavior and appearance, as well as their interactions with others on the scene, can have powerful effects on self-evaluation, motivation, and exertion. Such effects are mediated by the social comparison process wherein individuals compare their own performance, accomplishments, and well-being to those of co-participants. Upward comparisons are those made with persons who are perceived to be superior along certain dimensions, and downward comparisons are those made with persons who are perceived to be inferior. The social comparison process is most likely to arise when the parties identify with one another on the basis of common cultural backgrounds and life situations. In short, when people share similar hopes, anxieties, disappointments, and doubts, they are more likely to become important sources of feedback for one another with respect to their emotions and behaviors.

For example, the decision to begin an exercise program, the ability to stick with it, and the progression to a higher, more demanding regimen of exercise are all subject to the social comparison process, not just to the direct support of others. Indeed, once it is recognized that there are distinct stages involved in initiating and maintaining an exercise program, then it is necessary to consider the kinds and sources of support that people may need at different stages, as well as the different kinds of social influences that may operate through the social comparison process. Those planning group exercise programs must therefore compose the group carefully. It must be done in a way that optimizes the likelihood that members will see one another as similar peers, and on this basis can make both upward comparisons with individuals who model greater proficiency, and downward comparisons with individuals who face greater obstacles to exercise or who are less fit.

In sum, in both the physical activity and mental health sciences, the challenge facing those planning programs that mobilize support is to create new settings or capitalize on existing opportunities for the expression of relevant types of support among similar peers. These expressions may be communicated through direct interaction and dialogue and through the more covert social comparison process. They may occur in a diversity of activity settings and in social contexts ranging from the dyad to the large group.

Mobilizing Social Support

The preceding discussion suggests that social support can be marshaled in many ways, from many sources, and in many settings. With respect to the source, there are two important considerations, one concerning whether an individual or a group is mobilized, and the other concerning whether this individual or group is already part of the natural network or is introduced from the outside. This two by two matrix can be illustrated in the context of an exercise program for men who have recently suffered a myocardial infarction.

The program can be introduced in the hospital as a routine aspect of medical care, taking the form of a cardiac group composed of other men who have suffered a heart attack. An alternative is to assign a personal exercise coach to each patient or to set up a buddy system composed of pairs of patients who are matched according to the gradient of stress they can tolerate. Both program designs call for the introduction of new associates from outside the patients' natural social networks, typically associates who are in some sense fellow sufferers and who require support to achieve a common goal.

Another alternative is to enlist one or more people in the patient's social circle, providing them with the guidance they need to intensify and specialize their support for the exercise regimen. For example, if the wife is cast in the role of exercise coach, she may need instruction about how to manage the regimen in a way that is neither overprotective nor too demanding. Moreover, she and other family members may be called upon to modify certain household routines that otherwise may have prevented adherence to the regimen of exercise. For example, to allow Dad to take a walk before dinner, it may be necessary to postpone the family's evening meal and move forward the children's extracurricular activities. After dinner, Dad can take responsibility for the dishes while Mom takes her evening stroll.

Yet a fourth strategy of marshaling support involves the creation of a cardiac exercise group in the workplace, composed of co-workers who may exercise regularly at a given time and place at work, and who may even compete with one another or with employees at another company to attain personally optimal levels of cardiovascular fitness. In fact, it has been suggested that men are particularly responsive to competitive schemes of this sort (Hackett, 1978).

Elsewhere, I have described a range of initiatives in the mental health field that are aimed to optimize support either by supplementing the focal individual's network with one or a set of new peer ties or by capitalizing on existing relationships (Gottlieb, 1988). Although it is not clear when circumstances warrant one approach rather than another, several factors should be considered. When new ties are grafted from the outside they are typically people in the same situation as the focal individual and therefore are relevant sources of empathy and targets of social comparison. Yet these interventions demand the extra work entailed in determining the strongest basis for pairing strangers or for composing the group so that the supportive process is optimized. The advantages of enlisting natural ties as sources of support are that these relationships are already important to the focal individual and probably have an influential role either in maintaining undesirable behaviors or in reinforcing desirable ones. However, program planners have expressed reservations about manipulating the social fabric in which people are embedded, and they have often found that their interventions are resisted because they uproot established patterns of interaction.

Conclusion

The examples cited in this chapter indicate some of the ways in which the direct expression of support and the beneficial effects conferred by the social comparison process can facilitate positive health behaviors, including various forms of physical activity. The chapter also underscores a larger theme, namely that social relationships provide the crucible for integrating physical activity into the patterns of everyday life. This idea takes on extra importance in light of Fitness Canada's definition of the concept of active living as "a way of life in which physical activity is valued and integrated into daily life" (Fitness Canada, 1991, p. 4). By selectively drawing on people's existing social ties, and by creating occasions for people to form new social ties, those planning physical activity programs can boost motivation, exertion, self-evaluation, fitness, and health.

There is much room for creativity in developing these occasions because physical activity can occur wherever people interact, including in the schools, the workplace, and the many public settings of a community. But it is not just a matter of creating settings for physical activity but of shaping programs in ways that encourage particular forms of dialogue, experience swapping, modeling, and mutual aid. It is a matter of prompting physical activity through capitalizing on the human motive to affiliate, to share, and to care about and be cared about by others. People should be drawn to physical exercise as much by the magnetic power of the social field they find there as by the attraction and rewards of the physical activity. When seen in this light, physical activity is not only a form of social recreation but also a recreation of the social dimension of life.

References

Barrera, M., Jr. (1986). Distinctions between social support concepts, measures, and models. *American Journal of Community Psychology*, **14**, 413-446.

Barrera, M., Jr., Sandler, I., & Ramsay, T. (1981). Preliminary development of a scale of social support: Studies of college students. *American Journal of Community Psychology*, **9**, 435-447.

Berkman, L.F., & Syme, S.L. (1979). Social networks, host resistance, and mortality: A 9-year follow-up study of Alameda County residents. *American Journal of Epidemiology*, **109**, 186-204.

Brown, G.W., & Harris, T. (1978). *Social origins of depression*. New York: The Free Press.

Caplan, G. (1974). Support systems. In G. Caplan (Ed.), *Support systems and community mental health*. New York: Basic Books.

Cassel, J. (1974). Psychosocial processes and stress: Theoretical formulations. *International Journal of Health Services*, **4**, 471-482.

Cobb, S. (1976). Social support as a moderator of life stress. *Psychosomatic Medicine*, **38**, 300-314.

Cohen, S., Mermelstein, R., Kamarck, T., & Hoberman, H.M. (1985). Measuring the functional components of social support. In I.G. Sarason & B.R. Sarason (Eds.), *Social support: Theory, research, and applications* (pp. 73-95). Dordrecht, The Netherlands: Martinus Nijhoff.

Cutrona, C.E., & Russell, D. (1987). The provisions of social relationships and adaptation to stress. In W.H. Jones & D. Perlman (Eds.), *Advances in personal relationships* (Vol 1). Greenwich, CT: JAI Press.

Fitness Canada. (1991). *Active living: A conceptual overview*. Ottawa: Government of Canada.

Gottlieb, B.H. (1982). Social support in the workplace. In D.E. Biegel & A.J. Naparstek (Eds.), *Community support systems and mental health* (pp. 37-53). New York: Springer.

Gottlieb, B.H. (1988). Support interventions: A typology and agenda for research. In S. Duck (Ed.), *Handbook of personal relationships: Theory, research, and interventions* (pp. 519-542). Chichester, England: John Wiley & Sons.

Gottlieb, B.H., & Pancer, S.M. (1988). Social networks and the transition to parenthood. In G.Y. Michaels & W.A. Goldberg (Eds.), *The transition to parenthood: Current theory and research*. New Rochelle, NY: Cambridge University Press.

Hackett, T.P. (1978). The use of groups in the rehabilitation of the postcoronary patient. *Advances in Cardiology*, **24**, 127-135.

Heitzmann, C.A., & Kaplan, R.M. (1988). Assessment of methods for measuring social support. *Health Psychology*, **7**, 75-109.

Heller, K.A., Swindle, R.W., Jr., & Dusenbury, L. (1986). Component social support processes: Comments and integration. *Journal of Consulting and Clinical Psychology*, **54**, 466-470.

House, J.S., Landis, K.R., & Umberson, D. (1988). Social relationships and health. *Science*, **241**, 540-545.

Procidano, M.E., & Heller, K. (1983). Measures of perceived social support from friends and from family: Three validation studies. *American Journal of Community Psychology*, **11**, 1-24.

Sarason, I.G., Levine, H.M., Basham, R.B., & Sarason, B.R. (1983). Assessing social support: The Social Support Questionnaire. *Journal of Personality and Social Psychology*, **44**, 127-139.

Tardy, C.H. (1985). Social support measurement. *American Journal of Community Psychology*, **13**, 187-202.

Wilcox, B., & Birkel, R.C. (1983). Social networks and the help-seeking process: A structural perspective. In A. Nadler, J.D. Fisher, & B.M. DePaulo (Eds.), *New directions in helping*. (Vol 3, pp. 235-255). New York: Academic Press.

31

The Stay-At-Home Parents' Network: Social Support for Active Living

Tammy Horne

The purpose of this chapter is to describe the development of a social support network for mothers at home who are interested in physical activity and other wellness and leisure issues. The Stay-at-Home Parents' Network operates in two rural Alberta communities, Bonnyville and Rocky Mountain House. The project's purpose is to enable mothers at home to increase their participation in moderate physical activity (e.g., brisk walking, easy cycling, swimming, social dancing, low impact aerobics, active games with children). In the recent Campbell's Survey of the Well-Being of Canadians (Stephens & Craig, 1990), 53% of full-time homemakers were classified as inactive, according to their daily energy expenditure on various leisure activities. This prevalence of inactivity was high compared to managers and professionals (42%), blue collar workers (46%), students (20%), and retirees (44%). The only less active group was sales and clerical workers (54%). Alberta Health (1987), in comparing the activity of homemakers with other groups of women, reported similar results.

Recent federal statistics indicate that 42.7% of mothers with children under 3 and 34.9% of mothers with children ages 3 to 5 are at home full time (Statistics Canada, 1990). Moderate fitness gains by many inactive people can significantly reduce population-attributable risk for premature mortality, especially with respect to heart disease, in both women and men (Blair et al., 1989).

Coupled with homemakers' relatively low activity levels is a scarcity of fitness, wellness, and leisure programs targeted to the needs of parents at home with small children, especially in rural communities. Limited child care options make it difficult for parents to attend programs that are available.

In April 1991, a baseline survey of 630 mothers was conducted in four rural Alberta communities, including Bonnyville and Rocky Mountain House. Mothers were classified as active (activity twice or more per week) or inactive mothers (activity once per week or less). Compared to inactive mothers ($n = 157$), active mothers ($n = 473$) reported

- more social support from important others, particularly spouse or partner and other mothers;
- higher self-efficacy and less difficulty in overcoming barriers such as time constraints due to family commitments, lack of self-discipline, lack of babysitting, or cost;
- a more positive attitude toward participation and a belief that physical activity is fun; and
- a stronger intention to be active in the future (Horne, 1991).

These findings are consistent with previous research on differences between physical activity participants and nonparticipants (Brawley & Horne, 1989; Fitness and Amateur Sport, 1983; Sallis et al., 1989; Wankel, 1985, 1987, 1988; Wankel, Craig, & Stephens, 1990).

From these findings, it is evident that social support issues are important to at-home mothers' participation in physical activity. Both perceived support from important others and barriers related to support (e.g., family commitments, babysitting) differentiated active from inactive mothers.

The importance of social support is consistent with other physical activity research. Several reviews (Dishman, 1986; Martin & Dubbert, 1985; Wankel, 1987) have concluded that social support interventions are positively related to activity adherence in structured settings such as fitness classes. Also, recent population studies (Hovell et al., 1989; Sallis et al., 1989) have found that modeling (family and friends exercising), family and friend support, and neighborhood environment (safety, convenience, seeing others exercise) were all positively related to self-reported walking. Lack of company was a barrier to participation. Recent studies of the relationship between women's roles and physical activity participation (Verhoef & Love, in press; Verhoef, Love, & Rose, in press) have found that perceived lack of time predicted both presence and amount of activity. Mothers were less active than women without children, especially young mothers. Number of children was inversely related to both whether and how often women were active. Perceived social support predicted whether women were active, but not how often.

Social support can function in several ways to influence health behavior by enhancing

- access to information;
- feelings of positive self-identity, self-esteem, and control;
- positive social influences; and
- tangible resources (Cohen, 1988).

The Networks are structured to fulfill these functions.

Specific, physical activity-related objectives of the Networks were to increase

- positive attitudes and related beliefs about outcomes participation in moderate physical activity,
- confidence (self-efficacy) and related beliefs concerning barriers to participation,
- perceived social support for participation,
- future intention to participate, and
- self-reported weekly frequency of participation.

The focus on moderate physical activity is consistent with the concept of active living (Fitness Canada, 1988, 1991), as is the belief that physical activity is not just a healthy behavior in itself, but an integral part of a holistic approach to well-being. To this end, the Networks use physical activity as a catalyst to encourage discussion and organization around other wellness and leisure interests.

The achievement of the Networks' physical activity-related objectives will be evaluated by comparing results from annual telephone surveys conducted from 1991 to 1993. Results from the two test communities will be compared with those from two similar communities that do not have Networks. Even though Network membership will involve only a small proportion of people surveyed, the increased awareness of active living resulting from Network publicity and related promotions may encourage mothers to be active in other contexts such as in family outings or on their own. Network members will be contacted for qualitative telephone interviews about their experiences with their Network.

Philosophy of Network Development

It was very important that the Alberta Centre for Well-Being (ACFWB) and local service organizations be seen as resource agencies rather than as the Network organizers. Specific Network processes and activities are organized by the mothers.

The process undertaken to organize the two Networks is consistent with several tenets of community development (Cary, 1970; Labonte, 1989; Minkler, 1990). These include

- identifying and meeting local needs through grass roots participation and the use of local resources;
- starting where people are and working with, not for, them;
- respecting that local people, not outsiders, are the experts on their own issues; and
- making outside advice and assistance available when requested by local people.

Furthermore, public involvement is essential for local acceptance and sustainability of community health promotion programs (Canadian Public Health Association, 1988; Health and Welfare Canada, 1986; Lefebvre, Lasater, Carleton, & Peterson, 1987).

Principles from social marketing (Hastings & Haywood, 1991; Kotler & Roberto, 1989; Lefebvre & Flora, 1988; Novelli, 1990) are also evident in the process of Network organization. Analysis of consumer needs is central to program planning. Programs must be relevant to the target group for which they are intended, and consumer involvement is essential at all stages of programming.

Initiating Network Development

Test communities were selected on the basis of the willingness of parks and recreation departments to provide support to the Networks in their initial stages, and of public health units to provide a list of phone numbers of households containing children under age 6, for survey purposes. The first Network activity in each community was a public meeting in May 1991 for interested at-home parents. Parks and recreation departments, public health units, and regional Be Fit for Life centers assisted in planning the meetings. The role of those agencies was to provide space, refreshments, and child care; publicize the meetings through local media contacts, posters, and word-of-mouth; and discuss how they could serve as local resources to the Network.

Each meeting was held in the morning, so as not to compete with children's afternoon naps. Nine mothers attended in Bonnyville and 16 in Rocky Mountain House. The concept of the Network was introduced, then mothers discussed a format for sharing interests and schedules, what physical activities they could organize as group events for Network members, and how such activities might be implemented.

A form was developed to determine interests and schedules. This form contained space for

- favorite activities,
- fitness level,
- preferred days and times,
- child care and transportation needs,
- willingness to help other parents with child care and transportation, and
- other health-related topics of interest.

The mothers identified swimming and walking as initial favorites for summer. The Bonnyville mothers discussed a rotational babysitting system for swimming whereby some mothers would watch the children while the other mothers swam. Mothers responsible for babysitting would change weekly.

In both communities, the local parks and recreation departments agreed to sign up new participants by phone. Public health units agreed to publicize the Network through their well-baby and preschool programs, and the regional Be Fit for Life centers expressed interest in providing workshops upon request.

A volunteer committee of mothers was formed in each community to ensure that organization would occur at the local level. Four mothers formed each committee, with one acting as local coordinator. The coordinator position involved keeping the membership informed of upcoming events of both the Network and local agencies (e.g., public health, Family and Community Support Services). Membership lists were distributed every other month.

The local coordinator is also a liaison with the ACFWB. She reports all Network activities, problems, and plans. Such information is necessary both for research and for ensuring that resources are available to each community as needed. For instance, the ACFWB researcher could share the ideas from Rocky Mountain House with the coordinator of the Bonnyville Network, provide camera-ready posters for photocopying, or assist in contacting local newspapers with publicity information. Local coordinators receive honoraria as research assistants in return for providing information to the ACFWB researcher on the Networks' progress and activity attendance.

In terms of Cohen's (1988) social support functions, the public meeting involved mainly information sharing and socializing with similar others. The mothers also did some initial planning toward a process for sharing positive health behavior (physical activity) and providing resources to each other to overcome barriers to participation.

Public meetings were held in the spring in hopes that nice weather would encourage outdoor activities such as walking and cycling. However, it was difficult to plan Network events during summer because of vacations. Therefore, group events did not occur regularly until fall. Furthermore, members were reluctant to use the Network membership list to informally contact each other until they had a chance to meet in a group setting.

Attendance at specific group events has been low (usually 4-9 people per event). Events have included

- low impact aerobics at the home of one member who was a fitness instructor,
- moms' and tots' skating,
- park walks and picnics with kids,
- family swimming,
- children's play groups,
- bowling,
- tobogganing,
- pottery-making, and
- workshops on self-esteem, parenting, massage, clothing styles, skin care, and environment-friendly household products.

The Network in each community grew from 7 or 8 members in the early summer to 14 to 16 members by the end of fall (1991).

Another initial difficulty involved the volunteer committee. Mothers were unable to schedule group meetings, so much of the organizing fell to the local coordinators. The ACFWB researcher maintained frequent contact with the coordinators (about every 2 weeks) during the summer and early fall to discuss ideas and problems. The ACFWB also assisted the coordinators to organize three additional public meetings in each community to further discuss ways of getting more people involved. Since the beginning of 1992, Network members have begun to play a stronger role in working with the coordinators to organize events. For example, one mother might initiate an activity and another might handle any related publicity.

The major social support functions involved in Network participation are

- shared physical activity,
- information sharing on various wellness and leisure topics,
- setting up activities so that barriers to participation are minimized (e.g., doing activities with kids to minimize child care needs), and
- continued socializing with other at-home mothers.

Social Marketing Concerns

It is essential that all information and publicity concerning the Stay-at-Home Parents' Network fits with members' vision of it. Developing this fit involved several discussions among the ACFWB researcher, the local coordinators, and Network members. For example, the Network was originally called the Homemakers' Wellness Network. Bonnyville Network members pointed out that the word *homemaker* is often associated with caregivers such as the Red Cross. They felt that some mothers would think the Network was for those people, rather than for mothers at home with children.

Mothers also thought the word *wellness* was ambiguous, meant different things to different people, and could limit the scope of potential Network activities. The mothers suggested the name Stay-at-Home Parents' Network because it sounded supportive and was broad enough to include many different activities. The Rocky Mountain House group adopted the name for their Network.

Media publicity was another concern. The Networks were running free announcements in the community events section of the local weekly newspapers. This section is not highly visible and readers often missed announcements. The Bonnyville Parks and Recreation Department arranged for free Network announcements in a more prominent section, with town-sponsored activities. In Rocky Mountain House, free announcements for town activities were not available, so the ACFWB researcher paid for advertising for 2 weeks.

Another social marketing issue was the development of posters to publicize upcoming Network events. Initially, draft posters for upcoming activities were designed by the ACFWB. These posters were presented to the local coordinators, who sought feedback from Network members. The Bonnyville Network requested the addition of a cartoon and a slogan that could become identified with the Network. They submitted several examples, and poster mock-ups were created, from which the mothers then chose one. Rocky Mountain House adopted the same poster.

A related social marketing concern was poster wording. The mothers did not want to use the words "join the Network" because in their experience, joining programs usually meant work rather than recreation. The mothers preferred the words "meet other parents," and the posters were revised accordingly. Mothers also preferred "public meeting" to "public forum," as they thought that the latter term reminded people of politics. Mothers also wanted the poster to mention that Network events were not limited to physical activity but could include get-togethers to make crafts or discuss other topics of interest. They felt that mothers who engaged in less active events might participate in physical activity once they got to know the other mothers. Finally, mothers wanted the poster to state that children were welcome at events.

The concerns and preferences of rural at-home mothers needed to be addressed to maintain current members' interest and to attract new members. This participatory process ensured that materials were relevant to the target group, consistent with social marketing principles.

The Bonnyville Stay-at-Home Parents' Network started a newsletter describing upcoming group activities, interests of individual members, and events offered by service agencies (e.g., parenting and stress management workshops at Family and Community Support Services). The newsletter was produced every 4 to 8 weeks and mailed or hand delivered to all Network members. It was accompanied by the membership list. The Rocky Mountain House Network was sent copies of Bonnyville's newsletter and started its own.

The Bonnyville Network was also featured in the Bonnyville Nouvelle in January 1992. In this article, the local Network coordinator provided information on Network activities and plans.

Additional publicity for both Networks has been generated through an ACFWB study, funded by the Canadian Fitness and Lifestyle Research Institute, to evaluate a message promoting active living to at-home parents. The message is targeted to currently inactive mothers, as identified by the 1991 baseline survey, and includes information about the Network. Since completion of that study, the message has been generally available in Bonnyville and Rocky Mountain House through various service agencies.

Working Toward Local Autonomy

The Networks in both Rocky Mountain House and Bonnyville have been successful in getting activity space donated by community organizations. Rocky Mountain House has had weekly access to space at the Youth Centre in the Rocky Mountain House Arena since summer 1991, donated by the Rocky Mountain House Parks and Recreation Department. Space in Bonnyville was initially difficult to find. In late November 1991, the parks and recreation department donated the Farmer's Market space in the Bonnyville Arena. In February 1992, the Network obtained space in the Bonnyville Parent and Child Centre gym. This gym space is much sought-after, and the Network was able to secure it by collaborating with a child care service in the Play and Learn Centre, which had the space booked but seldom used it. The gym space is paid for by Family and Community Support Services (FCSS).

One indication of the shift toward local autonomy is the changing structure of public meetings. In the beginning, the ACFWB researcher facilitated meetings and directed much of the discussion, encouraging mothers to generate ideas for potential Network activities. Meetings are now run by the mothers themselves, with the local coordinators facilitating the discussions as needed. The researcher will attend future planning meetings only if invited by the mothers.

In addition, local coordinators have taken charge of signing up new members. Members used to register through the local parks and recreation departments, which gave their names to the coordinators. The coordinators in both communities thought it would be easier to handle new members themselves, since they already fielded inquiries about Network activities and were responsible for distributing the membership lists. They also liked the personal touch of being the first contact for potential new members.

In 1992, both Networks received a few hundred dollars from their local Family and Community Support Services office. This infusion of local funds will allow the Networks to hold special events such as workshops with guest speakers. These should increase the Networks' profiles and attract new members, resulting in a wider variety of activities in the future.

There is also a $5 annual membership fee for each Network. This low fee ensures that the Network is financially accessible to all. If memberships increase because of a higher profile and a wider range of activities, the Networks will eventually have more resources of their own (through membership fees) and will be less dependent on outside funding sources.

Both Networks have now developed planning committees. In Rocky Mountain House, specific tasks have been taken on by each committee member—advertising, bookkeeping, speaker recruitment, refreshments, and phoning members about events.

The Bonnyville Network's organizational structure is based on program areas rather than administrative duties. One mother is responsible for physical activities, another for wellness-related workshops and the newsletter, and a third for the children's play group.

The present role of the ACFWB researcher is mainly that of program evaluator. In addition to measuring progress with respect to the original objectives, the 1992 and 1993 evaluation surveys will assess ongoing needs. These findings will be shared with the local planning committees so they can ensure that new program offerings correspond to locally identified needs. Thus the survey information will provide a database for future local planning.

In summary, the Networks are run by mothers, for mothers, to ensure that programs are relevant to participants. The Networks incorporate the social support functions outlined by Cohen (1988). Furthermore, the presence of the Networks signal to mothers in those communities that there is social support for active living and other leisure and wellness interests. The knowledge that support is available may be as important as the actual exchange of resources (see Gottlieb, chapter 30). Gottlieb has also suggested that repeated and pleasurable contact with co-participants who share an interest in an activity creates favorable conditions for developing personal relationships, so that the boundaries between support groups and personal networks become more fluid. To the extent that this process increases contact among Network members, active living and other leisure and wellness interests should be facilitated.

Acknowledgment

This project is funded by the Recreation, Parks, and Wildlife Foundation of Alberta and by the University of Alberta Central Research Fund.

References

Alberta Health. (1987). *Promoting the health of Albertans*. Edmonton, AB: Province of Alberta.

Blair, S.N., Kohl, H.W., Paffenbarger, R.S., Clark, M.S., Cooper, K.H., & Gibbons, L.W. (1989). Physical fitness and all-cause mortality: A prospective study of healthy men and women. *Journal of the American Medical Association*, **262**, 2395-2401.

Brawley, L.R., & Horne, T. (1989). *Refining attitude–behavior models to predict adherence in normal and socially supportive conditions*. (Research Rep. No. 8706-4042-2099). Ottawa, ON: Canadian Fitness and Lifestyle Research Institute.

Canadian Public Health Association. (1988). *Strengthening community health means strengthening communities*. Ottawa, ON: Author.

Cary, L.J. (1970). *Community development as a process*. Columbia, MO: University of Missouri Press.

Cohen, S. (1988). Psychosocial models of the role of social support in the etiology of physical disease. *Health Psychology*, **7**, 269-297.

Dishman, R.K. (1986). Exercise compliance: A new view for public health. *Physician and Sports Medicine*, **14**, 127-145.

Fitness and Amateur Sport. (1983). *Canada Fitness Survey*. Ottawa: Government of Canada.

Fitness Canada. (1988). *A framework for active living and health*. Ottawa: Government of Canada.

Fitness Canada. (1991). *Active living: A conceptual overview*. Ottawa: Government of Canada.

Hastings, G., & Haywood, A. (1991). Social marketing and communication in health promotion. *Health Promotion International*, **6**, 135-145.

Health and Welfare Canada. (1986). *Achieving health for all: A framework for health promotion*. Ottawa: Government of Canada.

Horne, T. (1991). *The utility of the theory of planned behaviour in predicting moderate physical activity for a sample of rural Alberta homemakers*. Paper presented at the Canadian Association for Psychomotor Learning and Sport Psychology, London, ON.

Hovell, M.F., Sallis, J.F., Hofstetter, C.R., Spry, V.M., Faucher, P., & Casperson, C.J. (1989). Identifying correlates of walking for exercise: An epidemiologic prerequisite for physical activity promotion. *Preventive Medicine*, **18**, 856-866.

Kotler, P., & Roberto, E.M. (1989). *Social marketing: Strategies for changing public behavior*. New York: Free Press.

Labonte, R. (1989, March). Community and professional empowerment. *Canadian Nurse*, pp. 23-28.

Lefebvre, R.C., & Flora, J.A. (1988). Social marketing and public health intervention. *Health Education Quarterly*, **15**, 299-315.

Lefebvre, R.C., Lasater, T.M., Carleton, R.A., & Peterson, G. (1987). Theory and delivery of health programming in the community: The Pawtucket Heart Health Program. *Preventive Medicine*, **16**, 80-95.

Martin, J.E., & Dubbert, P.M. (1985). Adherence to exercise. *Exercise and Sport Sciences Reviews*, **13**, 137-167.

Minkler, M. (1990). Improving health through community organization. In K. Glanz, F.M. Lewis, & B.K. Rimer (Eds.), *Health behavior and health education: Theory, research, and practice* (pp. 257-287). San Francisco: Jossey-Bass.

Novelli, W.D. (1990). Applying social marketing to health promotion and disease prevention. In K. Glanz, F.M. Lewis, & B.K. Rimer (Eds.), *Health behavior and health education: Theory, research, and practice* (pp. 342-369). San Francisco: Jossey-Bass.

Sallis, J.F., Hovell, M.F., Hofstetter, C.R., Faucher, P., Elder, J.P., Blanchard, J., Casperson, C.J., Powell, K.E., & Christenson, G.M. (1989). A multivariate study of determinants of vigorous exercise in a community sample. *Preventive Medicine*, **18**, 20-34.

Statistics Canada. (1990). *Women in Canada*. Ottawa: Government of Canada.

Stephens, T., & Craig, C.L. (1990). *The well-being of Canadians: Highlights of the 1988 Campbell's Survey*. Ottawa: Canadian Fitness & Lifestyle Research Institute.

Verhoef, M.J., & Love, E.J. (in press). Women's exercise participation: The relevance of social roles compared to nonrole related determinants. *Canadian Journal of Public Health*.

Verhoef, M.J., Love, E.J., & Rose, M.S. (in press). Women's social roles and their exercise participation. *Women and Health*.

Wankel, L.M. (1985). Personal and situational factors affecting exercise involvement: The importance of enjoyment. *Research Quarterly for Exercise and Sport*, **56**, 275-282.

Wankel, L.M. (1987). Enhancing motivation for involvement in voluntary exercise programs. *Advances in Motivation and Achievement: Enhancing Motivation*, **5**, 239-286.

Wankel, L.M. (1988). Exercise adherence and leisure activity: Patterns of involvement and interventions to facilitate regular activity. In R.K. Dishman (Ed.), *Exercise adherence and public health* (pp. 369-396). Champaign, IL: Human Kinetics.

Wankel, L.M., Craig, C.L. & Stephens, T. (1990). *Social psychological factors associated with different patterns of physical activity involvement*. Paper presented at the World Congress on Sport for All, Tampere, Finland.

32

Coping in Physical Activity: The Role of Seeking Social Support

Peter R.E. Crocker

Regular involvement in physical activity can be an uplifting physical and emotional experience. Benefits may include enhanced cardiovascular functioning, improved strength, increased flexibility, weight control, skill development, stress control, new friendships, and improved psychological well-being (Bouchard, Shephard, Stephens, Sutton, & McPherson, 1990; Morgan & Goldston, 1987). Achievement of these benefits requires the management of personal and environmental challenges. Potential barriers to activity such as lack of skill and fitness, fatigue, and family and job conflicts compel the participant to develop mental and physical coping skills. These include not only physical and technical skills to perform the activity, but also effective communication, problem-solving, and emotional control. The successful use of coping skills will help the individual maximize the benefits from physical activity participation.

Researchers have suggested that social support is a coping resource that can increase involvement in physical activity. For example, individuals beginning exercise programs prefer to exercise with others (Heinzelmann & Bagley, 1970). Attendance is also higher for those who exercise in groups than for those who try to exercise alone (Massie & Shephard, 1971). Other studies have found that active spousal support significantly improves adherence to exercise (Andrew et al., 1981; Oldridge, 1982). Active manipulation of social support resources in the exercise environment increases frequency of exercise (King & Frederiksen, 1984), and improves exercise adherence (Martin et al., 1984; Wankel, Yardley, & Graham, 1985). Despite this evidence, the social support mechanisms underlying changes in exercise attendance and frequency are not well understood. Since all the aforementioned studies have defined and manipulated social support in different ways, it would be difficult for the practitioner to understand how to increase the benefits of social support in specific settings.

This chapter has several purposes. First, I integrate social support into the general framework of stress, appraisal, and coping. From this perspective, social support is an external coping resource that individuals can call upon to help manage threatening or challenging situations within physical activity settings. Second, I address the function of seeking social support, with illustrative examples of how participants may use social support for emotional or effectual reasons. Third, I review recent research focusing on how individuals with physical disabilities cope during physical activity. Last, I discuss implications for the practitioner.

Stress, Appraisal, and Coping

Deciding to engage in physical activity entails a complex process of cognitive evaluation of individual goals, perceived costs and benefits, and coping options and resources. Take the example of a woman choosing to attend an aerobic exercise class to lose weight and meet new people. This involvement, however, has financial, social, and physical costs such as program, babysitting, and transportation fees; reduced family contact; and exercise fatigue. She must evaluate whether she has the coping resources to manage these demands. Stress will occur if the perceived demands exceed the woman's perceived resources (Lazarus & Folkman, 1984).

How the participant copes with physical-activity-related demands changes stress (Crocker, Alderman, & Smith, 1988; Smith, 1980). Activity choice, adherence, and emotional experience depend somewhat on the type of coping strategies used in a particular situation. For a person who is uncertain how to perform a dance pattern, using a distress-reducing strategy such as behavioral withdrawal will produce far different results than using a problem-solving strategy such as asking a fellow exerciser for assistance (i.e., seeking social support).

Coping skills and resources involve not only action-oriented (behavioral) skills but also thought-related (cognitive) skills or the combination of both. Behavioral coping strategies include learning the activity movement skills, changing physical effort levels, and communicating physically and verbally. Cognitive strategies may include planning, denial, self-blame, and mental relaxation. Many coping efforts use both cognitive and behavioral skills. For example, solving a problem involves the cognitive skills of problem definition, generating possible solutions, and anticipating consequences. It also requires the individual to have behavioral skills to perform the selected solution. Effective coping will require efficacious use of both cognitive and behavioral skills.

Coping resources can also be envisioned as internal or external. Internal resources are skills within and directly under the control of the participant. These resources do not require the support of external agents or facilities. External resources, on the other hand, are not always available or controllable by the individual. These resources include relatives, friends, fellow participants, and exercise leaders. Other tangible external resources are equipment, facilities, and monetary sources.

Figure 32.1 is a simple flow diagram of a hypothetical exercise setting that illustrates how the appraisal and coping process works. The participant is a single parent who has decided to engage in an aerobic exercise class to control weight and make friends. However, she faces the challenge of finding a baby-sitter for her two young children for the duration of the exercise program. She evaluates her coping options and decides she can either get more information from others about baby-sitting services or not sign up for the class. She also evaluates her external and internal coping resources. She has no immediate family to assist her but she does have two close work friends with children. She can also seek information from the instructor and other participants. She believes she has the communication, planning, and problem-solving skills to ask others for this assistance. The result of this cognitive appraisal process is to ask one of her friends to baby-sit for the first few exercise classes and to seek information from the other participants.

There is a consensus among theorists that an important distinction exists between *problem-focused* and *emotion-focused coping* (Carver, Scheier, & Weintraub, 1989; Endler & Parker, 1989; Lazarus & Folkman, 1984). Problem-focused coping refers to cognitive and behavioral efforts to change a situation. These strategies include problem solving, planning, seeking information, learning new skills, and increasing efforts. In the example of the single parent, the strategy of seeking information from others changes the potential conflict between caring for her children and taking part in the exercise program.

Emotion-focused coping involves efforts to reduce emotional arousal and distress. Strategies include mental and behavioral withdrawal, seeking social support for emotional reasons, denial, and acceptance. These strategies are useful when the person is unable to change the situation. They may, however, become an obstacle to long-term benefits. For example, withdrawing from a class because of some conflict may provide short-term emotional relief. However, the withdrawal causes the frustration of important personal goals, such as losing weight and making new friends, resulting in long-term distress.

Social Support as Coping Assistance

Thoits (1986) argued that the benefits of social support can be better understood if reconceptualized as coping assistance. In this sense, social support is portrayed as an external coping resource that an individual can use to manage challenging or threatening situations. Social support can have both problem-focused and emotion-focused functions.

Applying social support as a problem-focused strategy would entail changing the physical activity setting or the individual to remove or alter the situation evaluated as threatening. Take the case of an individual having problems performing a movement pattern during exercise class. The instructor or a fellow participant may provide social support by helping the individual learn the movement pattern. This assistance helps the individual manage the exercise demands by actively changing and improving his or her ability. This type of assistance in physical activity is very powerful since perception of physical competence contributes to one's general sense of self-worth (Fox, 1988) and underlies intrinsic motivation (Deci & Ryan, 1985).

Emotion-focused coping assistance would consist of actions or thoughts to help the individual reduce or manage distressing feelings. Leaders or other participants may help the individual reinterpret the situation so it is perceived as less threatening. Using the previous example, another fellow exerciser may tell the individual that some movement patterns are complex and that difficulties are typical at first. Thoits (1986) stated that another's empathic understanding provides reassurance that these experiences are normal and may help to reduce self-criticism.

There is some utility in describing the functions of social support within a coping framework. Thoits (1986) stated,

In sum, significant others can suggest techniques of stress management or can participate directly in those efforts, thereby facilitating and strengthening a person's own coping attempts. These actions can

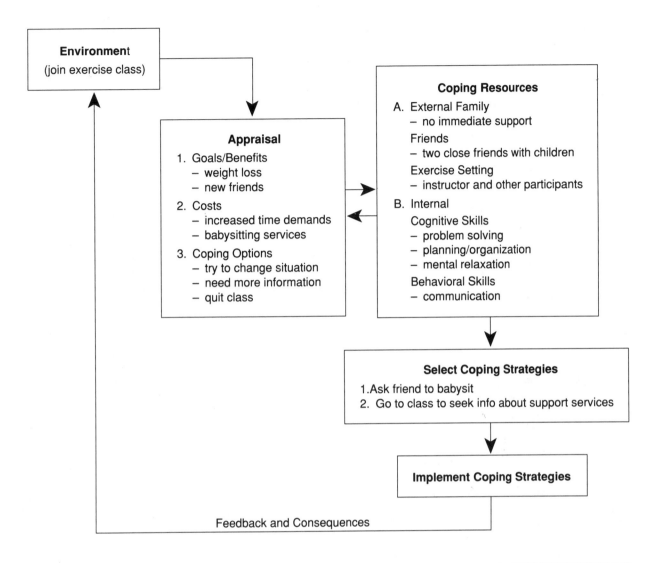

Figure 32.1 Simplified schematic flow chart of appraisal–coping process. The example involves a hypothetical case of a single parent joining an exercise class.

alter threatening aspects of the situation, threatening emotional reactions to the situation or both. (p. 419)

There are many actions that can be taken in physical activity settings to provide social support that serves both problem- and emotional-focused functions of coping. The practitioner may attempt to structure the physical activity situation to maximize these mechanisms of emotional and instrumental support. These two processes are consistent with the functions of social support noted in the definition offered by Gottlieb (chapter 30). However, as Gottlieb has noted, social support involves a transactional process in which the person operates in a dynamic situation entailing social structures (e.g., community exercise centers or sport club organizations) and social relationships (e.g., other participants, exercise leaders, coaches, and significant others). The practitioners can increase the availability of social support

resources by structuring the environment to increase social contact and place individuals with similar exercise, cultural, and life experiences together.

Seeking Social Support as an Active Coping Strategy

Organizing the physical activity setting to optimize the benefit of social support is an admirable goal for practitioners. The facilitative effects of social support, however, may not occur if the person does not actively seek or readily accept available social support resources. Generally, social support entails significant others' bolstering an individual's coping resources to manage stress and facilitate participation in physical activity. Often, this social support process acts as a passive coping skill. That is, the bolstering of coping resources occurs only if another person seeks out the individual and provides the required resources. In some cases, the well-meaning helper may give unwanted advice, producing more aversive effects than if there were no social support. A better situation would be the individual's seeking social support resources. In this case, the person has more control over the environment and is likely to seek the required assistance.

The seeking of social support represents only one of several potential active coping strategies to gain situational and emotional control in physical activity settings. Several interesting questions arise.

- How often do people seek social support compared to other coping strategies?
- What is the relationship of seeking social support to other types of coping strategies?
- How is seeking social support related to affective (emotional) experiences, expectation, and behavior?

Some of these questions were explored in recent research (Bouffard & Crocker, in press; Crocker & Bouffard, 1990, 1992) on how individuals with physical disabilities cope during physical activity. The findings related to the concept of seeking social support are highlighted.

Numerous strategies are available to manage threatening or challenging situations. The use of these strategies depends on the appraisal of environmental demands, the efficacy of individual resources, the availability of external resources, and coping options. The mere presence of social support resources does not mean an individual will choose to use these resources. Social support resources may be appraised as unsuitable or undesirable in a particularly stressful physical activity setting. Other strategies such as increasing effort and planning may be more appropriate to manage the situation.

Dr. Marcel Bouffard of the University of Alberta and I have been conducting research on how individuals involved in physical activity cope with potentially threatening or challenging situations (Bouffard & Crocker, in press; Crocker, 1991, in press; Crocker & Bouffard, 1990, 1991, 1992). This research has involved two distinct populations, individuals with physical disabilities and able-bodied competitive athletes. Only the research on the disabled will be discussed. The studies involving individuals with physical disabilities have sought to establish what coping strategies individuals use and whether individuals use the same coping strategies over time. Specific studies have also evaluated the relationship between coping and measures of affective experience, specific cognitive appraisal, and expectations for future behavior.

Our early research (Crocker & Bouffard, 1990) focused on the relationship between coping and the expectation of future participation in physical activity. We hypothesized that the use of problem-focused strategies would be positively related to expectations of future participation. Forty-nine people with spinal cord injuries and 21 amputees watched three videotaped scenarios representing frequent barriers to participation in physical activity. These barriers were being ignored by the able-bodied participants, being ignored by the instructor, and selection of an inappropriate activity. After each scenario, the subject completed a checklist containing numerous coping strategies and then indicated his or her expectation of future participation in the same physical activity.

The coping strategies were classified into several dimensions such as planful problem solving, distancing, self-controlling, escape or avoidance, reappraisal, and social support. The dimension of seeking social support (labeled *assertive communication* in the study) was captured by several items that reflected seeking information and ways of getting others to change the situation.

The findings indicated that seeking social support was reported more often than the other coping dimensions. Furthermore, it was significantly related to expectation of future participation in physical activity. In general, results indicated a positive relationship between using problem-focused strategies (assertive communication, planful problem solving), and expectation of future participation. On the other hand, if people believed they would use emotion-focused strategies more, they were less likely to say they would participate again. These findings make sense because if an individual does not attempt to change a barrier to physical activity, then future participation is unlikely. An effective way to change an activity situation is to seek social support for instrumental reasons from the person responsible.

The paradigm used in the previous study is limited in assessing how individuals cope with physical activities. First, subjects must use inferential processes that may reflect what they believe they would do rather than what they actually would do (Nisbett & Wilson, 1977). Second, subjects' response to the first situation in the video may produce a response set for the next two situations. Third, the social support scale did not differentiate between problem-focused and emotion-focused seeking of social support. To overcome these shortcomings, a longitudinal study was designed to examine appraisal, coping, and affective experience to perceived challenge in actual physical activity settings in three separate situations over 6 months (Bouffard & Crocker, in press; Crocker & Bouffard, 1992). Social support was assessed by separate instrumental and emotional scales.

In this study, each subject was asked on three occasions to report the most challenging physical activity of the preceding week. Cognitive appraisal scales were used to assess four appraisal variables related to goals or reasons for involvement in the particular physical activity. These variables were developing health and fitness, learning a skill, demonstrating competence, and gaining social approval.

Self-reported affect was measured by the Positive Affect Negative Affect Schedule (PANAS) (Watson, Clark, & Tellegen, 1988). Positive affect reflects one's level of pleasurable engagement with the environment, whereas negative affect is a general factor of subjective distress. Coping strategies were assessed using a modification of the COPE instrument, which contains conceptually distinct coping scales (Carver, Scheier, & Weintraub, 1989). Eleven scales were used, five problem-focused coping scales (active coping, planning, suppression of competing activities, restraint coping, seeking instrumental social support), three emotion-focused coping scales (seeking emotional social support, positive reinterpretation, turning to religion), and three other scales (focus on and venting of emotions, behavioral disengagement, mental disengagement). Based on pilot testing, small changes in the wording of some coping items were made to improve clarity.

The findings indicated that seeking social support for instrumental (problem-focused) reasons and social support for emotional reasons were highly positively correlated. Further, both social support scales were positively related to positive affect. The strength of these relationships varied across situations with correlations ranging form $r = .30$ to $r = .51$. Social support was also significantly related to the appraisal of social approval. That is, the more important it was to receive social approval in the activity, the more likely the individual was to seek social support.

The findings also showed that seeking social support was used less often than other problem-focused strategies such as planning and active coping. For example, the scale means for active coping and planning on the first occasion were 13.7 and 11.9, respectively (scales could range from a low of 4 [used very little] to 16 [used very much]). Seeking social support for instrumental and emotional reasons had means of 8.4 and 7.7, respectively.

Another interesting finding was that most people did not cope in the same way over challenging physical activity settings (Bouffard & Crocker, in press). The absence of a consistent coping pattern may be adaptive in the long term. Researchers (e.g., Lazarus & Folkman, 1984; Meichenbaum, 1985) have suggested that people who cope effectively do not use a consistent coping style across situations. An effective strategy used in a previous encounter with a challenging situation may no longer be right since the ''same'' situation is now different because the individual has changed through learning.

Several conclusions are warranted based on these studies. Seeking social support is but one of several coping strategies that individuals may use to manage threatening or challenging situations in physical activity. In the first study, many subjects reported they would use assertive communication to change the situations involving barriers to exercise. In the second study, involving participants in challenging activities, seeking social support was not used as often as other problem-focused strategies such as problem solving, planning, and effort. It is not necessary to seek social support in every physical activity setting. Therefore, the absence of social support resources may not lead to decreased participation and exercise adherence in many cases.

It would be erroneous to conclude that seeking social support is not important in physical activity. The active use of social support will depend on the dynamic transaction between the individual and the environment. The availability of social support to bolster the individual's coping resources is valuable in some activity settings and inappropriate and possibly counterproductive in others. In some situations, the use of small amounts of social support in combination with other coping strategies may be the difference between an individual continuing in the activity or disengaging. A diverse coping repertoire, which includes seeking social support, is needed to manage the numerous stressors the individual faces in physical activity settings.

The preceding discussion of the importance of coping skills to manage activity demands suggests that practitioners may need to integrate coping skills training into physical activity settings. Teaching participants effective ways to seek social support may have many benefits. It would allow individuals to share experiences, to form networks to solve problems, and to form interpersonal relationships (see Gottlieb, chapter 30; Horne, chapter 31). The combination of learning coping skills and physical activity skills will also promote a more holistic approach to active living and well-being.

Integrating coping skills training into regular activity settings will require that instructors receive specialized training. This should not be construed as a drawback but as a natural progression of health care training. Instructors are often required to have certification in first aid and cardiopulmonary resuscitation (CPR) to deal with acute health care problems. Coping skills training can be envisioned as a long-term health care skill. Teaching coping skills may slow down the dropout rate in exercise settings, estimated by Dishman and Dunn (1988) to be about 50% after 6 months. Keeping more individuals physically active will have more long-term health benefits. Research in the sporting domain has shown that training in coping skills reduces stress-related thoughts and affects and often improves skill performance (Crocker, Alderman, & Smith, 1988; Mace & Carroll, 1989). The potential for benefits to individuals involved in recreational and leisure activity exists.

Summary and Conclusions

The active seeking of social support can be incorporated into a general stress and coping framework. Seeking social support may be for problem-focused reasons such as gaining information and active assistance to change a troubling situation. Social support can also be pursued for emotion-focused reasons such as seeking social approval and sympathy. Both instrumental and emotional functions may strengthen the individual's coping resources to help manage threatening or challenging physical activity. Seeking social support, however, represents only one of a number of potential coping skills and resources an individual can employ. Teaching coping skills, such as seeking social support, in combination with physical activity skills will give participants a more complete coping repertoire to manage activity demands.

Acknowledgment

This paper was supported in part by funding from the Canadian Fitness and Lifestyle Research Institute.

References

Andrew, G.M., Oldridge, N.B., Parker, J.O., Cunningham, D.A., Rechnitzer, P.A., Jones, N.L., Buck, C., Kavanagh, T., Shephard, R.J., Sutton, J.R., & McDonald, W. (1981). Reasons for drop-out from exercise programs in postcoronary patients. *Medicine and Science in Sport and Exercise*, **13**, 164-168.

Bouchard, C., Shephard, R.J., Stephens, T., Sutton, J.R., & McPherson, B.D. (Eds.) (1990). *Exercise, fitness and health: A consensus of current knowledge*. Champaign, IL: Human Kinetics.

Bouffard, M., & Crocker, P.R.E. (in press). Coping by individuals with physical disabilities to perceived challenge in physical activity: Are people consistent? *Research Quarterly for Exercise and Sport*.

Carver, C.S., & Scheier, M.F. (1990). Origins and functions of positive and negative affect: A control-process view. *Psychological Review*, **97**, 19-35.

Carver, C.S., Scheier, M.F., & Weintraub, J.K. (1989). Assessing coping strategies: A theoretically based approach. *Journal of Personality and Social Psychology*, **56**, 267-283.

Crocker, P.R.E. (1989, October). *Ways of coping by athletes: Relationship to appraisal and emotion.* Paper presented at the annual meeting of Canadian Society for Psychomotor Learning and Sport Psychology, Victoria, BC.

Crocker, P.R.E. (1991, November), *Measuring coping strategies to performance difficulties by competitive athletes.* Paper presented at the annual meeting of Canadian Society for Psychomotor Learning and Sport Psychology, London, ON.

Crocker, P.R.E. (in press). Ways of coping with stress by competitive athletes. *International Journal of Sport Psychology*.

Crocker, P.R.E., Alderman, R.B., & Smith, F.M.R. (1988). Cognitive affective stress management training with high performance youth volleyball players: Effects on affect, cognition, and performance. *Journal of Sport and Exercise Psychology*, **10**, 448-460.

Crocker, P.R.E., & Bouffard, M. (1990). Ways of coping by individuals with physical disabilities to perceived barriers to physical activity. *CAPHER Journal*, **56**, 28-33.

Crocker, P.R.E., & Bouffard, M. (1991). *Challenge in physical activity by individuals with physical disabilities: Ways in coping, appraisal, and mood.* Final report submitted to the Canadian Fitness and Lifestyle Research Institute.

Crocker, P.R.E., & Bouffard, M. (1992). Perceived challenge in physical activity by individuals with physical disabilities: The relationship between appraisal and affect. *Adapted Physical Activity Quarterly*, **9**, 130-140.

Crocker, P.R.E., & Gordon, S. (1986). Emotional control training for soccer players. In J. Watkins, T. Reilly, & L. Burwitz (Eds.), *Sport science* (pp. 187-191). New York: E. & F.N. Spon.

Deci, E.L., & Ryan, R.M. (1985). *Intrinsic motivation and self-determination in human behavior*. New York: Plenum.

Dishman, R.K., & Dunn, A.L. (1988). Exercise adherence in children and youth. Implications for adulthood. In R.K. Dishman (Ed.), *Exercise adherence: Its impact on public health* (pp. 155-200). Champaign, IL: Human Kinetics.

Endler, N.S., & Parker, J.A. (1989). Multidimensional assessment of coping: A critical evaluation. *Journal of Personality and Social Psychology*, **58**, 844-854.

Folkman, S., & Lazarus, R.S. (1985). If it changes it must be a process: Study of emotion and coping during three stages of a college examination. *Journal of Personality and Social Psychology*, **48**, 150-170.

Fox, K.R. (1988). The self-esteem complex and youth fitness. *Quest*, **40**, 230-246.

Heinzelmann, F., & Bagley, R.W. (1970). Response to physical activity programs and their effects on health behavior. *Public Health Reports*, **85**, 905-911.

King, A.C., & Frederiksen, L.W. (1984). Low-cost strategies for increasing exercise behavior: Relapse preparation training and social support. *Behavior Modification*, **8**, 3-21.

Lazarus, R.S., & Folkman, S. (1984). *Stress, appraisal, and coping*. New York: Springer.

Mace, R.D., & Carroll, D. (1989). The effects of stress inoculation training on self-reported stress, observer's rating of stress, heart rate, and gymnastics performance. *Journal of Sports Sciences*, **7**, 257-266.

Martin, J., Dubbert, P.M., Katel, A.D., Thompson, K.J., Raczynski, J.R., Lake, M., Smith, P.O., Webster, J.S., Sikora, T., & Cohen, R.E. (1984). The behavioral control of exercise in sedentary adults: Studies 1 through 6. *Journal of Consulting and Clinical Psychology*, **52**, 795-811.

Massie, J.F., & Shephard, R.J. (1971). Physiological and psychological effects of training: A comparison of individual and gymnastic programs with a characterization of exercise drop-out. *Medicine and Science in Sports*, **3**, 110-117.

Meichenbaum, D. (1985). *Stress inoculation training.* Toronto: Pergamon.

Morgan, W.P., & Goldston, S.E. (Eds.) (1987). *Exercise and mental health.* Washington, DC: Hemisphere.

Nisbett, R.E., & Wilson, T.D. (1977). Telling more than we can know: Verbal reports on mental processes. *Psychological Review*, **84**, 231-259.

Oldridge, N.B. (1982). Compliance and exercise in primary and secondary prevention of coronary heart disease: A review. *Preventive Medicine*, **11**, 56-70.

Smith, R.E. (1980). A cognitive-affective approach to stress management training for athletes. In C. Nadeau, W. Halliwell, K. Newell, & G. Roberts (Eds.), *Psychology of motor behavior and sport–1979* (pp. 54-73). Champaign, IL: Human Kinetics.

Thoits, P.A. (1986). Social support as coping assistance. *Journal of Consulting and Clinical Psychology*, **54**, 416-423.

Wankel, L.M., Yardley, J.K., & Graham, J. (1985). The effects of motivational interventions upon the exercise adherence of high and low self-motivated adults. *Canadian Journal of Applied Sport Sciences*, **10**, 147-156.

Watson, D. (1988). The vicissitudes of mood measurement: Effects of varying descriptors, time frames, and response formats on measures of positive and negative affect. *Journal of Personality and Social Psychology*, **55**, 128-141.

Watson, Clark, L.A., & Tellegen (1988). Development and validation of brief measures of positive and negative affect: The PANAS scales. *Journal of Personality and Social Psychology*, **54**, pp. 1063-1070.

33

The Role of Social Support in Late Life Physical Activity

Sandra O'Brien Cousins

In response to growing concerns about the poor quality of life often accompanying the aging process, scientists have been searching for the contextual features of certain populations that may help to explain health status and health behaviors. Among the most prominent relationships between socioenvironmental factors and optimal health is a statistically powerful construct called *social support*.

Social support has been a useful measure in epidemiological research despite its having a variety of meanings including *family size*, *frequency of in-person contact*, and *living arrangements* (Strain & Payne, 1992). Several studies have already demonstrated that social support is an underlying requirement for optimal health (Pilisuk & Minkler, 1985), reduced psychological distress (Holahan & Moos, 1981), positive health behaviors (Hibbard, 1988), and reduced mortality in elderly populations (Blazer, 1982). Sarason, Pierce, Shearin, Sarason, and Waltz (1991) summarized evidence that it is *perceived* support, and not *received* support, that is predictive of coping effectiveness.

Exercise scientists are only beginning to appreciate the significance of social support in physical activity settings. The socializing characteristics and affiliative benefits of sport and exercise participation have been emphasized as important personal incentives for physical activity involvement (Duda & Tappe, 1989; Rudman, 1989). Positive relationships between social support and involvement in physical activity have been found in earlier studies (Andrew et al., 1981; Gottlieb & Baker, 1986; Langlie, 1977; Wankel, 1984). In a study on exercise adherence, Danielson and Wanzel (1977) found that women were more likely to attend fitness classes if they were accompanied by a companion. Wankel (1984) improved adherence in exercise settings by creating a buddy system.

Social support of exercise is thought to be an important environmental cue because some aging adults who plan to meet their fitness requirements with regular physical activity may well encounter

- disapproval from their spouses (Andrew et al., 1981; Dishman, 1986; Snyder & Spreitzer, 1973; Tait & Dobash, 1986),
- lack of peer involvement (Hauge, 1973),
- discouragement by the immediate family (Spreitzer & Snyder, 1973), and
- inadequate encouragement from physicians (Dishman, 1986; Gray, 1987; Powell, Spain, Christenson, & Mollenkamp, 1986; Weschler, Levine, Idelson, Rohman, & Taylor, 1983).

It is ironic that although physical activity settings may be among the most important sources of social contact and support in the lives of older adults, other forms of social support must apparently already exist for the potential of these activity settings to be tapped. For active living to occur, it appears that environmental sources of social support may be an essential prerequisite.

Despite acceptance that a moderate level of physical activity promotes health in older adults (O'Brien & Vertinsky, 1991), available evidence worldwide suggests that too many aging adults are falling short of health-promoting levels of exercise. Ruuskanen and Heikkinen (1992) report that 20% to 30% of Finnish adults over age 65 are totally sedentary. Stephens, Craig, and Ferris (1986) note that 59% of men and 69% of women over the age of 60 in Canada are classified as "sedentary" because they expend less than 1.4 kilocalories per day on leisure-time physical activity. Data collected on more than 19,000 Americans indicate that only 4% of adults over age 65 participate regularly in vigorous activities such as hiking, tennis, skiing, and skating (Brooks, 1988). Moreover, an age-related decline in participation rates is universally found in cross-national research, with women exhibiting less vigorous activity than men at all ages (Robinson, 1988).

It is my objective to examine the relationship between social support and leisure-time physical activity in the elderly. I hypothesize that the declining levels of physical activity accompanying old age are linked to, and possibly caused by, declining levels of companionship and encouragement. Understanding the effect of various social reinforcements and restraints on physical activity holds promise for community-level intervention because fostering social networks is relatively cost-effective and implementation is relatively easy.

Defining Social Support

The scientific assessment of social support is a recent endeavor requiring and generating operational definitions (Esdaile & Wilkins, 1987). Cassel (1976) has described social support as the gratification of a person's basic social needs and Cobb (1976) has defined it as information leading a person to believe that he or she is cared for, esteemed, and part of a network.

Social network originally described a specific set of linkages among a defined set of persons (Mitchell, 1969). Israel (1982) has defined social network as "person-centered" with reference to structural and measurable features of the network such as size and number of links in the network structure, the nature of the linkages (frequency, intensity of interactions), and the functions that networks provide (affective support, tangible aid, and services). Contemporary research has categorized social support as either practical (instrumental) or emotional (expressive) (Tausig & Michello, 1988), but interest is now shifting to characteristics of individuals and the determinants of social support to better understand the mechanisms through which social support serves its protective function (Hobfoll, Ritter, & Bloomfield Shoham, 1991; Sarason, Sarason, Hacker, & Basham, 1985).

The General Social Survey conducted by the Government of Canada in 1985 examined social support in the practical context of *help given* and *help received* (Statistics Canada, 1987). Help received was associated with levels of individual function and physical ability to live independently in noninstitutional settings, therefore being "less able" was associated with higher levels of social support.

Defining Physical Activity

Physical activity, exercise, and sport are often used interchangeably, but exercise and sport are merely subsets of physical activity. Casperson, Powell, and Christenson (1985) define *physical activity* as any bodily movement produced by skeletal muscles that results in energy expenditure. Thus occupational activity, domestic chores, and movements associated with one's needs for daily living are included in the meaning of physical activity. However, for research purposes *leisure-time physical activity* has often been used to describe the voluntary, nonwork activities of adults (Taylor et al., 1978).

The Social Contexts of Support

A sociological perspective might advocate categorizing social support in terms of the social context in which support is found. In the physical activity setting, *microcontext* for social support might refer to spouse, family, friends, teammates, and co-workers who informally offer or withhold encouragement about exercise behavior. Community organizations, facilities, and programs may be thought of as contributors to the *mesocontext* with regard to social support for physical activity participation. *Macro* support systems may be formalized as more global social contracts, resources, and policies. Particip-ACTION Canada, Fitness Canada, and the Secretariat for Fitness in the Third Age are among some of the social programs available at the national level in Canada to support elderly adults in more active lifestyles.

The realization that social support may be needed at all three contextual levels simultaneously is occurring at a time when the conceptualization and measurement of social support is, of necessity, becoming more refined. In the past, global measures of social support have been applied with mixed success; more recently, situation-specific criteria of social support are recommended as more effective statistical predictors (Krause, 1986).

Assessing Social Support

The measurement of a multidimensional construct such as social support is difficult, if only because there are now a legion of available instruments that tap into emotional support, tangible support, informational support, and support provided to others at both perceptual and enacted levels. Gottlieb (1991) identifies several assessment devices, noting that the most popular measure of enacted support is Barrera, Sandler, and Ramsay's (1981) Inventory of Socially Supportive Behaviors (ISSB).

Social support, expressed as a *quantity*, has been measured objectively as the number of social contacts one has or the number of phone contacts or visits from friends in the past week. The *quality* of social support has been more subjectively assessed with perceptual rating scales about the adequacy of one's support network. It is probably important at this stage of scientific understanding to pursue both quantitative and qualitative avenues of assessment whenever possible.

The Importance of Social Support to Physical Activity

The Social Support–Active Lifestyle Connection

As evidence mounts regarding the significant health-promoting role of exercise, sport, and play in mental, social, and physical health, social scientists are provoked to ask why so few adults are actively participating.

The first route of explanation hypothesizes that early socialization and habituation to an active lifestyle foster early competency in physical skill (Brooks, 1988). This line of inquiry seeks evidence that childhood social support and encouragement to explore movement and develop vigorous play patterns create a powerful and lifelong force that determines what individuals value and strive for (O'Brien Cousins, 1993).

An extension of this early and habitual activity hypothesis more generally regards the larger circumstantial situation of specific populations and how current social context may influence lifestyle behaviors. For example, gender, age, health, education, marital status, cultural milieu, and geographic setting are considered to be important features of the social environment that influence perceptions, beliefs, and ultimately habitual lifestyles (O'Brien Cousins, in press).

The Role of Social Support in Late-Life Physical Activity

The socializing characteristics of physical activity, exercise, and sport appear to be among the key reasons older adults participate. Intense socialization is proposed to be fundamental to the older-adult recreational experience (Shivers, 1992; Takala, 1992). Possibly men more than women depend on physical activity for social support. From research on quality of life in the elderly, Grimby and associates claim that ''emotional problems and social isolation seemed to be more closely related to reduced physical activity, fitness, and performance in men than in women'' (Grimby, Grimby, Frandin, & Wiklund, 1992, p. 86).

However, many older women lacking companionship apparently seek out active recreational settings to supplement their social needs. Ishii-Kuntz (1990) examined how predisposing, enabling, and need factors influence elderly women's participation in voluntary organizations and senior centers. A nationwide probability sample provided data that indicated that age, race, and health status influenced older women's active participation. Elderly widows were more likely to be involved in voluntary organizations than married women, with loneliness being a major factor leading to participation in senior centers.

A recent study of 327 Vancouver women over the age of 70 found perceived social support to be one of the significant determinants of their exercise behavior (O'Brien Cousins, 1993). Women who had the highest levels of energy expenditure on self-reported physical activity (upwards of 2,500 kcal per week) reported the highest levels of social support for exercise participation. Social support was assessed using a four-item composite indicator with 5-point Likert scales ranging from

4 (low support) to 20 (high support). The most active women in the study claimed they

- had physician support for vigorous activity,
- had families who were athletic in middle age,
- felt encouragement by at least one other person to maintain above-normal physical ability, and
- had friends who were currently interested in physical fitness activities.

In all categories, women who were older reported lower levels of social support for exercise. In this same study, social support was lowest in those who were separated, divorced, or single, whereas married women perceived the most overall social support to exercise.

Physical Activity as Social Networking

Recreation centers, senior's groups, sport clubs, and even shopping malls provide positive settings for socializing and physical activity (Graham, Graham, & MacLean, 1991). Within these settings, both formal and informal structures can provide instrumental aid, information, and advice. In addition, such settings supply one of the biggest benefits of leisure activity—companionship (Tinsley, Teaff, Colbs, & Kaufman, 1985). Finding companionship for activity seems to occur more frequently among males (Curtis & White, 1984), and women apparently are less likely to take advantage of these existing community networks for participation in physical activity and sport. And when they do, women are unfortunately not always welcome as equal participants (Cole, 1991). However, it is not apparently women's choice to exercise alone. From young adulthood on, females are found more often in caregiving and domestic situations that may limit their ability to formalize social networks outside the home environment.

According to a national survey on women who have disabilities, physical limitations and medical concerns were not considered to be their limiting factors to activity participation. ''The primary changes that would encourage greater participation in physical activities were accessible facilities that are closer to home, knowledgeable instructors, people with whom to participate, and more available information on programs'' (Fitness Canada Women's Program, 1990, p. 35). Social support may be lacking for older women with limitations, because almost half of the women surveyed said they alone were responsible for getting involved in activity, whereas family and friends were influential in activating only 13% of respondents.

The Role of Physical Activity Leadership Support

Physical activity has been found to become less structured and more casual with age (Stephens & Craig,

1990). Ironically people may become more independent from leadership support in the exercise setting at the very life stages where they may also feel that they are at increased risk in exercise. However, casual participation does guarantee a sense of personal control over the pace of an activity and does reduce perceptions of risk by removing social pressures to "keep up" (O'Brien & Burgess, 1992).

Females participate at about half the rate of males in organized sport and participate at about twice the rate of males in supervised exercise programs. It could be interpreted that women are more cautious and concerned about exercising safely, whereas men seek support for challenge and excitement in higher risk settings.

The Role of Companionship and Community Opportunity

Social support and group cohesiveness have been studied with a view to understanding why people begin physical activity, why some maintain their involvement, and why others stop participating altogether. Dishman (1990) has noted that after 6 months, more than half of adults who begin an exercise program have already dropped out. As might be expected, people who do not adhere to a specific fitness or sport setting are less personally attracted to the group's task and to the group as a social unit (Carron, Widmeyer, & Brawley, 1988). The literature underscores the need for an awareness of how the social and physical environment can affect the elderly individual's sustained involvement in group activity (Barris, 1987). Overall, the results of current research confirm the importance of social support, including instructor feedback and praise during exercise (Martin et al., 1984).

Curtis and White (1984) identified that finding others to participate with was a problem for more than 20% of elderly women, and they were the age group that most found the lack of companionship a barrier to participation. Older women had twice as much difficulty as men the same age in finding companionship, yet they reported that time conflicts in activities were only half the problem that men reported.

The Role of Spousal Support

It has been hypothesized that women who have active life companions, active partners, or active spouses are more likely to be physically active themselves (Snyder & Spreitzer, 1973). Having a spouse who is indirectly involved in sports is thought to reinforce earlier encouragement from one's parents and to increase one's perceived ability to be involved as an adult (Spreitzer & Snyder, 1976).

In analyzing family influence on sport involvement, Snyder and Spreitzer (1973) found considerable similarity and mutual reinforcement of activity patterns in couples. Other research suggests that "women who take part in sport perceive a very high degree of support from their nominated or significant male" (Tait & Dobash, 1986). Compared with men, women age 45 and older report less support from their spouse and declining encouragement to be active with advancing years (Stephens & Craig, 1990).

One of the few available studies on the role of spousal support to exercise adherence provides data only on men. Myocardial patients were studied for drop-out rate from an exercise program over a 7-year period (Andrew et al., 1981). Of all the determinants being considered, spousal approval was the most significant. The drop-out rate of those with little or no support from their wives was 3 times greater than that of men with positive spousal encouragement.

The Role of Physician Support

The cautionary warnings that one must always consult a physician before taking up physical activity may be doing more harm than good.

> Certainly anyone who is doubtful about one's personal state of health should consult a physician. In principle, however, there is less risk in activity than in continuous inactivity. In a nutshell, our opinion is that it is more advisable to pass a careful medical examination if one intends to be sedentary in order to establish whether one's state of health is good enough to withstand the inactivity. (Astrand, 1986, p. 4)

Evidence suggests that ordinary people will not get extraordinary advice from a physician about how to start an exercise program. Moreover, the "see your physician" prescription may prevent many adults from ever getting started because a chain of dependency is then formed. If becoming more physically active depends on visiting the doctor, many older adults will not follow through. Even if an individual does go for a checkup, physicians often do not discuss their attitudes and knowledge about exercise with their patients.

Health promoters have begun to examine the interest and competency of physicians to provide encouragement for their patients' activity patterns. It has been noted that physicians who have graduated since the late 1960s are more likely to believe in the importance of regular aerobic exercise, but overall only about one-quarter of physicians have been found to think engagement in aerobic activity three times a week is very important to health (Wechsler et al., 1983). Internists are more likely to ask about exercise behaviors than general practitioners (53% vs. 31%) and all physicians are more likely to ask about smoking, alcohol, and other drugs than they are about diet, exercise, and stress (Wechsler et al., 1983). One in five physicians is optimistic about his or her ability to help patients increase exercise, yet only 3% to 8% of physicians thought they were successful in helping patients achieve changes in various health behaviors.

Surveys of physicians in Massachusetts and Maryland indicated that just less than 50% of primary care physicans routinely inquire about their patients' exercise practices (Wechsler et al., 1983). Furthermore, only 27% of the physicians thought that exercise was "very important" for the average person. Thus "a large proportion of physicians are not fully convinced of the value of exercise for health" (Powell et al., 1986, p. 18). Whether physician inquiries include in-depth questions about intensity, duration, or frequency of exercise is not known. If physicians question younger individuals differently than older ones about exercise, they may be undermining support for more active living in some communities.

Considerations for the Future

Evidence is rapidly accumulating that social support is indeed a significant force in assisting individuals to initiate activity, to adhere to activity once started, and to increase enjoyment of the activity experience. Older adults, especially older women, may be most in need of a helping hand in this regard. Available research on older adult physical activity and perceived levels of support suggests that the two issues are related. Further study is needed to uncover the types of social support that will stimulate more aging adults to reap the rewards of physically active lifestyles. At the same time, we need to know more about the characteristics of currently active adults and the mechanisms by which they obtain, or maintain, high levels of endorsement for physical activity late into life.

Although activity levels appear to be improving at all ages, it is apparent that older men and women persist in underestimating their physical abilities and limiting their activity choices to a few involvements that are deemed to be socially acceptable and age appropriate. Social incentives need to be explored to challenge the self-fulfilling prophecy and ultimately empower older adults to venture into less passive activities that may offer new opportunities and new skills. To foster broader and more vigorous physical activity participation at all ages, society must be willing to share its sport and recreation resources with its oldest taxpayers and allow them moments of priority to enjoy these facilities as full participants, rather than as spectators. This means that administrators must be willing to share the nation's expertise by providing the best of support staff, including coaches and fitness leaders, to address the challenge of creating the richest experiences possible for citizens at their oldest life stage.

Acknowledgments

The author wishes to acknowledge Dr. Patricia Vertinsky of the University of British Columbia, Dr. Art Quinney and Dr. Brian Nielson of the University of Alberta, and the Social Sciences and Humanities Research Council of Canada for their instrumental and emotional support.

References

Andrew, G.M., Oldridge, N.B., Parker, J.O., Cunningham, D.A., Rechnitzer, P.A., Jones, N.L., Buck, C., Kavanagh, T., Shephard, R.J., Sutton, J.R., & McDonald, W. (1981). Reasons for dropout from exercise programs in postcoronary patients. *Medicine & Science in Sports & Exercise*, **13**(3), 164-168.

Astrand, P.O. (1986). Exercise physiology of the mature athlete. In J.R. Sutton & R.M. Brock (Eds.), *Sports medicine for the mature athlete* (pp. 3-13). Indianapolis, IN: Benchmark.

Barrera, M., Jr., Sandler, I.N., & Ramsay, T.B. (1981). Preliminary development of a scale to measure social support: Studies on college students. *American Journal of Community Psychology*, **9**, 435-447.

Barris, R. (1987). Activity: The interface between person and environment. *Physical & Occupational Therapy in Geriatrics*, **5**(2), 39-49.

Blazer, D.G. (1982). Social support and mortality in an elderly community population. *American Journal of Epidemiology*, **115**(5), 684-694.

Brooks, C. (1988). A causal modeling analysis of sociodemographics and moderate to vigorous physical activity behavior of American adults. *Research Quarterly for Exercise & Sport*, **59**(4), 328-338.

Carron, A.V., Widmeyer, W.N., & Brawley, L.R. (1988). Group cohesion and individual adherence to physical activity. *Journal of Sport & Exercise Psychology*, **10**, 127-138.

Casperson, C.J., Powell, K.E., & Christenson, G.M. (1985). Physical activity, exercise, and physical fitness: Definitions and distinctions for health-related research. *Public Health Reports*, **100**, 126-131.

Cassel, J. (1976). The contribution of the social environment to host resistance. *American Journal of Epidemiology*, **104**, 107-123.

Cobb, S. (1976). Social support as a moderator of life stress. *Psychosomatic Medicine*, **3B**(5), 300-314.

Cole, C. (1991, July 18). No more women, left-handed golfers swear. *The Edmonton Journal*, pp. 1-2.

Curtis, J.E., & White, P.G. (1984). Age and sport participation: Decline in participation or increased specialization with age? In N. Theberge & P. Donnelly (Eds.), *Sport and the sociological imagination* (pp. 273-293). Fort Worth, TX: Texas Christian University.

Danielson, R., & Wanzel, R. (1977). Exercise objectives of fitness program dropouts. In D. Landers & R. Christina (Eds.), *Psychology of motor behavior &*

sport (pp. 310-320). Champaign, IL: Human Kinetics.

Dishman, R.K. (1986). Exercise adherence and habitual physical activity. In W.P. Morgan & S.N. Goldston (Eds.), *Exercise and mental health* (pp. 57-83). Washington, DC: Hemisphere.

Dishman, R.K. (1990). Determinants of participation in physical activity. In C. Bouchard, R.J. Shephard, T. Stephens, J.R. Sutton, & B.D. McPherson (Eds.), *Exercise, fitness, and health: A consensus of current knowledge.* Champaign, IL: Human Kinetics.

Duda, J.L., & Tappe, M.K. (1989). Personal investment in exercise among middle-aged older adults. *Perceptual Motor Skills*, **66**(2), 543-549.

Esdaile, J.M., & Wilkins, K. (1987). Social support and social networks as promoters of physical and psychological well-being in arthritic and rheumatic disorders. *Health Services and Promotion Branch Working Paper No. HSPB 88-15.* Ottawa: Health & Welfare Canada.

Fitness Canada Women's Program. (1990). *Physical activity and women with disabilities: A national survey.* Ottawa: Government of Canada.

Gottlieb, B.H. (1991). Social support and family care of the elderly. *Canadian Journal on Aging*, **10**(4), 359-375.

Gottlieb, N.J., & Baker, J.A. (1986). The relative influence of health beliefs, parental and peer behaviors, and exercise program on smoking, alcohol use, and physical activity. *Social Science & Medicine*, **22**, 915-927.

Graham, D.F., Graham, I., & MacLean, M.J. (1991). Going to the mall: A leisure activity of urban elderly people. *Canadian Journal on Aging*, **10**(4), 345-358.

Gray, J.A.M. (1987). Exercise and aging. In D. Macleod, R. Maughan, M. Nimmo, T. Reilly, & C. Williams (Eds.), *Exercise: Benefits, limits and adaptations* (pp. 33-48). New York: E. & F.N. Spon.

Grimby, G., Grimby, A., Frandin, K., & Wiklund, I. (1992, May-June). *Physically fit and active elderly have a higher quality of life.* Paper presented at the Third International Conference for Physical Activity, Aging, and Sports, University of Jyvaskyla, Finland.

Hauge, A. (1973). The influence of the family on female sport participation. In D.V. Harris (Ed.), *DGWS research reports: Women in sports.* Washington, DC: AAHPER Press.

Hibbard, J.H. (1988). Age, social ties, and health behaviors: An exploratory study. *Health Education Research*, **3**(2), 131-139.

Hobfoll, S.E., Ritter, C., & Bloomfield Shoham, S. (1991). Women's satisfaction with social support and their receipt of aid. *Journal of Personality & Social Psychology*, **61**(2), 332-341.

Holohan, C.J., & Moos, R.H. (1981). Social support and psychological distress: A longitudinal analysis. *Journal of Abnormal Psychology*, **4**, 365-370.

Ishii-Kuntz, M. (1990). Formal activities for elderly women: Determinants of participation in voluntary and senior center activities. *Journal of Women & Aging*, **2**(1), 79-97.

Israel, B.A. (1982). Social networks and health status: Linking theory, research, and practice. *Patient Counseling & Health Education*, **4**(2), 65-79.

Krause, N. (1986). Social support, stress, and well-being among older adults. *Journal of Gerontology*, **41**(4), 512-519.

Langlie, J.K. (1977). Social network, health beliefs, and preventive health behavior. *Journal of Health & Social Behavior*, **18**, 244-260.

Martin, J.E., Dubbert, P.M., Katell, A.D., Thompson, J.K., Raczynski, J.R., Lake, M., Smith, P.O., Webster, J.S., Sikora, T., & Cohen, R.E. (1984). Behavioral control of exercise in sedentary adults: Studies 1 through 6. *Journal of Consulting & Clinical Psychology*, **52**(5), 795-811.

Mitchell, J.C. (1969). The concept and use of social networks. In J.C. Mitchell (Ed.), *Social networks in urban situations: Analysis of personal relationships in Central African towns.* Manchester, England: Manchester University Press.

O'Brien Cousins, S.J. (1993). *The determinants of late-life exercise in women over age 70.* Unpublished doctoral dissertation, University of British Columbia, Vancouver, BC.

O'Brien Cousins, S.J. (in press). The life situational determinants of exercise in women over age 70. *Proceedings of the international conference on physical activity, aging, and sport.* Jyvaskyla, Finland: University of Jyvaskyla.

O'Brien, S.J., & Burgess, A.C. (1992). Perspectives on older adults in physical activity and sport. *Educational Gerontology*, **18**, 461-481.

O'Brien, S.J., & Vertinsky, P.A. (1991). Unfit survivors: Exercise as a resource for aging women. *The Gerontologist*, **31**(3), 347-358.

Pilisuk, M., & Minkler, M. (1985). Social support: Economic and political considerations. *Social Policy*, **15**(3), 6-11.

Powell, K.E., Spain, K.G., Christenson, G.M., & Mollenkamp, M.P. (1986). The status of the 1990 objective for physical fitness and exercise. *Public Health Reports*, **101**, 15-21.

Robinson, K, (1988). Time expenditures in sport across 10 countries. *International Review of Sport Sociology*, **2**, 67-84.

Rudman, W.J. (1989). Sport as a part of successful aging. *American Behavioral Scientist*, **29**(4), 453-470.

Ruuskanen, J., & Heikkinen, E. (1992, May-June). *A community-based intervention program of physical exercise promotion and counseling for the elderly. Program and abstracts: Physical activity and sports for healthy aging* (p. 87), University of Jyvaskyla, Finland.

Sarason, B.R., Pierce, G.R., Shearin, E.N., Sarason, I.G., & Waltz, J.A. (1991). Perceived social support and working models of self and actual others. *Journal of Personality & Social Psychology*, **60**(2), pp. 273-287.

Sarason, B.R., Sarason, I.G., Hacker, T.A., & Basham, R.B. (1985). Concomitants of social support: Social skills, physical attractiveness, and gender. *Journal of Personality & Social Psychology*, **49**(2), 469-480.

Schoenborn, C.A. (1986). Health habits of U.S. adults, 1985: The "Alameda 7" revisited. *Public Health Reports*, **101**, 571-580.

Shivers, J.S. (1992, May-June). *Physical recreational experiences in successful aging.* Paper presented at the Third International Conference for Physical Activity, Aging, and Sports, University of Jyvaskyla, Finland.

Snyder, E.E., & Spreitzer, E. (1973). Family influence and involvement in sports. *Research Quarterly*, **44**(2), 249-255.

Spreitzer, E., & Snyder, E.E. (1976). Socialization into sport: An exploratory path analysis. *Research Quarterly*, **47**(2), 238-245.

Statistics Canada. (1987). *General social survey analysis series: Health and social support, 1985.* Ottawa: Minister of Supply & Services.

Stephens, T., & Craig, C.L. (1990). *The well-being of Canadians: Highlights of the 1988 Campbell's Survey.* Ottawa: Canadian Fitness & Lifestyle Research Institute.

Stephens, T., Craig, C.L., & Ferris, B.F. (1986). Adult physical fitness in Canada: Findings from the Canada Fitness Survey I. *Canadian Journal of Public Health*, **77**(4), 285-290.

Strain, L.A., & Payne, B.J. (1992). Social networks and patterns of social interaction among ever-single and separated/divorced elderly Canadians. *Canadian Journal on Aging*, **11**(1), 31-53.

Tait, J.L., & Dobash, R.E. (1986). Sporting women: The social network of reasons for participation. In J.A. Mangan & R.B. Small (Eds.), *Sports, culture, society.* New York: E. & F.N. Spon.

Takala, P. (1992, May-June). *The meaning of physical activity during old age.* Paper presented at the Third International Conference for Physical Activity, Aging, and Sports, University of Jyvaskyla, Finland.

Tausig, M., & Michello, J. (1988). Seeking social support. *Basic & Applied Social Psychology*, **9**(1), 1-12.

Taylor, H.L., Jacobs, D.R., Schucker, B., Kinedson, J., Leon, A.S., & Debacker, G. (1978). A questionnaire for the assessment of leisure-time physical activities. *Journal of Chronic Diseases*, **31**, 741-755.

Tinsley, H.E.A., Teaff, J.D., Colbs, S.L., & Kaufman, N. (1985). A system of classifying leisure activities in terms of the psychologial benefits of participation reported by older persons. *Journal of Gerontology*, **40**(2), 172-178.

Wankel, L.M. (1984). Decision-making and social-support strategies for increasing exercise involvement. *Journal of Cardiac Rehabilitation*, **4**, 124-135.

Wechsler, H., Levine, S., Idelson, R.K., Rohman, M., & Taylor, J.O. (1983). The physician's role in health promotion—a survey of primary-care physicians. *New England Journal of Medicine*, **308**, 97-100.

34

Reaching the Hard To Reach

34.1
Active Living Programs for the Elderly in Rural and Isolated Communities
Norah C. Keating

34.2
Active Living Programs for Low Socioeconomic Individuals
Shannon E. Etkin

Editor's Note:

This chapter presents the content of a panel session at the conference. The two sections address active living for specific populations for whom there are significant real and perceived barriers for involvement. The sections are presented in one chapter since there is significant commonality.

34.1

Reaching the Hard To Reach: Active Living Programs for the Elderly in Rural and Isolated Communities

Norah C. Keating

Isolated. Rural. Elderly. These words hardly create a vision of people who have integrated physical activity into daily life. In fact, many people who write about recreation and leisure of seniors worry that older people participate less in leisure than do younger people (Mobily et al., 1984), that their activities require little physical exertion (Strain & Chappell, 1982), and that they lack skills in the creative use of leisure time (Kivett & Orthner, 1980). Rural seniors are seen as especially disadvantaged in their pursuit of active living because they are often a long way from commercial recreation facilities, are geographically isolated, and adhere to a work ethic that allows little time for leisure (Kivett & Orthner, 1980; Leitner & Leitner, 1985).

An aging population means that we must reconsider the focus of our interest. If we are to provide informed services to seniors, we must understand something of their backgrounds, interests, and needs in relation to active living. McPherson (1986) has said that we are beginning a new domain of inquiry and practice that requires an understanding of the aging process and of the interests and needs of the elderly.

The Variety of Rural Seniors

When I was first doing my training in gerontology, one of my professors said that with aging we become "more so." What he meant was that with age we develop our individual characteristics and idiosyncrasies and become more unlike one another. This has become my foremost assumption in working with older people: Never assume that they are similar to one another. I'd like to use that assumption in discussing rural seniors and the variety of ways they may or may not be involved in active living. To begin I will provide some background on the lives of rural seniors in Canada, and then I will introduce three people who illustrate some of the differences professionals might encounter in work with rural seniors.

A hundred years ago, there was little variety among rural residents in Canada. Especially in the west, most were young men involved in agriculture, fishing, or mining. There were many more young people than old, because older people were not seen as essential to building a new country nor were they strong enough to endure the harsh environment. In fact, in the 1890 census retired people were placed in the category of *nonproductive*, along with Indian chiefs, members of religious orders, paupers, inmates in asylums, and students (Keating, 1991).

In those early days, rural Canadians had an active lifestyle by necessity because they had to deal directly with the natural environment. This way of living led to the development of a strong work ethic and to the rejection of activities that did not involve physical labor. There were no pensions or mandatory retirement and people worked as long as possible. Leisure was to be avoided, for to be caught loafing was cause for embarrassment (Bauder & Doerflinger, 1967).

By the middle part of this century, there had been dramatic changes in rural life across Canada. Continued technological improvement in primary industries such as farming, and labor shortages in cities meant that more than 1 million people left rural areas (Hodge & Collins, 1987). Because the majority of these migrants were young, their departure contributed to the aging of the rural population. At the same time that people were leaving farming, urban people began to move out of the cities into recreation areas and small towns. The result was that the population of rural Canada increased as did the range of occupations and backgrounds of its residents. Many of the newcomers had lives that were not focused on subduing a harsh physical environment, and they may have been the first group of rural residents who had an interest in active leisure. Both the movement of people out of farming and the migration to rural areas had changed the rural countryside and the milieu in which rural residents were involved in active living (Hodge & Collins, 1987; Keating, 1991). By the late 20th century, rural Canada's residents had become very diverse in age and background.

In the last 100 years, rural Canada has also become ethnically diverse. Between 1871 and 1971 most immigrants came from Europe (Bond, 1986). Many of these immigrants settled in rural areas of the country that still reflect a strong ethnic bias. One example is a group of farmers who came from the Netherlands to northern Alberta in 1911. Today second, third, and fourth generation farmers still farm in the much-expanded community and 96% of the residents are still of Dutch background and "reformed" religion (Neerlandia Historical Society, 1985). Because of their special family and religious values and their approaches to work, seniors in such communities may have quite different expectations regarding active living than do descendents of Irish fishermen in Newfoundland or of Mennonites in southern Ontario.

In the last decade about half of all immigrants to Canada have arrived from Asia (Bond, 1986). Most of these immigrants come to Ontario, British Columbia, Quebec, and Alberta (Statistics Canada, 1990). It will be increasingly important for planners to be aware of the ethnic mix in their communities and to learn about the values of those who are potential clients. An increase in the size of the native population (Ponting, 1986) and their increased interest in the restoration of their lands and heritage will also add to the mosaic of rural elders.

Finally, both geographic and cultural isolation also contribute to diversity among rural seniors. Some rural seniors live close to urban centers in southern Canada and others are at a great distance from population areas. In fact, outside of a narrow band of population near the United States border, the typical rural community in Canada is isolated and often dependent on a single industry such as mining or logging (Flynn, 1987). So, for example, both the village of Morinville, 20 km outside of Edmonton, and the village of South Indian Lake, 600 km north of Winnipeg, have small populations and could be considered rural. Yet Morinville is on the doorstep of a large metropolitan center, but South Indian Lake is at a great distance from many services considered essential by urban Canadians.

In addition to being geographically remote, communities may also be culturally remote. Mennonite settlements in central Ontario, Hutterite colonies of southern Alberta, native communities of the Northwest Territories, and fishing villages in Newfoundland are examples of culturally remote areas that have forms of social life that are rare elsewhere (Stalwick, 1983). Many such remote populations have high proportions of elderly residents, a reflection of their social marginalization (Maclouf & Lion, 1983). Planning active living programs for seniors in a remote northern community will require different skills and cultural understanding than will planning programs for seniors in villages in southern Ontario.

This brief review of the history of rural Canada provides some illustration of the variety of rural seniors.

With increasing changes in rural Canada, this variety is likely to increase. In the rest of this section I will focus on approaches to active living of seniors living in an isolated rural community. I will use three seniors who live in a village in British Columbia to illustrate some of the issues in the lives of isolated rural seniors that influence their active living.

Kaslo is located on Kootenay Lake in the interior of British Columbia about 600 km east of Vancouver. It was established in the 1890s to serve the silver-mining boom sweeping the Kootenays. When mining declined at the end of World War I, fruit farming and logging began. Kaslo residents are now employed in logging, sawmilling, and tourism. Kaslo has a population of 1,100 (The Canadian Encyclopedia, 1985).

Deborah Benard was born and raised in Vancouver. For 30 years she worked for the province of British Columbia. The last 10 years before she retired at age 62 she was an assistant deputy minister. She and her husband, Richard, retired at the same time. Richard had been a senior executive with a large insurance company. He grew up in a small town in Ontario and was looking forward to retiring to the countryside. Six months ago they moved to the village of Kaslo.

Stan Thompson was a miner's son, born about 10 km from Kaslo. Stan's family eked out a living by mining and subsistence farming. Stan is now 78 and still farms the family homestead where he has lived all his life. For 50 years he has also been the bartender in the Kaslo hotel. Stan has never married but has a large extended family living in the Kaslo area.

Approaches to Active Living by Rural Seniors

Rural Canada has a history of heavy emphasis on work and hardly seems to be the milieu in which a high value would be placed on leisure activities. Stan Thompson represents a rural resident who has worked hard all his life. He is also typical of early western residents in that he has always been a bachelor. In contrast, the Benards are like other urban migrants to the countryside. They have always had time available for leisure and do not have a negative attitude toward nonwork activities. In fact, they retired early and moved to Kaslo to pursue an active retirement. These three people illustrate some of the great diversity in backgrounds, interests, and opportunities for leisure that are now being recognized by leisure experts (Leitner & Leitner, 1985).

How do such rural seniors decide about the level and type of leisure activities in their lives? We know that rural and urban seniors do not have different levels of activity (Strain & Chappell, 1982). However, the types activities rural seniors do and the reasons they do them may be unique because of the opportunities available in rural communities. Some leisure theorists have argued there may be more spillover from work to leisure for isolated rural residents because of limited leisure opportunities in these communities. The idea of spillover is that people carry their skills and attitudes from work to leisure (Zuzanek & Mannell, 1983) and that work determines both the amount and type of leisure activities (McPherson, 1990). An example of spillover is a farmer who volunteers as a judge at agricultural fairs.

In contrast, others believe that leisure compensates for elements of life that are missing on the job (Zuzanek & Mannell, 1983). Opportunities for compensation are often very limited in isolated communities. Although the farmer could extend her knowledge of farming to taking part in agricultural fairs, she will not find an orchestra in Kaslo where she can play the clarinet.

What are the work-leisure relationships of the three seniors described earlier? The Benards have always seen their leisure activities as compensation for their sedentary work lives. In Vancouver, they were active in leisure pursuits that were organized through membership in a fitness club. They played squash, attended aerobics classes, and swam. The Benards would not find compensation for a sedentary work life in organized recreation in Kaslo. Fortunately, their retirement strategy was to live in a place where activity could be built into their daily lives, thus reducing the need for compensation.

In contrast, Stan Thompson has never distinguished between his work and leisure activities. His "active leisure" has always been working on the farm when he is not at his job in town. Although Stan's farm activities are clearly different and more active than his town job, he did not choose the farm life but grew up with it. For him, activities involved in running the farm may provide compensation but that compensation is unplanned and not seen as leisure.

The Benards and Stan Thompson are very different rural seniors. Their active leisure choices are related to their work but in quite different ways. The Benards made a distinct and conscious shift from an active leisure life that was urban, facility-based, and compensatory to an active lifestyle that does not rely on organized activities. This decision was made at a relatively young age. They are almost a generation younger than Stan Thompson. In contrast, Stan does not consciously think about active living. He is also unlikely to be interested in facility-based activities because none have been available to him. Unlike the Benards, if he takes part in leisure activities he is likely to be attracted to those that do not require much physical exertion. He is much older than the Benards and sees himself as having an active life. To him, fishing is a lot more attractive and feasible than cross-country skiing. A person such as Stan Thompson who comes from an impoverished background and has always held two jobs may not see a place for leisure in his life. Stan seems most likely to be seen as one of the people described in the title of this paper as *hard to reach*.

Adopting New Leisure Activities

What are the professional issues we need to address in designing and implementing programs for isolated rural seniors? Gerontologists (Kivett & Orthner, 1980) have said that characteristics of older people include adherence to a strong work ethic, limited finances and transportation, limited social roles, lack of skills in creative use of leisure time, geographic isolation, and physical frailty. Paradoxically, these characteristics are likely to make active living difficult but very important because they might increase feelings of isolation.

For the most part the Benards are quite unlike this average older person. They have retired early, have a secure income, travel extensively, and have excellent skills in identifying and taking part in leisure activities. However, the Benards do live in an isolated rural area and both have health problems. Deborah has hypertension and Richard has some chronic knee problems developed from years of jogging and other high-impact aerobic sports. Stan Thompson seems more like the rural senior who needs active living programs but is not likely to use them. He has strong work values, limited finances, and lives in an isolated area. He no longer drives but counts on neighbors and friends to take him to the few places he needs to go. However, Stan is also in good health and is perfectly happy with infrequent fishing trips, which are his only leisure activity.

Which of these seniors could benefit most from active living programs? The answer to this question depends in part on whose perspective is taken in determining benefit. From the point of view of a recreation professional, all three seniors described here might benefit from such programs. Programs could help Deborah and Richard Benard replace lost work and friendship roles. Even though they have chosen to move to Kaslo, they may begin to regret their decision if they cannot become integrated into the community or develop the lifestyle they want. Stan Thompson has not lost social roles but is at risk of loss because of his age. He may soon be forced to retire from his job and is finding it increasingly difficult to run the farm.

Even if we believe that it is appropriate to intervene in the lives of rural seniors, it is important to try to determine which rural seniors are likely to adopt active living pursuits. While both the Benards and Stan Thompson could benefit from some new activities, strategies to encourage their involvement and the likelihood of their becoming involved may be quite different. Although all are involved in some active pursuits, the Benards made a major move to adopt new activities in retirement, while Stan Thompson has continued with his preretirement approach.

To consider the question of how rural seniors might become involved, I have borrowed a framework that outlines conditions that influence the likelihood of taking on new activities (Brandenburg et al., 1982). The process begins with the individual's preoccupations and interests, and ends with adoption of an activity if certain conditions are met. These conditions include opportunity, knowledge, favorable social milieu, and receptiveness.

Preoccupations and Interests

The Benards' main focus in life is to become integrated into their new community and to develop their new retirement lifestyle. They live close to the center of the village and they walk or cycle to do all their errands. In the short time they have been in Kaslo, they have planted a large garden and learned to split wood for the fireplace. They feel that they are in better shape and have less stress than they have had for years. They are exploring recreation possibilities on the lake and are looking forward to winter skiing and snowshoeing.

Stan Thompson has had no abrupt shift in his lifestyle. His interests remain in retaining friendships with people he has known all his life through working in the hotel. His major concerns are about what might happen to him if he becomes ill and unable to work. Although he has a large extended family of brothers and sisters and their children and grandchildren, he worries about being a burden to them. One of his major sources of enjoyment is spending time with his family.

Opportunity

Opportunity is seen as the presence of favorable conditions in the near environment. In villages such as Kaslo, some opportunity factors are more important than others. For example, geographic accessibility is the reason cited most often for seniors' lack of involvement in leisure activities (Strain & Chappell, 1982). Kaslo is far from other towns and has few formal recreation services of its own. On the other hand, Kaslo is becoming a tourist area because of its natural beauty and outdoor recreational opportunities.

The Benards and Stan Thompson have access to the same number of limited facilities, although Stan lives out of town and thus is further away. However, all three prefer activities in the natural environment. Stan is much more limited in his opportunity to take part in such activities because of his age and work commitment. Time and health are often given as reasons for nonparticipation in recreational activities (Strain & Chappell, 1982). Clearly opportunity is not a sufficient reason for adoption of an activity. These three seniors living in the same community have very different patterns of recreation despite similar options for involvement.

Knowledge

Knowledge about an activity is the second condition of its adoption. People gain knowledge through prior experience with the activity, having read or been told about it, or seeing a demonstration. Since the current cohort of seniors was not raised expecting to have active leisure (McPherson, 1978), many older people don't know about recreational activities. Nonetheless, in a community as small as Kaslo, Stan will know about most activities. He has a large family and works in a very public job. The Benards will also find out about active living opportunities because they are looking for those in their lives. In small, integrated communities it seems unlikely that lack of involvement in an activity could be traced to not knowing about it. There are few secrets in a community of 1,100.

Social Milieu

Seniors are most likely to adopt and continue an activity if their closest reference group supports the activity (Keating, 1991). For example, when a 60-year-old friend of mine took up jogging, several of her friends told her that she was crazy because a woman of her age was likely to die on the trail. Her response was to tell them she would be happy to die with her sneakers on. She then set out to find a new social group by training for the Seniors Games with other physically fit seniors. She didn't give up her other friends but stopped talking to them about her fitness regime. My friend's experience is an example of a societal norm that exercise is risky for seniors (Mobily, 1982).

Stan Thompson has two close reference groups: his extended family and a lifelong network of friends whom he has known through his job in Kaslo. If Stan chose to become involved in a new activity, he could find someone he already knew who would be understanding and supportive. Yet because Stan is well known, it might also be difficult for him to do something new. Comments like "What has gotten into you?" or "Have you taken leave of your senses?" can put a damper on the most intrepid of seniors. Unlike my city friend, it would be hard for Stan to find people who do not know him but who are involved in an activity in which he might like to participate.

Deborah and Richard have no local network, although community members are well aware that they have arrived. However, marriage partners are an important aspect of the social milieu (Dorfman, Heckert, Hill, & Kohout, 1988). Yet the Benards are also disadvantaged in terms of social milieu because they have no family members or old friends nearby (Alberta Recreation and Parks, 1988; Scott & Roberto, 1987). A question for recreation planners concerning the Benards is whether the lack of supportive social network will hinder their involvement in active living or whether, like my friend who joined the Seniors Games, they will find a group with whom to participate.

Receptiveness

The final condition to involvement in an activity is receptiveness or willingness to enter into a new experience. Some people have argued that receptiveness is more important than social milieu in determining whether someone will take up a new activity. For example, in a study of Newfoundland seniors, Doucette (1987) found that seniors who took up a new art or craft activity felt that they had entered a distinct life phase marked by events such as retirement or relocation. All saw the shift as having deep personal significance and requiring new approaches to life. The adoption of new activities is one strategy used to adjust to the change.

A longstanding desire to do something may also be the basis of this receptiveness. The Benards have planned their move for years and are open to new experiences. We don't know whether Stan has a longstanding desire to do something else, although he is worried about his health and his future. He may be more receptive to new activities as he anticipates changes in his life.

Another aspect of receptiveness is a belief in the value of active living. Many seniors think that their everyday activities provide sufficient exercise. These same seniors may have grown up with sporadic physical education programs in high schools where regular exercise for women was frowned upon (Mobily, Leslie, Lemke, Wallace, & Kohout, 1986). Deborah Benard was raised in just such a milieu. It was only through her contact with younger colleagues that she became involved in a fitness club and has come to value physical activity. Deborah is unusual—current estimates are that only about 30% of those aged 65 to 74 and 14% of those over 75 years of age are involved in regular activities that include aerobic activity as well as flexibility, strength, and balance (Teague & Hunnicutt, 1989). Stan Thompson also believes in physical activity but thinks that his farming gives him enough exercise. Experts would say that he may be wrong. Research on groups of seniors who saw themselves as more active than others has shown that when these seniors were monitored, the findings did not support their ideas of how vigorous they were (Mobily, 1982).

Adoption of an Activity

This analysis of the interests, opportunities, knowledge, and social milieu of three isolated rural seniors provides information to determine what might influence Deborah, Richard, and Stan to adopt active living pursuits. Active living professionals must decide how much to intervene if they believe that the active living choices of such seniors are not optimal.

Issues in the Marketing and Targeting of Active Living Programs for Rural Seniors

Three issues are especially relevant in thinking about interventions to reach the hard to reach. The first is that organized activities will appeal only to some seniors at some times. The second is that small cohesive communities provide opportunities for active living that are unavailable in urban centers. The third is the notion that seniors become "more so" as they grow older.

It's All in the Timing

Although we assume that organized activities will appeal only to some seniors at some times, finding out who is likely to be receptive to active living is not always easy. People who are entering a new life stage, who are looking forward to taking part in long-anticipated activities, or who have a belief in the value of active living are likely to be easily recruited.

Deborah and Richard Benard will be easy to reach because they are receptive and used to dealing with new situations. They are probably as open to new adventures as they have been in years. Capturing people at these turning points can be very satisfying for programmers and participants alike. The active lifestyle they develop in their new community will be an important basis for how they live the rest of their lives.

The truly hard to reach are more like Stan. Changes in Stan's life have been gradual, although he will probably be forced to retire soon. Intervening in lives of seniors like Stan requires professionals to think about both the strategies they might use and the ethics of intervention. Some of the strategies to reach such seniors use informal networks such as family. Others are more direct. Stan might be invited to participate in spillover activities such as talking to schoolchildren about the early days of farming in Kaslo or having small numbers of children visit him on the farm for some hands-on experience. The ethical issue is whether the professional has a right to intervene. In many circumstances we are willing to accept the idea of encouraging people to do something "for their own good." Each professional has to determine the dividing line between facilitating and cajoling. Calling Stan to ask him to talk to a group of students may be facilitating, but calling him three times may be undue pressure. There are times in anyone's life when they are not only hard to reach but unwilling to be reached.

Small Is Beautiful

Small, cohesive communities are both easier and more difficult places to develop active living pursuits than are larger centers. They are easier because such communities have preexisting informal networks of friends and family. One approach to active living not commonly used by professionals is to use these existing informal networks to introduce active living. In a small community, every informal event of any size is well publicized. Thus a professional might help organize activities at the church picnic, encourage physically active events at a family reunion, or use family networks to help motivate a senior member to make some changes in his lifestyle. Stan is well integrated into family and social networks. The task for the professional is to think about how or whether to use his network to get him involved.

Life in rural areas includes contact with people of all ages. Most rural seniors favor activities that include people of all ages (Strain, 1979), although many rural communities provide the majority of their programs for seniors through organizations such as seniors centers. This approach is unlikely to result in a wide age range of participants. An alternative is for programmers to think about activities that will appeal to people of various ages. One example is a fitness program that was recently organized and advertised for the "not so young and not so fit." The ad resulted in a class of 25 people from age 35 to 85. All shared inactive lifestyles and wished to do more. They developed a sense of camaraderie as they monitored their increasing fitness levels throughout the course.

A prevalent point of view is that one of the deterrents to active living is the lack of facilities in small communities. An essential aspect of determining the need for a recreation facility is to assess the receptiveness to people of all ages to the use of the facility. The Benards would use a recreation center because they are willing to take part in all opportunities for active living. They are also likely to be equally active if no such facility exists. Stan Thompson might be persuaded to join a curling club if he could afford the fees, be part of a group of friends, and become skillful enough to enjoy the sport. But it is just as likely that he would drop out after a few games. Facilities are likely to be used by the easy to reach but are unlikely to provide the key to reaching the hard to reach.

Becoming "More So"

In the last decade there has been a dramatic shift in attitudes of professionals toward aging. When I first started teaching courses in aging, I found that many of my students had very negative attitudes. Many thought that older people were frail, ill, poor, and inactive. During those early years I invited many seniors into my classes to help students confront their stereotypes. My favorite guest was a man who said that the best thing about retirement was having to pay only half price on the ski lifts at Banff. Ironically, other gerontologists and I may have done our job too well. The current stereotype appears to be just the opposite of the earlier one. We now have television programs called "The Best Years," a seniors gymnastic group at my university called the U of Agers, and Jane Fonda looking eternally youthful in her fitness tapes.

It seems reasonable to assume that if people have 60 or 70 or 80 years to develop their idiosyncrasies and interests, they will not be very similar to each other.

Older people are both youthful and frail, inactive and fit. The best strategy to encourage active living among such a diverse group is to think of interventions that are not based on age but on interest and ability. A fishing derby will attract everyone from young children to seniors like Stan. Cross-country ski races will leave out Stan but attract Deborah Benard as well as some teenagers and other adults.

Conclusion

Some rural seniors are hard to reach, some easy to reach, some unwilling to be reached. Active living professionals must hone their skills in determining which seniors have which attitudes. There are no overall prescriptions in reaching the hard to reach. Some will be reached through creative provision of formal and informal opportunities, some by being swept along by a concerned network of family and friends, and some not at all. Though we may truly believe that all rural seniors could benefit from health promotion activities, it is both futile and unwise to attempt to reach such a goal. Our responsibility is to provide options; theirs is to take them up or not.

References

Alberta Recreation and Parks. (1984a). *A look at leisure #18: Recreation patterns of older adults.* Edmonton: Government of Alberta.

Alberta Recreation and Parks. (1984b). *A look at leisure #19: Community type variations in recreation patterns.* Edmonton: Government of Alberta.

Alberta Recreation and Parks. (1988). *1988 general recreation survey.* Edmonton: Government of Alberta.

Bauder, W., & Doerflinger, J. (1967). Work roles among the rural aged. In E. Youmans (Ed.), *Older rural Americans: A sociological perspective* (pp. 22-43). Lexington: University of Kentucky Press.

Bond, J.B. (1986, May). *Aging: A cultural perspective.* Keynote address at the annual meeting of the Alberta Association on Gerontology, Lake Louise, AB.

Brandenburg, J., Greiner, W., Hamilton-Smith, E., Scholten, H., Senior, R., & Webb, J. (1982). A conceptual model of how people adopt recreation activities. *Journal of Leisure Studies,* **1,** 263-276.

The Canadian Encyclopaedia (1st ed.). (1985). Edmonton, AB: Hurtig.

Dorfman, L., Heckert, D., Hill, E., & Kohout, F. (1988). Retirement satisfaction in rural husbands and wives. *Journal of Rural Sociology,* **53**(1), 25-39.

Doucette, L. (1987, October). *Aging in the context of regional culture: A study of late-life creativity.* Paper presented to the annual meeting of the Canadian Association on Gerontology, Calgary, AB.

Flynn, D. (1987). Rural life in Canada: Surviving the empty northland and the American river presence. *The Rural Sociologist*, **75**, 388-394.

Hodge, G. (1984). *Shelter and services for the small town elderly: The role of assisted housing*. Ottawa: Canada Mortgage and Housing Corporation.

Hodge, G., & Collins, J.B. (1987). *The elderly in Canada's small towns*. Vancouver, BC: The Centre for Human Settlements, University of British Columbia.

Humboldt Community Survey Committee. (1976). *Humboldt community survey*. Humboldt, SK.

Keating, N.C. (1991). *Aging in rural Canada*. Markham, ON: Butterworths.

Kivett, V.R, & Orthner, D. (1980). Activity patterns and leisure preferences of rural elderly with visual impairment. *Therapeutic Recreation Journal*, **13**, 44.

Leitner, M.J., & Leitner, S.F. (1985). Leisure in later life: A sourcebook for the provision of recreational services for elders. *Activities, Adaptation & Aging*, **7**(3/4), 1-23.

Maclouf, P., & Lion, A. (1983). *Aging in remote rural areas: A challenge to social and medical services*. (Eurosocial 24). Vienna: European Centre for Social Welfare Training and Research.

McPherson, B.D. (1978). Aging and involvement in physical activity: A sociological perspective. In F. Landry & W. Orban (Eds.), *Physical activity and human well-being* (pp. 11-125). Miami, FL: Symposia Specialists.

McPherson, B.D. (1986). Sport, health, well-being, and aging: Some conceptual and methodological issues and questions for sport scientists. In B.D. McPherson (Ed.), *Sport and aging* (pp. 3-23). Champaign, IL: Human Kinetics.

McPherson, B.D. (1990). *Aging as a social process: An introduction to individual and population aging* (2nd ed.). Toronto: Butterworths.

McPherson, B.D., & Kozlik, C.A. (1987). Age patterns in leisure participation: The Canadian case. In V. Marshall (Ed.), *Aging in Canada: Social perspectives* (pp. 211-227). Markham, ON: Fitzhenry and Whiteside.

Mobily, K.E. (1982). Motivational aspects of exercise for the elderly: Barriers and solutions. *Physical & Occupational Therapy in Geriatrics*, **1**(4):43-54.

Mobily, K.E., Leslie, D.K., Lemke, J.H., Wallace, R.B., & Kohout, F.J. (1986). Leisure patterns and attitudes of the rural elderly. *The Journal of Applied Gerontology*, **5**, 201-214.

Mobily, K.E, Leslie, D.K, Wallace, R.B, Lemke, J.H., Kohout, F.J., & Morris, M.C. (1984). Factors associated with the aging leisure repertoire: The Iowa 65+ rural health study. *Journal of Leisure Studies*, **16**, 338-343.

Neerlandia Historical Society. (1985). *A furrow laid bare*. Neerlandia, AB: Neerlandia Historical Society.

Ponting, J.R. (1986). Assessing a generation of change. In J.R. Ponting (Ed.), *Arduous journey: Canadian indians and decolonization* (pp. 394-409). Toronto: McClelland and Stewart.

Scott, J.P., & Roberto, K. (1987). Informal supports of older adults: A rural-urban comparison. *Family Relations*, **36**, 444-449.

Stalwick, H. (1983). *Canadian perspective on aging in remote rural areas: A challenge for sociomedical services*. Paper presented to the International Expert Group Meeting on Aging in Remote Areas, Limoges, France.

Statistics Canada. (1987). *The nation: Age, sex, and marital status* (Catalogue No. 93-101). Ottawa: Minister of Supply and Services Canada.

Statistics Canada. (1990). *Immigrants in Canada. Selected highlights*. Ottawa: Minister of Supply and Services Canada (Housing, Family, and Social Statistics Division).

Strain, L.A. (1979). *Outdoor recreation for rural senior citizens*. Winnipeg, MB: Natural Resources Institute, University of Manitoba.

Strain, L.A., & Chappell, N.L. (1982). Outdoor recreation and the rural elderly: Participation, problems, and needs. *Therapeutic Recreation Journal*, **16**(4), 42-48.

Teague, M.L., & Hunnicutt, B.K. (1989). An analysis of the 1990 public health service physical fitness and exercise objectives for older Americans. *Health Values*, **13**(4), 15-22.

Zuzanek, J., & Mannell, R. (1983). Work–leisure relationships from a sociological and social psychological perspective. *Journal of Leisure Studies*, **2**, 327-344.

34.2

Reaching the Hard to Reach:
Active Living Programs for Low Socioeconomic Individuals
Shannon E. Etkin

The title of this presentation demonstrates the professional mind-set that provides the basis for much of the angst that service providers and service providers and service recipients face in trying to provide and access active living programs. The title contains two premises, one explicit, the other implicit.

1. Low socioeconomic individuals are hard to reach.
2. The target group is to be a recipient of the program.

These two premises give the message that people of low socioeconomic status are difficult to attract to the programs that we design for them. The fault lies with the target group, not the service providers.

The title conveys the way many service providers of active living programs think. A different mind-set exists in the application of basic standards of program design when it comes to designing programs for low-income groups.

In this paper I will outline the false assumptions often made by professionals in planning delivery of active living programs to recipients from backgrounds different from their own. I will take a look at the barriers that reduce the participation of people with lower incomes. I will then present strategies to reduce the barriers and enhance participation. I hope the reader will then be in a position to examine his or her own practices and reflect upon the nature of change that is needed to provide diverse populations fair and equitable access to active living programs.

A double standard often exists in providing services to individuals of differing socioeconomic status. The double standard is so ingrained in most organizational cultures that we are unaware of our service discrimination.

For example, a community center was developing a program for a low-income population that previously was poorly served. The staff person responsible for the initiative complained when only a couple of people showed up. When the supervisor inquired as to how the program was promoted, the staff member responded that posters were put up and brochures were available. The supervisor acknowledged the difficulty in getting those people out to programs and commented that they were not interested in getting fit. The staff member was not held responsible for the poor turnout.

Consider the contrasting approach taken at another center developing a new program. Promotion of the program through posters was not considered adequate. The supervisor talked to the appropriate staff member about the need to develop a marketing plan that considered what publications the target group read, where they gathered, and what potential established groups the center could collaborate with. I should mention that this program was being offered to an upwardly mobile economic group. The second approach recognized this group had choices to make about use of their leisure time. The supervisor understood that if the program was not properly designed and marketed to meet the clients' needs, participation rates would be low. Another part of the message was that this client group would voice their dissatisfaction about inappropriate programs to the center's leadership. Such action could affect the staff person's employment.

These two examples illustrate the bias that often overrides good planning and design when the target group is an "outsider." When programs for outsiders fail, too often we blame the target group rather than consider whether the failure was due to the plan, beliefs, misconceptions, and actions of the service providers.

We know that disenfranchised persons have much less power and assertiveness in challenging program leaders to make the changes needed to meet their needs. This inequality in power works to the disadvantage of lower income people seeking access to programs.

Tryfit

In my work with Family Service Association of Metropolitan Toronto I thought it would be possible to develop an effective program model for provision and delivery of active living programs to low-income families. I hoped this model program would help combat the myths and biases that exist around service provision to people of lower socioeconomic status.

The project was developed with the cooperation of the senior staff of Bolton Camp, two farsighted individuals then working with the Ontario Ministry of Tourism and Recreation, and the City of Toronto Parks and Recreation Department. The YMCAs of Metropolitan Toronto joined the project midstream and became valuable partners.

Tryfit combined physical activity programs with functional educational programs in an appropriate setting. Staff were trained to work with the client group and were part of a multidisciplinary team. The client group, low-income mother-led families, were involved in many aspects of the project design and given opportunities for personal growth and development. The project ran for 13 weeks. It included support groups and buddy systems, baby-sitting, and goal setting. Several evaluations of the program clearly showed its success in attracting low-income families and maintaining high participation rates. Studies also showed participants increased their levels of fitness and well-being.

How Aware Are We?

"I'm not garbage" was one of the cries heard from a woman participating in Tryfit. She was desperate for us to understand the trap that she was in and that we are not fully aware of.

It is easy for the health and fitness professionals to say, "Of course she is not garbage." But what do we really know of this mass of people we label as disadvantaged, poor, or of low socioeconomic status? Do we, the practitioners, operate on damaging stereotypes that reduce the appeal of that group? Do we feel uncomfortable with them; do we spend less time with them; do we avert our eyes and feel that they have no place in our decision making? Do we treat them like garbage?

How aware are we of who the hard to reach are? Statistically, the highest representation of individuals who are most disadvantaged are single mothers and their children, and single women age 50 to 65. The working poor, whether married or single are also part of this category labeled low socioeconomic. But do we really know who these people are?

Do we know of the teenage mother who has two children, was beaten by her husband, and was shunned by her family? Do we know of the family with at least a dozen children—most adopted because the parents could not stand to see a child in pain—in which the father suffers a debilitating injury and loses his job? Do we know of the bright articulate, middle-aged woman left with only a designer handbag because her husband has left her, destroying her financial underpinnings? Do we know of the Jamaican immigrant, a mother supporting seven boys, living in a housing project, whose spirit

won't be defeated nor will her dream that the future will be better for her sons?

The common denominator for the target group is poverty but the individual differences are as great as those of any group of people categorized by economic level. Not recognizing the differences has allowed us to fall into several traps.

One trap is associating low socioeconomic status with negative descriptors: dirty, unmotivated, hopeless, stupid, illiterate, immoral, unsavory. We develop our own self-fulfilling prophecies, based on our assumptions, that protect our integrity and our position when the hard to reach don't show interest in our programs.

Our professional training also sets up certain traps. Two stand out immediately.

1. After years of training we think we know the answers. It thus becomes harder for us to ask people what they want and instead we give them what we believe they need.
2. We tend to view our disciplines as having an exclusivity. This leads us to be professional chauvinists. Recreationists are often disparaged by social workers as being lightweights, and the social workers are seen as talking the day away by recreationists. We hide behind our standards to protect our integrity and self-esteem, risking those we could serve.

The trap expands as our own cultural biases come into play. Increasingly in Canada, especially in our large urban centers, we must become more aware of the effect of our cultural biases on the design and delivery of programs to people from nondominant cultures. A lack of awareness and understanding of different cultural beliefs can lead to exclusion from programs. Certain religious groups may not participate in swim programs, not because the group is unaware of the program or because they are not interested, but because mixing males and females in swim attire is considered inappropriate.

It can be easy to fall into a trap because of our misperceptions of the people we believe we are trying to serve. To be more effective we must develop a better understanding of the barriers that limit the participation of low-income groups in active living programs.

Barriers to Participation

Poverty and Materialism

"Serving Disadvantaged Women," a report from the Ontario Ministry of Tourism and Recreation, highlights the effect of poverty on the participation of women in active living programs. The conclusions reached were supported in discussions with women attending Bolton Camp and Tryfit.

The key statistics and conclusions reached were as follows:

- 43% of single mother families live in poverty.
- Disadvantaged women are less apt to follow beneficial health regimens (they exercise less, smoke more, and are more often overweight).
- These women have more time constraints due to shift work, day-care travel time, and lack of convenient transportation.
- These women do not view themselves as one of the middle-class, active, and fit people who are projected in much of advertising.

Poverty is a barrier to participation in many subtle as well as obvious ways. Participation in sports like skating, nordic skiing, and aerobics classes can be relatively low cost especially when equipment is made available. But if instructors declare the need for ''proper'' attire, people with little money to spend on fashion will feel embarrassed and out of place at these activities. We tend to get caught up in materials and technology, seeking such gear as sports shoes that sound as though they are composed of materials that belong in the space shuttle, microfibers so our skin can breath, and artificial ice. The simple programs such as walking that can improve fitness are rarely offered in courses. Yet, these may be the types of programs that disadvantaged individuals feel most comfortable with.

We love to

- build wave pools that are costly to construct and operate, necessitating fee increases;
- build recreational palaces and forget hiking and footpaths; and
- reduce access to lakes and rivers (often because the water is polluted) and spend money on snow-making machines.

All of these actions reduce the ease of access to active and healthy lifestyles for people in poverty.

Planners, politicians, and professionals in active living must reduce their fascination with material and technology and refocus on simple, cost-efficient practices to encourage healthier communities. We must also, as you will find in the next chapter, move beyond our own narrow fields and join wider groups of professionals in related areas.

Professionalism

The development and acquisition of knowledge within specific fields has its merits but too often is used to build fences, maintaining power and authority for a select group. People who are disadvantaged need services that are as complete as possible. If they fear getting involved in an active living program because of low self-esteem then we must ensure that the primary service provider works with social service and health care providers to optimize the potential success of active living programs.

Recreation schedules usually give priority to organized events—the swim teams and hockey teams—providing a chance for our children and our professional staff to show their competence. Less emphasis is placed on open gym times or family sports that will better meet the needs of some low-income groups.

Staff certification and minimum qualifications are also used as a systematic way to prevent access to staff positions by people from low-income groups. Often we ask for a bachelor's degree when there is nothing inherent in having that degree that makes a person better qualified for the position. Perhaps a positive attitude to the target group and an appropriate certificate would be sufficient in some instances. The use of assistant leaders from the target group also may encourage more participants. We might have to institute our own training programs and appropriate recruitment strategies to encourage potential instructors from low-income groups. The fewer staff that come from the target groups the more difficult it will be to involve these groups.

Alienation

We all want to exercise control over our environment. Loss of control makes us uncomfortable and nervous. As our self-esteem becomes challenged, fear builds up. Loss of control over events leads to alienation and shifting of responsibility from ourselves to others. The economically disadvantaged live in a different subculture from those who are not from low-income groups. There are differences in language, beliefs, goals, and shared realities. Teens in a housing project preferred not to go on a hiking trip, much to the instructors' and administrators' surprise. The staff could not understand the fear these tough, streetwise teens had of the wilderness. I have had camp staff shocked at the language used by some mothers from disadvantaged groups. The staff became alienated from the group they were supposed to help because they could not understand how the participants' communication patterns were connected to their culture.

Senior staff running a seniors active living program were distraught when expanding service to a new ethnic group. Staff thought members of the group lied to ensure they would get into the program. The clients claimed lower income levels and certain maladies to enhance their chances of acceptance into the program. They did not see what they were doing as wrong. Staff, however, did not understand that for these people refusing to accept ''no'' as an answer and embellishing upon ones' needs was the only way the could survive in their country of birth. A lack of knowledge of our clients' cultures causes us to look negatively on some of their actions.

Consider the advertising that we generally see advocating healthy living. Clean-cut men and women, "perfect" models wearing the latest sport fashions, tell us it is great to be involved. They can be hard to relate to, especially by the poor and hard to reach.

We have forgotten that the middle-class norms of many of our practitioners and policy-makers are not necessarily the norms of other groups in society. Unfortunately, we tend to rank other norms as not just different, but inferior. This prejudices our interactions and alienates the groups we label as hard to reach.

Inflexibility

Offering services that are inflexible in such areas as hours of service leads to many problems of access by low-income persons. Providing programs only with a fixed length prohibits peoples on fixed incomes from joining the programs because they might not, for example, be able to afford 10 weeks. Requiring full payment several months in advance for programs limits access too.

I have worked with mothers who wanted to send their children to resident camp but only if the mothers could come along to keep an eye on their children. The families were from the Middle East and could not risk being separated from their children. Our program was not set up to accommodate their needs. Registration for many parks and recreation programs with limited capacity starts at 8:00 a.m. Hourly workers and single parent families are disadvantaged in this process. Many service providers are still falsely living in an era where most families had two parents, one of whom did not work outside the home. A municipal children's summer day camp runs only 9 days out of every 10. How do dual working families cope with finding care on the 10 day?

Fear

This fourth barrier can be most intimidating. The fear of interacting with people who are different from you, the fear of being in a new situation, and the fear of failure are common to both the service providers and the target group. Low-income women we have worked with are leery of new situations and new people. Many have been burned before and have little trust of those who have another good idea to sell them. Staff at a recreation center were afraid of the mess that the children would create while their moms were in a program. There was fear of how the regular members would feel about having these people around. It took 12 weeks for staff to become comfortable with the low-income families.

When we take a look at the collective impact of these barriers on low socioeconomic individuals and on the providers of active living programs we can better understand the wide rifts that exist and why each group feels the other is hard to reach.

It is possible to develop strategies that will overcome these barriers and lead to more successful programming with low-income groups. These new strategies will be explored in the following section.

New Strategies for Success

The strategies for success will build upon factors that will lower the barriers just described. The program design factors must, of necessity, deal with the needs and attitudes of both the target group for service provision and the service providers. Dealing with only one side of the equation will doom the outreach to failure.

Environment

Programs must be offered in a setting and with staff that ensure the target group will feel comfortable and secure.

The success of the Tryfit model was aided in part because of the environment in which it was taking place and the context in which people doing the outreach were known. The common intersection for mothers participating in Tryfit was Bolton Camp. The mothers or their children had previously attended Bolton Camp. They felt secure with the staff and the programs at the camp. This security allowed them to risk attending a new program. Mothers' comments to this effect and the inability of community centers to draw more than two or three participants to their programs demonstrate this environmental importance. Other factors to consider in developing programs for low-income families are the same as those for similar programs directed to mainstream groups. But we have to understand the subculture within which the target group operates.

If a group is fearful of going to a new place to try a program, we must offer the program in a place they are comfortable.

Empowerment

Successful programs will be ones that allow for ownership by the target group. We must be prepared to give up control to the participants to foster commitment. In both senior and adult programs, participants appreciate choices in program components, times available, and targets to reach. It means the professionals must see the world from the perspective of the participants. Tryfit mothers asked for programs on Friday night, traditionally a down time. It made sense to the mothers because it was the only way they could afford to go out on Friday night. Empowering clients actually will decrease the stress on service providers as the chances for success are enhanced.

Building on Participants' Strengths

Programs for low-income groups must emphasize and build upon the positive aspects of the individuals' lifestyles. A very overweight woman showed up for a Tryfit class. She could move only with much difficulty. The instructor could easily ignore her or, as in this case, applaud her for showing up. Many of the people from low-income groups that I have worked with want to give back to others in similar circumstances. Programs that provide participants the opportunity to serve others while benefiting themselves will enhance the overall success of active living programs. Tryfit gave mothers the opportunity to become fitness leaders and take responsibility for promoting the program. The participants benefited and the staff's job was made easier.

Holistic Approaches

We must develop our programs from the bottom up, incorporating as many factors as possible to increase the number of needs that will be met in one program. This factor is probably more significant for attracting lower income groups into active living programs than for other socioeconomic groups. Economically disadvantaged individuals and families I have worked with tend to have more impediments to participating fully in an active lifestyle. Programs that allow for many of their needs to be met at one time will be more successful. Active living programs that give weight to the socialization, respite, health, and self-esteem issues of the participants along with the need for physical activity will attract more disadvantaged people.

Two programs further illustrate the importance of a holistic approach.

The Tryfit demonstration project came up with the following positive results:

- 85% of participants completed 13 weeks,
- 82% felt an improved level of fitness,
- 76% made positive changes in their eating habits,
- 95% recorded an increase in energy attributed to the program, and
- 80% improved their level of cardiovascular fitness.

But the anecdotal comments of the mothers are more revealing. They spoke of the importance of the support of the group in maintaining their participation, the positive effect on their children, and the new friendships formed. They indicated, too, their willingness to be involved in continuing the project so more families could benefit from it. The fitness leaders were applauded for the positive and caring atmosphere they created.

Guests at Illahee Lodge, a residential recreational program, with which I have been affiliated, for low-income and isolated seniors, listed the warmth of the staff and the experience of making new friends as reasons for partaking in the program. All of the activities from swimming to shuffleboard, dancing to crafts were important but only insofar as they helped participants attain higher order needs, such as belonging to a group that cared about them.

The seniors at Illahee Lodge and the mothers in Tryfit participated in those programs not so they could run faster, jump higher, or outperform another person but because participation in the programs met important life quality needs.

Conclusion

To effectively provide a good range and quality of active living programs to that group generally labeled as having low socioeconomic status requires a new state of mind from the professionals charged with providing service.

It is easy to discuss the barriers and the strategies needed to overcome them. However the planners, decision makers, and practitioners must not only talk the talk but they must walk the walk, too!

- A York region school trustee speaking in favor of a year-round school plan stated that a recreational service provider said such a plan would be a boon to families, giving them uncrowded access to the ski slopes. In response, a mother asked what families he was referring to—she and her friends could not afford a ski holiday, and instead relied on park land for walks and public beaches for swimming during their holidays.
- A local recreation center was asked why a family could swim cheaper during general swim than family swim if the center wanted to promote family activity. The center's staff replied that they had always priced it like that.
- Health and Welfare Canada sponsored a television commercial urging us to get out and ski. The advertisement showed mainstream professional-looking skiers, downhilling in the latest fashions.
- Natural neighborhood skating rinks have been closed, forcing us to use artificial rinks with restrictive times and rules that limit opportunities rather than enhance them.
- The emphasis on million-dollar athletes and the public costs of sports such as bobsledding and luging (Canada sent more support personnel than athletes to the Olympics) must be addressed if we are truly serious about opening up opportunities for active living and improving the well-being of disadvantaged groups.

Cost barriers, including child care must be addressed. Access to public park lands, clean waterfronts, and bicycle trails are all part of the issues that must be faced nationwide.

But while those issues are being examined, local service providers can reach the hard to reach if they make a real commitment that those individuals have a right to the services. The strategies have been examined in this paper. Programs exist that do meet the needs of disadvantaged individuals. Tryfit, Bolton Camp, and Illahee Lodge are but three of them.[1]

Finally, providers of active living programs must ask themselves the question, "Who really are the hard to reach?" If, as I suggest, it is the service providers, then it is incumbent upon the leadership to confront the issues outlined in the arenas afforded to us. We must exert pressure on the political, educational, and professional bodies to ensure our responsibility to the entire community is understood. The issue of poverty as a barrier must be addressed and blame removed from those of reduced means. We must see the roles we have played in maintaining the barriers and recognize the need to provide the tools for low-income people to participate more fully in active living programs. The hard to reach can be reached.

Note

1) Information about Illahee Lodge, Bolton Camp, and Tryfit can be obtained from the Family Service Association of Metropolitan Toronto, (416) 922-3126.

Part V

The Active Living Concept:
Critical Analysis and
Challenges for the Future

Active living—What is it? Why is it? And what is its value for practice, policy, and research? These are questions being addressed by those who have long been associated with physical activity, fitness, health, and the active living movement. There is a need for critical appraisal of this concept because of its relative novelty, because of its potential impact on government policy, and most of all because it may guide professional practice in physical activity, fitness, and health. Part V allows for just such a critical examination.

Makosky describes the concept of active living and presents the advantages of pursuing and promoting such a concept. Bouchard follows this discussion with a critical examination of the concept of active living from the biological perspective. Bouchard cautions that careless application and promotion of the active living concept may occur to the detriment of advances already made in establishing the health benefits of vigorous exercise and physical activity. Echoing these and other cautions, McPherson critiques the active living concept from the sociopsychological perspective. McPherson suggests that all stakeholders, be they researchers, policymakers, communities, and social marketers in the field, should strive to effectively communicate ideas and information to avoid the very real possibility that active living will be nothing more than a slogan or rhetoric. In critiquing the active living concept, Edwards raises some important and forthright questions for researchers, policymakers, and practitioners. Edwards's perspective demands action on the part of the reader and aptly closes this self-questioning.

35

A Critical Examination of the Active Living Concept

35.1
The Active Living Concept
Lyle Makosky

35.2
Active Living From the Biological Sciences Perspective: A Word of Caution
Claude Bouchard

35.3
Active Living: Concept, Variable, Rhetoric, or Slogan?
Barry D. McPherson

35.4
Active Living: A Critical Examination
Peggy Edwards

Editor's Note:

This chapter presents the content of a plenary panel session at the conference. It presents the concept of active living and then offers a critique of the concept from three perspectives. The editors have placed four papers into the same chapter so that the continuity and integration of the concept is maintained.

35.1

The Active Living Concept
Lyle Makosky

The purpose of this paper is to describe the concept of active living and what it could mean for you and for the citizens of our countries. I am confident the authors of the following discussion papers will do an excellent job critiquing active living as it relates to their areas of expertise.

All of the conference participants have heard or read something about the concept of active living. Some, in fact, have helped develop the concept. But for many, active living remains a vague notion—or worse, a misunderstood concept. Therefore, I will explain the concept before addressing why it is needed and where it could take us in the future.

The Concept of Active Living

It is commonly accepted that physical activity plays an important role in shaping individuals' lives as well as our wider social systems. Physical activity is important not only because it enhances a person's cardiovascular capacity, endurance, strength, balance, and flexibility, but also because it can provide us with a sense of inner harmony as well as insights about ourselves and the world around us.

Active living recognizes that. It appreciates both the physiological and the social, mental, emotional, and spiritual aspects and benefits of physical activity. It emphasizes the linkages between the mind, body, and spirit, and the interaction of the individual with others and the environment.

This is clearly a different way of looking at physical activity. Active living moves away from the notion that physical activity is good for only your body to the idea that it is good for the whole person. It is a humanistic and subjective view of physical activity rather than a mechanical view. It recognizes that physical activity contributes to an increased sense of well-being and quality of life, not simply more muscle, a flatter stomach, or greater endurance.

As you can appreciate, active living is very much a personal experience. Whether it involves biking to work or building a house, taking part in a community skate-athon or competing in the Olympics, gardening or walking a baby carriage, physical activity allows us to test our limits and experience beauty, creativity, power, and a sense of belonging.

In fact, with active living the experience is as important as the outcome. Establishing the meaning and value of physical activity is a subjective process that is rooted in personal experience. And the experience can vary dramatically from person to person, even with the same activity. It's comparable to two people traveling across Canada together. Even though they look at the same landscape and have the same destination, their experiences of the journey may be completely different.

Active living is also a way of life in which individuals make useful, pleasurable, and satisfying physical activities an integral part of their daily routine. It recognizes that decisions as to how and when we engage in physical activity are affected by the state of the environment, our interactions with others, past experiences, changes in our lives, social norms, personal opinions about what constitutes "a good life," the physical space and role we are in at the moment, and a range of other factors.

At this time there is a danger of asking active living to have a tidy definition or to fit neatly in a box. Active living is not about a new formula, a fad, or a new advertising campaign. Active living is about our changing approach to physical activity and fitness, involving the meaningful integration of physical activity into every dimension of our life.

Active living encourages Canadians to be active in a way that suits their schedules, circumstances, and unique interests, needs, and skills. For some people, walking or wheeling may be a mode of transportation. For others, it is a form of exercise, an opportunity for socialization, or a way to get some fresh air and enjoy nature. It can be a way to meet other people or to find solitude, to release tension, or to stimulate the thought process.

Another intended characteristic of active living is that it be accessible to all, regardless of age, physical capabilities, or economic situation. Active living embraces the full spectrum of physical activity—from those involving minimal movement capacity to those that demand intensive, high-level training.

Active living is for all people, all times of the day, and all periods of life. It allows us to express who we are, either as individuals or as groups. The nature, form, frequency, and intensity of physical activity is relative to each individual's ability, needs, aspirations, and environment.

Active living is for all spaces and all places. It can be part of our lives at home, at school, in the community, and at the workplace—not just at the gym or on a bike path or tennis court. It does not have to be limited to the times or areas we have set aside specifically for leisure activities. All people have to do is imagine how they can be active in terms relevant to the space they are occupying or the task or role they are undertaking at any given time.

And, of course, active living is conducive to overall well-being, because a physically active way of life provides individuals the opportunity for health, happiness, and personal fulfillment. Active living accepts that an individual's interpretation of well-being is subjective and uniquely personal.

Most importantly, active living is not limiting. It is everything mentioned and more. It means different things to different people, and many of its benefits are subjective, intangible, and impossible to quantify.

The Need for the Active Living Concept

This concept—this new approach to understanding, appreciating, and promoting the benefits of physical activity—is not something that was just pulled out of the sky. It has been developed over the past several years through a collaborative effort involving Fitness Canada, the provincial–territorial governments, and fitness leaders. And it responds directly to a recommendation that came out of the 1986 Canadian Summit on Fitness.

A very clear message emerged from that summit: Fundamental change was required in our traditional view of fitness.

Delegates to this conference pointed out that the exclusive focus on cardiovascular endurance, flexibility, and muscular strength was extremely limiting. They emphasized that fitness was not just physiological fitness, but total fitness—physical, mental, social, and spiritual. They also tied fitness to daily living patterns and expressed a need for a more inclusive approach to promoting physical activity. And they recommended that individuals, industry, and social institutions work together to ensure that physical activity and optimal well-being become integral parts of life in this country—a Canadian cultural trademark.

The message that came out of the 1986 summit was a reflection of changing Canadian social conditions and evolving views about health, fitness, and physical activity.

For example, the views of many Canadians about health have changed over the past decade. Health now means more than simply not being ill. It is viewed as a state of complete physical, mental, and social well-being. It is seen as a basic and dynamic resource in our daily lives, influenced by our circumstances, our beliefs, our culture, and our social, economic, and physical environments.

The texture of Canadian society also is changing. Such factors as the deteriorating natural environment, the economic recession, and rapid changes in the composition of the population and the work force are affecting social norms and values. This is evident in the fact that Canadians today put more value on quality of life, and they are seeking different ways of defining that quality.

It is also reflected in changing attitudes toward physical activity. People are discovering the potential of physical activity to help them experience a greater well-being. And while vigorous activity is still important, there is a growing acceptance of the joys, values, and benefits of all kinds of activities. Indeed, increasing research shows that even modest levels of physical activity yield positive benefits throughout life.

In saying that, one doesn't want to detract from the obvious breakthrough the cardiovascular fitness approach made in the 1970s. This was an extremely important and fertile period in the evolution of the fitness movement, as increasing numbers of Canadians came to appreciate the benefits of being fit.

However, hindsight has shown us the limits of this approach. Quite simply, it did not appeal to everyone. The fitness boom became commercialized, glorifying an image of the young, white, heterosexual, attractive, and able-bodied person—an image that many Canadians did not identify with.

Still others were not attracted to the prescriptive, high-intensity approach to fitness in the 1970s. Such benefits as the joy of play, personal achievement and development, and social interaction were pushed to the side by the overwhelming emphasis on achieving fitness goals.

Some groups could not identify with the narrow cardiovascular fitness approach. For them, fitness was intimidating. It didn't meet their needs, and it had little relevance to their daily lives.

And finally, for some Canadians there were significant barriers—both real and perceived—to becoming involved in the physical fitness movement. These included a lack of opportunities to participate; an inadequate range of activities; insufficient equipment, facilities, and leadership; high costs; and a perceived lack of time (Stephens, 1983).

As a result of these factors, the increased participation rates recorded in the 1970s were concentrated in select pockets of the population. This was borne out by the 1981 Canada Fitness Survey, which revealed significantly higher participation rates among university graduates compared with Canadians with an elementary education, among managers and professionals compared with blue collar workers, and in specific regions of the country (Stephens, 1983).

The bottom line was that a new approach to fitness was needed. The approach needed to have a place for those who wanted to take part in vigorous activities such as jogging or aerobics classes, as well as those who looked to physical activities as a means of relaxation, as a way to spend time with their families and their friends. It needed to address those who wanted to proceed at a slower pace and those who needed to express their personal identity differently. It also needed to encompass those who viewed physical activity as a natural part of daily life, not as a special, segmented undertaking.

The Elements of Active Living

And so the concept of active living was developed. It is a concept that is rooted in the belief that the ultimate aim of physical activity should be individual well-being and quality of life. The concept includes many facets of life, it supports a broad range of outdoor and indoor activities, and it allows individuals to express their own thoughts, feelings, and aspirations through those activities.

In developing this concept over the past couple of years, three principal elements of active living have been identified:

(1) It is individual.
(2) It is social.
(3) It is inclusive.

Active Living Is Individual

Active living is a result of a conscious, personal choice. Why does someone walk to work instead of taking the bus or the car; bike with the family instead of watching television; take dance lessons instead of going to the movies? There is no set answer to these questions because the decisions are made by individuals, based on their current circumstances, past experiences, values, and aspirations. And the decisions are affected by such other factors as the time of the day, changes in the life cycle, the weather, and physical environments.

Active living acknowledges that experts can provide information and guidance in support of specific actions and that professionals have an important role in organizing programs. But it also acknowledges that individuals are best able to decide how to live actively and to judge the value of different activities. In this way, active living is empowering. It empowers individuals to make physical activity an integral part of their lives, on their own terms. It empowers them to make responsible choices about the types of activities they will participate in. And it says that they will not be judged for those choices or for their decision to act alone or with others.

Active Living Is Social

Engaging in physical activity is a personal choice, but it is also a matter of political decisions and culture. It is affected by the norms and values we share with others in society. Therefore, it is cultural in the sense that the activities we choose, how we integrate them, the meaning we draw from them, and the priority we place on them all say something about who we are as a people, about our cultural identity. It also affirms that through physical activity choices and strategies, individuals have the opportunity to change their environment.

In this social context, physical activity allows us to share, cooperate, collaborate, and compete with other individuals and sectors of society. We learn to respect differences among groups and to appreciate our values and customs, as well as those of other ethnic, religious, or political groups.

Active living also allows for participatory decision making, in which different sectors of society work cooperatively to improve opportunities for physical activity. Through this collaboration we can respond to the challenge issued at the 1986 Canadian Summit on Fitness, the challenge to make physical activity a Canadian cultural trademark.

Active Living Is Inclusive

Active living is based on the premise that anyone can enjoy and benefit from a physically active lifestyle, at any time, in any place, and in any way they find appealing. It recognizes that physical activity is a right for all, regardless of age, social or economic status, race, or religion. And it values a diversity of physical activity opportunities that individuals have access to and find useful and satisfying.

The challenge is to integrate physical activity into all ages, living spaces, and roles so as to eventually ensure its naturalness. For the present, inclusion must be promoted. Over time, this cultural characteristic will be celebrated as a natural one.

Implications and Challenges of Active Living

Active living will obviously have some important policy and program implications and will present some distinct challenges for the health, fitness, and recreation communities.

Our first challenge will be to ensure that the environment exists to allow Canadians to make informed, responsible choices about physical activity. Several steps must be taken to foster such an environment.

For example, there is a clear need for research that examines people in their totality. Active living links the body, mind, and spirit in action, so we need to study the physical activity experience in the larger context of human development.

Studying people in their totality will require a collective scientific effort. And the shift from a ''performance enhancing'' to a ''human development'' model will not be without consequences for the research agenda. It could, for example, imply that active living research might best be organized around issues that can be explored from a multidisciplinary perspective. It could also mean a restructuring of current research efforts, with more or less emphasis being assigned to specific areas.

But research is only one way we will meet the challenge of fostering the right environment for active living. We will also need to legitimize a spectrum of physical activities and norms of behavior that are broader in scope. We will need to eliminate restrictive social norms for specific populations, such as the elderly, women, persons with disabilities, and those who are economically or socially disadvantaged.

We will need to respect and celebrate differences in physical activity preferences among various cultural and racial groups. If personal choice and the respect of differences is valued, the manner of living or of being healthy for individuals cannot be dictated. We can't be prescriptive or judgmental. At the same time, the causal relationship between certain habits and activities and their health outcomes can't be ignored. With this in mind, more knowledge about the effect of physical activity on human health, knowledge that is relevant to the individual's circumstance, is required.

The existing notion of physical activity is one almost exclusively oriented toward skills and fitness. This notion will need to be revised, because of new evidence that even low-level physical activity has health benefits. And it will have to be revised to include not just the physical performance and outcomes, but the psychological, social, and personal experiences associated with the activity and its relevance to daily life.

The measures of physical activity will also need to be expanded beyond how many calories were spent and how intense the activity was. Other measuring sticks will be required, such as the level of psychic energy and personal satisfaction associated with the activity.

As leaders in the fitness community, our second challenge will be to work together to improve the diversity of opportunities for physical activity. Implementing active living will mean initiating and promoting a wider range of cooperative programs at all levels—local, regional, and national. It will mean encouraging social institutions to embrace the values of active living and to respond to the needs it creates. It will involve many sectors of society, including urban planners; community leaders; environmentalists; school boards; the business community; cultural groups; and, of course, medical, health, and fitness professionals.

It should be evident that inspired leadership will be required if we are to convince Canadians to embrace active living. This is perhaps our third major challenge, because it means issues of power will have to be addressed. The traditional, expert-driven fitness system will have to be broadened to ensure full public participation in decision making. It will have to involve all types of leadership—formal and informal, volunteer and professional, policy makers and practitioners.

The active living movement has important implications for fitness leadership. However, this will not mean a complete upheaval. There will always be a need for the traditional fitness leaders and appraisers—those who provide exercise counseling to individuals and groups who actively seek it out.

The needs and aspirations of many Canadians who are fitness and performance oriented still need to be met. So do the needs of those Canadians who are concerned about their cardiovascular health or about preventing coronary heart disease. The safe participation of Canadians in many forms of bodily movement can be met only by knowledgeable leaders, and they have a key role to play within the active living model.

However, the approach that many fitness leaders have adopted in the past might have to be expanded to take into account the personal choice and individual empowerment aspects of active living. Life experiences must command greater attention.

The active living leader is primarily an inspirer, an informed organizer, and an enabler. The challenge to these individuals will be to form alliances with other sectors of society that are involved or want to be involved in the active living movement.

The good news is that the multidimensional nature of physical activity can provide a sound basis for groups and social organizations to network and form new partnerships. In fact, this is already occurring. Through the new Active Living Environments initiative, leaders from different sectors and disciplines have started to talk to each other and to plan how they can work together. Civic planners and engineers are talking to cyclists, and conservation groups are working with parks and recreation programmers. This is an important and exciting development.

Active living can have a tremendous impact on our policy agenda and the strategies we develop to implement those policies. As a new way of thinking about physical activity, it will lead to innovative models, linkages, and partnerships, both at the community level and at the national level. It will have an effect on our language and attitudes and on how we allocate resources and evaluate results.

Another key challenge ahead of us is to effectively communicate the active living message to specific target groups. While the media can play a positive role in this regard, there are limitations to social marketing. Information and persuasive appeals can be effectively transmitted by mass media channels, but interpersonal networks are often more influential. Those networks can include fitness industry professionals, personnel managers, researchers, sociologists, business people, and homemakers.

Solid evidence supports the need for more personal, informal communication of the benefits of physical activity to specific target audiences. A case in point is the Action Sport experiment initiated in the United Kingdom in 1982 to demonstrate the value of sports leadership in increasing participation in sport and recreation by those who live in the inner city. This study indicated that the most effective way to reach the target group was through word of mouth, by local leaders as opposed to physical activity experts.

Among other things, this means we have to identify not only the most appropriate message for target groups, but also the most appropriate messenger—the individual or group that will best reach and have credibility with the target group.

Making Active Living a Canadian Cultural Trademark

One of the themes I have integrated into this paper is making active living a Canadian cultural trademark. If we are to achieve this objective, we must address some very specific and practical cultural obstacles.

For example, the use of competitive activities to integrate individuals into group or team structures is an acknowledged reality in Canada. These are often positive growth experiences, and they certainly have a place in the active living model.

However, not everyone enjoys the competitive environment. Our challenge is therefore to find and promote a wider range of cooperative, shared experiences that will expand the network of Canadians involved in active living. Folk and social dancing, community landscaping and gardening projects, t'ai chi, water-based recreational activities, hiking, and cross-country skiing represent a few examples of the many popular alternative activities that might be encouraged.

The commercialization of the body—the marketing of fitness based on heterosexual attractiveness—has also taken a toll on the cultural dimension of physical activity. We have to counter this imagery by reorienting physical activity toward some larger purpose than simply looking good. We have to promote such outcomes as pleasure, self-expression, the building of character, the discovery of others and of our environment, inner peace, personal accomplishment, and friendship.

Another cultural challenge we will have to overcome is the current emphasis on indoor winter activities. Historically, Canadians participated in a wide range of outdoor winter activities. At one time, snowshoeing, tobogganing, skating, and sleigh riding were widespread social and family activities. However, with technical improvements in construction practices and our ability to control indoor environments, much winter activity is now undertaken indoors.

We have to address this cultural pattern by reaffirming the pleasures of outdoor winter activities. We already have a number of successful experiments to guide us, including the decision by the National Capital Commission to flood the canal in Ottawa for skating, the development of cross-country ski trails in larger metropolitan areas, and the introduction of winter festivals in many communities.

Finally, a challenge implicit in active living is the need to work together to create and enhance physical environments that support and promote a wide range of physical activities.

Today, most Canadians live in large urban centers that often provide limited recreational space and few areas where people can experience the natural environment in surroundings they perceive to be safe and secure. In many neighborhoods, the fascination of architects with concrete and glass has led to a reduction in green space and natural walking routes, the very types of physical environments that are needed if Canadians are to embrace the active living concept.

On the bright side, there are indications that in these times of high government deficits and tax rates, the public is much more likely to support the development of facilities and infrastructures that offer broad and versatile applications than it is a large, single-purpose facility. In other words, the public will likely endorse the creation of bike paths and hiking and skiing trails before the construction of hockey arenas and football stadiums. And that bodes well for the active living movement.

Conclusion

One of my objectives in this paper was to develop an appreciation for the concept of active living as a different way of looking at physical activity.

Implementation of the active living concept will clearly require sweeping attitudinal changes among some sectors of society—and within the health, fitness, and recreation community. It will require us to answer some difficult questions.

- If active living is to be inclusive, how do we ensure that in making opportunities available to some individuals, we do not impinge on the rights of others?
- If the meaning of physical activity varies from person to person and within subcultures, how do we reach those who are different?
- If well-being is subjective, how do we measure and evaluate physical activity?
- How can active living become an integral part of life in communities, and what role does the community itself have in that process?
- How can active living be integrated into the schools and the workplace?

Answering these questions at the practical level may seem like a formidable task. However, I believe people are willing and ready to make the shift. And I believe that integrating physical activity into the daily lives of Canadians as proposed in the active living model will lead to genuine, positive social change.

In summary, active living is a way of life. It's not just exercise but a set of values that emphasize natural, ingrained physical activity based on lifestyles. Those values legitimize the subjective, personalized choices of physical activity that people make and the meanings they draw from them.

Active living includes all levels of intensity of physical activity including traditional forms of fitness and exercise. But we also seek to democratize physical activity, to popularize and demystify it, and to ensure it is accessible and relevant.

The basic qualifier is that the action includes physical activity or reasonable physical movement, but is not restricted to those that are exclusively or even predominantly physical activity based, as long as bodily movement is involved.

Yes, this raises questions of the activity threshold level, causal impact, and measurement models, but I would suggest that it is more important now to liberate and legitimize people and their personal inventiveness, their sense of play, and their intuitive desire to include physical movement as part of living naturally. That is, we should accept the lack of tidiness in the definition of active living and its use and reduce the inhibiting factor that results from judgments about whether people are acting "correctly."

As professionals and practitioners, it is our business to lead the movement, to create the environments and opportunities for all Canadians to experience living at its best, and to endorse active living as "natural living" not as "correct living."

References

Stephens, T. (1983). *Fitness and lifestyle in Canada.* Ottawa: Canada Fitness Survey.

35.2

Active Living From the Biological Sciences Perspective: A Word of Caution

Claude Bouchard

Active living is a slogan developed in recent years under the leadership of Fitness Canada with the support of affiliated agencies and associations. I have been asked to examine critically the concept and I will do so briefly from the point of view of the biological and clinical sciences.

At the outset, it is useful to remember that about 10% to 15% of adult Canadian men and women engage regularly in some forms of physical activity. The same surveys also tell us that about 45% to 50% of the adults living in Canada are occasionally active or regularly active for part of the year. We are therefore confronted with the challenge of convincing the 40% or so remaining adults, who are completely sedentary, that regular physical activity is an essential component of a healthy lifestyle. It is also relevant to recognize that about 35% of adult Canadians eat more calories than they expend and have consequently developed a body weight problem. Most of them are simply overweight, but 10% to 12% are obese.

Given these simple numbers, it is clear to me that although we have made remarkable progress in promoting regular physical activity and in furthering the understanding of the notion of fitness among Canadians, we still are confronted by a daunting task. Can we improve these population statistics with the advent of the active living program? I harbor great doubts about the effectiveness of the new slogan for the improvement of these and other relevant health statistics. Some of the reasons for my skepticism follow.

First, some believe active living represents a conceptual advance. I am not convinced at all that it is. In my judgment, it may be even less useful than previous concepts used to focus the public attention on physical activity, fitness, and health. The expression is equivocal in the sense that it does not fully describe what it intends to do. For some, the slogan will clearly stand for a physically active mode of life. However, for a good number of people, active living is not synonymous with a physically active lifestyle. In some circumstances, it could be perceived as the ratio of the number of hours awake to the hours asleep. To uninformed laypersons, active living could conceivably be defined in terms of the amount or proportion of time allocated to doing things intellectually or physically, or as an abundance of social interactions. There may even be more extreme and distorted perceptions of the intent of the slogan. To be a conceptual advance, active living should be easily and readily defined and recognized by all segments of the public with whom we are trying to communicate in our efforts to promote regular physical activity. From this point of view, active living has yet to demonstrate that it is a more effective slogan than others used in the past.

Second, active living has been defined so far largely in terms of fun, pleasure, feelings, and experiences. All these outcomes obviously are important and they should be an integral part of a physically active lifestyle. However, so far I have been unable to identify the underlying quantity or metric behind active living. I have yet to see the notions of frequency, intensity, or volume of activity associated with active living. This is not a trivial point. If active living has no clear underlying quantities, it will not be easily measured and evaluated. Therefore, needed information such as baseline measurements and changes following promotion campaigns, and variations by age, gender, social class, provinces, regions, and ethnic groups cannot be objectively obtained.

Third, the circumstances under which regular physical activity generates fitness and health benefits are better understood today than they were only a few years ago. Two main requirements are emerging from the growing body of knowledge on physical activity, health-related fitness, and health. On the one hand, frequent periods of activity (about four times a week and more), at moderate intensity (about 40% to 60% of maximum), and for 30 to 60 min per session generate a reasonable amount of energy expenditure to affect energy balance and provide a healthy stimulus for various physiological systems and metabolic pathways. On the other hand, occasional periods of exercise at higher intensities seem to be particularly beneficial for heart health. Regular physical activity as defined here translates into significant biological and health benefits as illustrated in Table 35.21. These benefits are known to be brought about by regular physical activity that has such volume and intensity characteristics. Regular physical activity can engender beneficial responses not only in the biological domain but also in the psychological and social dimensions. However, it is important to keep in mind that these psychological and social benefits are generally associated not only with regular physical activity but also with participation in a variety of activities including passive leisure activities and activities that have no apparent relationship with physical activity (e.g., travel, concert music, reading, etc.). I do not mean to imply here that regular physical activity is not beneficial from a psychosocial point of view. It clearly is. However, other forms of active leisure are thought to be equally advantageous to psychosocial health and well-being. In contrast, none of these other forms of leisure activities have the potential to impact as favorably on the health-related fitness components or on morbidity data and

mortality rate as regular physical activity when it attains desirable levels of frequency and intensity.

Fourth, my perception of the active living slogan is that it seems to consider the recent advances regarding the usefulness of moderately intense physical activity as a license to conclude that people should just do something, physical activity or not. If this is the premise upon which active living is being promoted, it is not valid. Moderate intensity physical activity has never meant a 5% to 10% increase in heart rate as a result of a marginally augmented metabolic demand. The foundation of a physically active lifestyle was briefly defined in the preceding paragraph. A minimal total amount of activity of moderate intensity should be the cornerstone of active living. Moderate intensity means that heart rate and energy expenditure should be increased to at least 40% of maximum values. This does not mean that we should embark on a crusade against games of bowls (pétanques), horseshoes, bowling, archery, meditation, and other low energy cost activities. They are all worthy leisure activities that should be encouraged and promoted, but they should be in addition to activities that have the potential to favorably influence fitness and health. We must be cautious and not inadvertently destroy the progress made over the past 25 years. The Canadian population understands now better than ever

Table 35.21 An Overview of the Effects of Regular Physical Activity on the Health-Related Fitness Components

Morphological component
- Favors energy balance
- Reduces upper-body fat and visceral fat
- Maintains or increases bone density
- Improves joint flexibility

Muscular component
- Improves muscle strength
- improves musclar endurance

Motor component
- Improves balance
- Improves coordination

Cardiorespiratory component
- Increases exercise tolerance
- Improves heart and lung functions
- Reduces blood pressure

Metabolic component
- Decreases blood triglycerides
- Increases blood HDL-cholesterol
- Improves insulin sensitivity of tissues
- Increases lipid oxidation
- Favors balance between lipid intake and lipid oxidation

what fitness is and how it can be improved. Now is not the time to lead the public into believing that any definition of *active* is appropriate. Promoting fun, pleasure, and *joie de vivre* is not necessarily the same as promoting a physically active lifestyle that may influence fitness and health. However, both approaches are not mutually exclusive. Ideally, one would like them embodied in a single program. Unfortunately, I do not find them both integrated in the active living slogan as it is currently being promoted.

Fifth, the message embodied in the active living documentation creates a distorted perception not only in the general public but also in the physical activity and fitness professional communities that may eventually be counterproductive. We run the risk of demobilizing the highly motivated fitness community by promoting, perhaps inadvertently, the notion that a physically active lifestyle is devoid of any meaningful volume and intensity requirements. It would be foolish to destroy for no valid reason the enormous investment we have collectively made in the fitness movement. Most people involved in the fitness movement all over the world still strongly believe that a healthy life free from impairment and disability is largely dependent on a sound body. In this context, regular physical activity, meeting the volume and intensity criteria I outlined previously, remains a useful component of a preventive lifestyle aimed at maintaining a sound body. The scientific and clinical literature about the relationships between physical activity, health, and health-related fitness is quite supportive of that view. No amount of rhetoric is likely to change that.

All forms of physical activity are important and should be taken into consideration in the broad context of fitness and health. They include physical activity associated with one's occupation, accomplishment of daily personal chores, and more importantly for the fitness community, leisure-time physical activity. The latter component is that of greatest interest because volume and intensity of activity can be modulated for fitness and health purposes. If we ever decide to do without these volume and intensity requirements, then we should be prepared to abandon traditional claims about contributing to fitness and health. Physical activity scientists and clinicians are taking great care to identify the true effects of regular physical activity and the circumstances under which it affects health and fitness. Unsubstantiated claims from greedy entrepreneurs or careless promoters rarely go unchallenged by the fitness community. We are placing ourselves in a very vulnerable position in this regard with the active living slogan as presently promoted. It does not need to be that way as fun, pleasure, and *joie de vivre* should not be incompatible with reasonable recommendations concerning volume and intensity of regular physical activity.

35.3

Active Living: Concept, Variable, Rhetoric, or Slogan?

Barry D. McPherson

Since the 1986 Canadian Summit on Fitness, many practitioners and scientists in Canada have encountered or utilized the term *active living*. Increasingly, the term has permeated the Canadian literature for fitness and exercise professionals. As well, the term is being used increasingly in policies, programs, and public communication messages, and new organizations and positions have been created within some provincial and federal government agencies to promote active living. To date, however, the term has not been used in the scholarly or scientific literature. Yet active living is being touted by some proponents "as a simple yet compelling and relevant concept" and as "an umbrella concept" (Focus on Active Living Secretariat, 1992). Unfortunately, many fitness, exercise, and recreation professionals have readily accepted and adopted the use of this term without giving serious thought to its meaning, its measurement, its policy relevance, or its viability as a promotional tool or slogan. Morever, no one seems to be questioning why the term was created or why it should be adopted and used by scholars or practitioners. Is the term being used as a substitute for *fitness, exercise, wellness,* or *physical recreation* now that recent evidence suggests that lower intensity activity is more appealing to the masses and may be more successful as a goal in terms of achieving long-term compliance?

To stimulate debate and discussion, this paper critically examines the term from conceptual, empirical, policy, and marketing perspectives. Throughout, more questions are raised than answers provided. Hopefully, by introducing these questions, practitioners, policy makers, and scholars will be motivated to search for common meanings for the concept, philosophy, or slogan. If questions like those posed in this paper are not addressed seriously and soon, active living as a concept, as a movement, or as a slogan may become a fad, thereby achieving nothing more than an intermittent degree of visibility similar to that of the "wellness" movement that emerged in the mid-1980s.

Active living as a concept will not survive if it lacks a precise, commonly accepted definition, if it cannot be operationalized and measured precisely and consistently, or if it cannot be located within an existing or reformulated paradigm of health and activity promotion that involves such related concepts as habitual physical activity, fitness, and health (Bouchard, Shephard, Stephens, Sutton, & McPherson, 1990). It will also fail if its policy relevance within the larger domain of health promotion is unclear, and if its usefulness as a slogan is unclear or proves to be ineffectual. More generally, the following are questions that merit further discussion and debate:

- Are we merely placing "old wine (i.e., total fitness) in a new bottle" as part of a new communication plan for the 1990s?
- Is the idea sufficiently understood and entrenched in our vocabulary that it will survive a change in government or in the leadership within the fitness or health promotion community?
- How can we communicate with others if a variety of meanings or perceptions exist about the term?
- Can the use of the term or the adoption of the philosophy or rhetoric lead to a meaningful change in attitudes, beliefs, values, and behaviors, thereby enhancing lifestyles and the quality of life?
- Will the term be adopted internationally, or is there something uniquely Canadian about the idea, as has been suggested by references to active living as a "Canadian cultural trademark"?
- To what extent, and in what way, does the term imply some minimum or maximum level of physical activity?
- Who are the stakeholders? Does the concept belong to the fitness community, the health promotion community, or the recreation community?

This critique is written in the spirit of posing and addressing such general questions. Professionals in health, recreation, and physical activity must consider, and then either answer or discard these and related questions. More importantly, both scientists and practitioners have a responsibility to participate fully in the critical analysis of new ideas or concepts rather than passively accept untested ideas and new processes. The objective of this article is to stimulate practitioners, scholars, and policy makers to consider whether and how active living can become a meaningful and useful concept that might contribute to practice, policy, research, and marketing in the domains of physical activity, recreation, and health promotion.

A Conceptual Perspective

Active living, as a concept, represents a smorgasbord of vague ideas and diverse meanings. As presently used, active living is not a "concept" because it lacks a general theoretical basis and a common definition. The term has far too many components or subelements—is it a philosophy, a scientific construct, a policy, a marketing slogan? Contrary to the claim of the Focus on Active Living Secretariat (1992), active living is not "a simple yet compelling and relevant concept." It is not simple. It may be compelling for some, but its use as a relevant and valid concept has not been tested and documented. Is the term any different from a mythical or dream-like lifestyle that might be promoted by the developers of a new upper-middle-class condominium project?

In the early stages of developing and refining concepts, breadth and diversity of opinion and meaning are common and necessary. This may be the stage we are at in 1992 with respect to active living. Ultimately, however, a precise and generally accepted definition must be derived if a concept is to become part of our permanent working vocabulary in science, in policy work, or in practice. Moreover, a definition must be comprehensible and usable by multiple stakeholders—scholars, the media, citizens, public communicators, service delivery and program planners, and policy makers from a variety of related but diverse agencies (e.g., those in health promotion, fitness, and recreation).

It is also essential to derive a precise meaning to determine whether observed behaviors, attitudes, beliefs, or values represent a particular phenomenon. That is, a precise definition is essential to clearly and completely define the attributes of the concept (i.e., both what is included and excluded), to avoid overlap in meaning or measurement with other related constructs (e.g., habitual physical activity, health promotion, fitness, physical recreation, sustainable development, wellness, vitality), and to facilitate reliable and valid measurement on both the individual and societal levels of analysis. This process involves comparing the meaning with well-defined existing concepts, eliminating possible overlap in content, and defining both what is and is not included within the meaning of the new concept. To initiate this critique of the meaning and use of active living, a brief discussion follows of why a thorough and critical process of conceptualization is needed at this time.

What Is a Concept?

Concepts can originate as products of our imagination, by observation and experience, or by logical derivation from a set of existing concepts. However a concept is derived initially, naming it is only the first step toward understanding and using the concept in research, policy, or practice. More important than naming a concept is the process of arriving at a specific meaning so that the concept can be distinguished from other phenomena, thereby facilitating understanding, measurement, and communication. To date, we have not gone much beyond naming a concept that is currently being used in a variety of forums and publications.

By definition, a concept is an abstract term that is used to describe phenomena that resemble each other in important and relevant ways (e.g., gender, VO_2, work). Generally, concepts are the building blocks of theories. Is active living a unique concept or does it include components that are common to existing concepts? Does the concept lead to the development of, or fit into, any existing paradigm, model, or theory?

A concept also needs to be operationalized. If it cannot be defined, it cannot be measured. If a concept cannot be measured in some way, how do we know whether, where, in what way, to what extent, and why the phenomenon is or is not present; whether it represents a universal or specific phenomenon; whether the phenomenon increases, decreases, disappears, or remains stable over time; or whether and in what way (e.g., as an independent, intervening, or dependent variable) the concept is related to other phenomena? Consequently, we need to construct variables to operationalize or measure the concept.

Ideally, variables should be culture free and represent continua (e.g., income). One problem with a term such as active living is that frequently it is viewed as a dichotomous phenomenon (e.g., inactive living vs. active living). To illustrate, the concept *democracy* implies that a political system is either democratic or not democratic, or that it applies only to some societies and at some point in history. Moreover, concepts like democracy can take different meanings in the same society. Ideally then, new concepts should be defined as general variables that can be measured along a continuum, by a single indicator or by multiple indicators. Hence, we should be developing general variables that measure both the quantitative (e.g., degree, frequency, intensity) and the qualitative components of active living, however the concept is ultimately defined. Moreover, if a variable is to be culture free and used globally, it should not be an exclusive Canadian cultural trademark.

What Is Active Living?

To date, many definitions of active living have appeared in a variety of government documents. An examination of these definitions certainly justifies the conclusion of the Secretariat on Active Living that it is an ''umbrella'' term and that it represents an ''open-ended'' approach (Focus on Active Living Secretariat, 1992). A serious flaw in these various statements is the use of definitive language written in the present tense. This implies or assumes that we know what active living is and how

and why it can lead to beneficial outcomes for individuals and for communities. There is no evidence to date that the definitive claims made by the rhetoric in these definitions have been verified. Consequently, the definitional statements constitute nothing more than philosophical statements, popular opinion, government rhetoric, promotional slogans, or dreams. An unquestioning reader of this literature might assume that a magic elixir had been discovered that could eliminate or cure some or all of the ills derived from sedentary living.

A content analysis of these various definitions reveals that they include many general and often unrelated elements or components. When the elements are combined, the definition is too vague, too complex, too comprehensive, and too imprecise to have much utility for practitioners, policy makers, scientists, social marketers, or community animators.

While all of the statements about active living seem to be based on the premise of enhancing the well-being and quality of life of Canadians, the components and mechanisms represent diverse objectives, processes, and dreams. Moreover, in some cases, because the mandates of government agencies vary, specific components are excluded or included for political rather than conceptual reasons. To illustrate, in Ontario, the Ministry of Tourism and Recreation (MTR) is responsible for *recreation* as well as *fitness*. Consequently, in the MTR document on active living, a definition of recreation is provided (''All those things a person or group chooses to do in order to make leisure time more interesting, more enjoyable, and more satisfying''). Since the mandate of MTR includes all forms of recreation, their document indicates that sculpting, playing bridge, watching television, attending picnics, and completing household tasks are examples of appropriate or ideal active living pursuits. Can we conclude that a home with clean windows and a weedless garden is an active living household? Does this MTR definition imply that active living does not or cannot occur at work? In a similar way, agencies with a health promotion mandate introduce or highlight, specific, but different, elements in their definitions of active living.

Turning to the issue of uniqueness and to the possible overlap with existing ideas, any discussion of the meaning of active living must resolve how the term fits with health promotion and with existing terms in the physical activity domain. In some definitions of health promotion, active living can be substituted for the word *health*, and the meaning of the sentence remains unchanged. The question then arises whether the definitions are sufficiently different to justify the existence and continued use of both health promotion and active living? Both concepts place a holistic emphasis on the integration of physical, mental, and social well-being. Is active living a subset of health promotion, or is health promotion a subset of active living? If there is overlap in meaning how can this redundancy be resolved to avoid confusion? Similarly, as a social movement, how does active living differ from "Health for All," "Wellness," "Sustainable Development," "Life—Be in It," or "Total Quality Living"? Thus, we must ask: What is new about active living, and how does it differ from previous attempts to encourage healthier lifestyles?

To address these questions we must decide not only what is to be included in the concept, but also what is to be excluded. Is passive leisure (e.g., reading) a component of active living? To what extent should affective and cognitive components be included, and how are these to be weighted in comparison to the behavioral or physical component? To illustrate, Fitness Canada implies that physical activity is the essential and primary element; however, the Ontario Ministry of Tourism and Recreation and the Health Promotion Directorate imply that all three elements are necessary and that one is not more important than the others. Similarly, to what extent does the active living concept include or exclude such related lifestyle factors as dietary habits, smoking, drinking, stress management, or driver safety? Other questions that come to mind from this type of analysis include the following:

- Should work be included, or are we discussing the nonwork segment of our lives?
- Will the concept have a similar meaning among a variety of age, gender, social class, language, ethnic, or regional groups?
- Should the concept emphasize the qualitative or quantitative facets of active living, or both?
- How is the concept related to existing concepts that are grounded in more established health, exercise, physical activity, or fitness paradigms?

The answers to these questions, once derived and generally accepted, will have profound implications for the precise measurement of the concept.

An Empirical Perspective

Total Quality Management (TQM) is one recent approach to evaluating the extent to which a business or organization is successful in achieving its objectives. An essential element of this approach is the use of *benchmarking*, on a variety of measures, to identify where we began and what we achieved at subsequent points in time. This process of benchmarking provides quantifiable and defensible answers as to whether a business is successful and whether customers are being served satisfactorily. We need to develop ways to benchmark active living if the term is to survive and become a useful tool in the measurement of progress in our fight against sedentary living and unhealthy lifestyles.

Whereas a variety of nominal definitions have been proposed, virtually no attention has been given to why or how active living might be measured should we wish to know whether the phenomenon is present, to what extent it is present, where it is or is not present, and whether over time there is or is not a change in knowledge, attitudes, and behaviors that reflect the onset and continuation of a healthy lifestyle. From a research or program and policy evaluation perspective the term is fuzzy and ill-defined. Consequently, we are unable to establish baseline measures, to measure changes, or to initiate effective or meaningful needs assessment studies. We also are unable to evaluate the relevance or effectiveness of programs or policies designed to promote or enhance active living among individuals or within communities, regions, or nations. And we are unable to relate the concept within a larger theoretical framework to important and similar concepts.

We still do not fully understand the relationships between exercise, fitness, physical activity, and health where more precisely defined concepts and reasonably valid and reliable measurement techniques are available to scholars and practitioners. Therefore, is another concept such as active living needed, especially if we are unsure of its meaning, its measurement, and its relationship to a larger theoretical or conceptual framework? If the answer is yes, an explicit operational definition must be derived and validated. Some questions to address in the process of arriving at a valid and reliable operational definition for benchmarking follow:

- Can the concept be used as both an independent (the process) and a dependent (the product) variable?
- Should and can the concept be used at both the micro (individual) and macro (group, society) level of anlaysis?
- Should the concept be measured as a unidimensional or a multidimensional phenomenon?
- How can the subjective and objective components of the concept be measured and weighted?
- Must physical activity be included and, if so, what is the minimal acceptable level or type of involvement?
- When using the concept, what individual factors (e.g., psychological, biological, social, medical) or societal factors (e.g., economic, political, environmental, cultural) should be controlled as possible confounding factors?
- If cognitive and emotional components are included, how are they to be measured and weighted in comparison with the behavioral component?
- How does the concept, as a dependent variable, relate to such existing and potentially related dependent measures as well-being, quality of life, degree of independence, degree of physical activity involvement, life satisfaction, Total Quality Living, or morale? Does active living duplicate elements within some of these related constructs? If so, which ones?
- How can the concept be operationalized to measure low levels of active living as well as variations

over time in the amount, degree, type, intensity, quality, or meaning of active living?

A Policy Perspective

Within the larger framework of health, fitness, and activity promotion, it is not clear how, why, or where active living fits into public policy. Is it part of or separate from the healthy public policy movement? A well-articulated discussion of the meaning and relevance of active living within a broader public policy statement is urgently needed. Policy makers, program personnel, and communicators should not have to wade through a morass of rhetoric in search of valid and useful knowledge.

In an era of shrinking resources, public and private sector funds are more likely to be generated and allocated for programs or research when there is definitive knowledge that the money will make a difference and that the programs and research are unique and essential. As well, funds are more likely to be allocated in response to the demands of visible and vocal pressure groups (e.g., those who act on behalf of the chronically unemployed, abused children, seniors, natives). Thus, does the current thrust toward promoting and facilitating active living constitute a sufficiently persuasive argument to justify the creation of new resources or the reallocation of existing scarce resources to ensure that policies are implemented and programs are effective, especially when active living must compete with "Health for All," "Vitality," and other programs promoting healthy lifestyle changes? Is an effective lobby group likely to emerge that will demand that resources be allocated for the promotion of active living lifestyles within some or all segments of the population?

Since those involved with the active living movement are not proposing to invoke mandatory changes in behavior (e.g., as we would for drug or alcohol use and abuse, or for the use of seat belts), it is unlikely that we can legislate conformity to active living. Unlike some aspects of health promotion, as a social change strategy we are involved in designing policies and programs to change voluntary rather than involuntary behavior.

At present, little or no research demonstrates that active living leads to cost savings in health care or to a higher quality of life for individuals or a community. That is, impact studies have not been completed, especially on a longitudinal basis. Moreover, evidence is lacking to demonstrate that active living can have or is having an impact in all regions, or that it can reach or is reaching members of marginal groups who are less physically active.

In general, being physically active is still not highly valued or practiced within most segments of society, especially among certain ethnic, racial, income, or occupational groups. Consequently, the level of awareness and understanding about active living needs to be heightened among politicians; among business, industry, and union leaders in the private sector; and among the general population. For the most part we still rely on generic mass communication programs to disseminate messages about health and active living. Alternatively, specific resources and unique programs are needed to reach marginal groups (e.g., the unemployed, women, ethnic minorities, older adults, the disabled), perhaps via empowerment at the individual and group level.

Most effective public policies involve acceptance and cooperation by a variety of stakeholders within the public and private sector. To date, the promotion of active living has been virtually the exclusive domain of one relatively small government agency, along with its affiliated partners in the provinces. To have a lasting and widespread effect, government agencies must work more closely with the private sector, with public communication personnel, and with the education, health, and community recreation segments of the public sector. For example, bonuses could be paid to employees who can document consistent active living habits (e.g., walking to work, climbing stairs instead of using an elevator, walking at lunch). Alternatively, disincentives (e.g., charging higher health or life insurance premiums for those classified as inactive; requiring a greater share of health benefits to be paid by the nonactive employee) could be invoked for those who are not active, who smoke, or who adhere to unhealthy dietary practices. Similarly, grants to municipal governments or to school boards could be based on the demonstrated effectiveness of active living programs or on documented growth in the number of active children, adolescents, and adults in the community.

In summary, effective programs and policies will be developed, initiated, and adopted only if clearly defined concepts and valid and clearly written research reports and policies are available. Only well-defined knowledge will be used in practice; vague statements and rhetoric will not be used appropriately and effectively, if at all.

A Social Marketing Perspective

Social marketing seeks to initiate changes in thinking and behavior by using marketing tools and techniques to promote ideas that have some significant potential social benefits. Thus, in health and activity promotion, three types of social products are usually marketed: beliefs, attitudes, and values. To be successful, the social marketing process must establish precise and measurable objectives and must measure whether the objectives have been met. That is, it must measure whether attitudes, values, or beliefs have changed and persist, and whether changes in behavior have occurred, in what direction, and to what degree.

In a 1991 address to the Australian Heart Foundation Heart Week Conference, A. Salmon stated that active living is a symbol of a national campaign to promote regular physical activity. Maybe active living is nothing more than a media symbol or slogan similar to "Just do it," "Quality is job one," or "Drink milk for health." At the minimum, then, a phrase has been created that serves as a slogan to encourage citizens to adopt what for many is an unknown lifestyle. Attempts to identify prospective participants must be initiated by first marketing and then selling active living. However, to be successful, the idea must be clearly defined and the benefits or advantages of the process or idea must be known, understood, and accepted. This is an extremely difficult task when dealing with a social idea such as active living, which is intangible, variable, unknown, and undefined.

Effective marketing also involves an understanding of the competition. Today, both the marketers and the prospective consumers may be confused as to how active living differs from wellness, from fitness (which most have rejected in the past), from the Heart Health Initiative, or from the new vitality promotional program. The consumer is increasingly bombarded with messages promoting healthier and more active lifestyles. Active living is yet another of these messages. In short, we need to determine whether active living is the most effective social idea to market within the health promotion world to realize permanent attitudinal and behavioral change.

To effectively market a new product, buyer readiness states must be understood (McDougall, Kotler, & Armstrong, 1992). Is the public ready for yet another activity-related idea or product? Moreover, clear and realistic objectives of the amount of change that is desired and realistic should be identified. That is, are we hoping to convert 10%, 20%, 40%, or 80% of the population to active living lifestyles? Furthermore, which segments of the population should receive the greatest attention in terms of the social marketing of this new idea?

To illustrate the difficulty of establishing such marketing objectives, note that most people respond in surveys that their health is good or excellent. Given this perception of excellence, attempts to change beliefs, attitudes, and behaviors is a hard sell, especially when an innate need or value is not recognized or accepted.

In short, we must fully understand all factors that may influence the amount and degree of cognitive and behavioral change. Consequently, is it a realistic goal to expect that the active living message will be received and adopted by all marginal groups? Or should priorities and unique strategies be established so that active living is promoted within specific marginal groups? If so, how are these marketing priorities to be established so that other marginal or disadvantaged groups do not argue that they are not being served?

Early in any marketing strategy, it must be determined whether the promotional techniques are being received and whether any degree of change, quantitative and qualitative, that has resulted since the initiation of a promotional campaign is permanent or temporary. Can we, as a result of the active living movement, document and evaluate changes in beliefs, attitudes, or behavioral intentions; in the amount of interaction with others about active living; in type, frequency, or level of activity involvement; or in the desired outcomes of active living (e.g., a higher quality of life, improved well-being)? Thus, before a marketing plan is formulated and evaluated, and before any of these marketing-oriented questions are addressed, a more precise definition of active living and appropriate measurement tools must be derived.

To illustrate further, in comparison with health promotion strategies involving drug use, impaired driving, tobacco use, and healthy eating, active living lacks a focus and a method whereby a change in beliefs, attitudes, or behavior can be measured, and whereby any change in behavior or attitudes can be attributed to the onset of a promotional campaign.

Conclusion

In a recent issue of *Health Promotion*, O'Connor and Petrasovits describe the three main pillars of the Heart Health Initiative as

> *a solid science base*, which has served to define the problem and point to solutions; *a policy*, which articulates agreed goals and strategies for action; and *the community* which, as the focus for heart health programs, defines their content and ensures their sustainability at the local level. (1992, p. 2)

In the case of both active living and the Heart Health Initiative, a fourth pillar, *social marketing*, should be added to realize changes in behavior and attitudes.

At all stages in the evolution of an active living movement, representatives of all four pillars must communicate, collaborate, and understand the goals and needs of the other groups if the term is to survive. Finally, as a word of caution to all stakeholders who intend to use the term active living, remember that only precisely defined terms and valid knowledge based on objective and reliable measurement techniques will be used and survive over time. Vague concepts and rhetoric cannot be used effectively to understand or change behavior, and such terms ultimately have a short lifespan. Herein lies the immediate challenge to all stakeholders: Time and creative energy must be devoted to a critical examination and resolution of the ambiguity and rhetoric surrounding the meaning, measurement, use, and effectiveness of active living as a concept, as a variable, and as a slogan, regardless of whether the ultimate use is for research, policy, or practice.

References

Action Sport. (1984). *The second annual report of the project directorate, 1983-84*. Birmingham, England: The Sports Council.

Bouchard, C., Shephard, R.J., Stephens, T., Sutton, J.R., & McPherson, B.D. (Eds.) (1990). *Exercise, fitness, and health: A consensus of current knowledge*. Champaign, IL: Human Kinetics.

Edwards, P. (1990). *A healthy city is an active city*. Copenhagen, Denmark: WHO Euro Healthy Cities Office.

Focus on Active Living Secretariat. (1992). *Active living: A compelling and relevant concept*. Ottawa, ON: Active Living Secretariat.

McDougall, G., Kotler, P., & Armstrong, G. (1992). *Marketing*. Toronto, ON: Prentice Hall Canada.

O'Connor, B., & Petrasovits, A. (1992). Science, policy and community: The three pillars of heart health. *Health Promotion*, **30**(4), 2-4.

Rigg, M. (1986). *Action sport: Community sports leadership in the inner cities—summary report*. Prepared for the Sports Council by the Policy Studies Institute, England.

Salmon, A. (1991). Address to the Australian Heart Foundation Heart Week Conference.

35.4

Active Living: A Critical Examination

Peggy Edwards

Most practitioners have little trouble with the idea of active living. It is a democratic idea that is concerned with equity, values, personal choice, and healthy, sustainable living. Practitioners are concerned about what to do with the concept. They are asking questions such as

- How is it different from what I've been doing all along? Is it just old wine in a new bottle?
- What does it mean to the farmer or fisherman who is already active on the job?
- What does it mean to the way I do my job as a recreation professional, as a public health nurse, as a teacher, as a fitness professional, or as a health educator?
- How does active living fit within the broad sociopolitical way we now view health and health promotion?
- How do I market this vague concept? It was a lot easier to tell people they need to be active for 15 minutes, 3 times a week.

These are tough questions that raise more questions, both for scientists and policy makers.

How is active living different, in a practical sense, from the physical activity and leisure programs we've always done? In some cases, there may be very little difference; the task may be to build on the good work already done and to look for new ways to broaden our reach. But there are some important variations, both in what active living is and how we might go about encouraging it.

- **Active living puts the emphasis on daily activities, including the energy expended in work and chores**. Despite this emphasis, most of what we know about the social and psychological benefits of physical activity relate to leisure-time activity. So, I challenge the researchers: What can you tell us about the active living needs and benefits for a farmer or a fisherman? I'm not asking about his physical needs; we know that he needs to compensate for repetitive work and heavy lifting. But will leisure-time activity improve his quality of life? And does it matter whether the activity is playing cards or jogging?

- **Active living focuses on moderation**. From a broad population health perspective, the work of Steven Blair and others may be the most important research we have seen in decades (Blair, Kohl, Paffenbarger, Cooper, & Gibbons, 1989). What Blair's research and the active living concept says to public health is simply this: The greatest public good will come from moving the sedentary individual into moderate activity—the equivalent of 20 minutes of brisk walking a day.

In practical terms, this means the public health professional's role in active living must be to advocate and facilitate active living opportunities for those who are not yet active—disadvantaged families, some immigrants and refugees, certain groups of blue-collar male workers, isolated seniors, and people who are mentally and physically challenged.

- **Active living emphasizes personal choice, letting people decide for themselves how they want to live actively**. Too often in the past, physical activity programs and leisure services have been forced on people, because professionals think it will improve people's lives. We label it empowerment and pat ourselves on the back. In reality, we can never empower someone else, because in doing so we strip them of their ability to choose. The job of professionals is to facilitate group development and to serve as a resource to groups who are empowering themselves.

This kind of approach—call it health promotion or community development—has been lacking in most traditional recreation and physical activity programming. Yet when it is tried, we learn a lot about the needs and aspirations of the people we work with. For example, last year in Toronto, a group of community centers asked teenage girls what kinds of activities they wanted to be involved in. The young women identified a "girls night out in the gym" as a preferred activity. But many said they would not attend because it was unsafe to walk home from the community center at night and many had child care responsibilities—caring for their own children or for siblings while their mothers worked.

Studies repeatedly show that youths want to take leadership roles in active living (Canadian Council on Children and Youth, 1985). Studies repeatedly show that children want to play sports for fun, that they fear failure in athletic competition, and that they drop out because their self-efficacy is so low, they believe they will fail (see Chapter 12). So why do the majority of schools still have a physical education curriculum that stresses traditional, competitive sports? Why do we have six-tiered competitive leagues that sit 7-year-olds on the bench and are dominated by adults who believe in winning at all costs?

- **Active living is different because it talks about values**. It encourages people to value the social, physical, mental, emotional, and spiritual aspects of active living.

Some of the architects of the active living concept like to compare it to a widely accepted definition of health "as a state of social, physical, and mental well-being." This is good but it is also out of date. In 1986, the World Health Organization Ottawa Charter on Health Promotion redefined health as "the ability of an individual or group to change and cope with their environment so as to realize their aspirations and needs" (WHO, 1986). They went on to define health promotion as the process of "enabling people to take control over and improve their health."

These broad sociopolitical definitions of health are a far cry from simply the absence of disease. They encompass individuals and groups taking control and realizing their positive aspirations for an improved quality of life. They take responsibility for health from the medical domain and place it squarely in the midst of sociopolitical action. Active living advocates can learn a lot from the experiences of

health promoters. The active living campaign is now where the antismoking campaign was 10 years ago. We had the health evidence and it was time for sociocultural and political action. We now have more than enough evidence about the health benefits of active living. Let's stop defining it and start doing it.

We know that high-quality, daily physical activity improves children's health, alertness, and in most cases their academic performance (Zitzelsberg, 1991). So why is Quality Daily Physical Education (QDPE) not the norm? And why have fewer than 400 schools qualified for the QDPE Award sponsored by the Canadian Association of Health, Physical Education, and Recreation? And why did the Ottawa Board of Education recently deal with a 5-week teachers' strike by canceling all extra-curricular physical activity? Because parents and active living leaders in the community have not posted their values.

The Canada Life Assurance Company has a controlled, precise, 10-year study that links an employee fitness program to reduced absenteeism, reduced staff turnover, and improved employee health. The improvements more than pay for the cost of the program (Walker & Cox, 1991). The Campbell's survey indicates that people with active living opportunities at work were most likely to maintain their activity levels (Canadian Fitness and Lifestyle Institute, 1990). Canada's 1985 Health Promotion survey shows that 80% of Canadians think that health should be promoted in the workplace. It also indicates that poor working women who need it the most are the least likely to receive active living and health promotion programs at work (Health and Welfare Canada, 1989). So why is it still a struggle to convince our own workplaces to enact active living policies and programs?

We know that about 70% of Canadians would like to walk or cycle to work. If half the workers in Canada who lived within walking distance of work left their cars at home, their efforts would save about 22 million liters of gasoline each year (Hawthorne, 1989). So why dont we have more bike lanes and walking paths? Why is there no political will to restrict the number of cars in our city centers? Because we've spent more time proving our point than we've spent in advocating for public policies that make the healthy choices the easy choices.

My closing message to scientists is this: Stop qualifying the overwhelmingly positive data on the relationship between psychological and social well-being and active living. Let's tell the public that what they know in their hearts is true. Give us more research on the relationship between activity and social well-being. Reach out to the huge body of literature in anthropology and the social sciences that will teach us more about how social support affects well-being.

I urge policy makers and practitioners to think broadly about what influences the quality of life of individuals and communities. It doesn't matter whether you start with active living, health promotion, fitness, or sustainable development. If your mutual goal is to enable people to improve their quality of life, collaboration is the only answer. If you want active living to become part of the culture, share it. Don't capitalize it or insist that you are the only ones that can determine whether a certain approach fits your definition. Let it go and work together to make it happen.

John McNight, a community developer from Chicago, said, "Let's have less studies and more stories." I know that everyone in this room has stories to tell about projects and personal experiences that demonstrate the potential of active living. Let's hear more of these stories—both the successes and the failures. Let's learn from each other about the practical ways to make active living a reality.

One last thing. Let's all learn to lighten up! Active living works because it is positive and fun. People swim, dance, walk, or whatever because active living improves the quality of their lives. Active all our lives; you had better believe it!

References

Blair, S., Kohl, H., Paffenbarger, R., Cooper, K., & Gibbons, L. (1989). Physical fitness and all-cause mortality: A prospective study of healthy men and women. *Journal of the American Medical Association*, **262**, 2395-2437.

Canadian Council on Children and Youth. (1985). *Choices and challenges: A status report on youth physical activity programs in Canada*. Ottawa: Author.

Canadian Fitness and Lifestyle Research Institute. (1990). *The well-being of Canadians: Highlights of the 1988 Campbell's Survey*. Ottawa: Author.

Hawthorne, W. (1989). *Why Ontarians walk; why Ontarians don't walk more*. Toronto: Energy Probe Research Foundation.

Health and Welfare Canada. (1989). *The active health report*. Ottawa: Author.

Walker, J., & Cox, M. (1991). *Canada Life 10: Corporate fitness ten years after*. Toronto: Canada Life Assurance Company.

World Health Organization. (1986). *Ottawa charter on health promotion*. Ottawa: Canadian Public Health Association.

Zitzelsberg, L. (1991). *Physical activity and the child: Review and synthesis*. Ottawa: Government of Canada.

36

Challenge to an Active Future: Limitations of our Current Knowledge Base

Roy J. Shephard

Except for the convinced Calvinist, the future is, almost by definition, indeterminate, and it is correspondingly difficult to suggest what may be the challenges facing the next generation of investigators promoting an active future. On the other hand, the less-inhibited individual may find the assignment relatively easy, since it is impossible to prove that even the most outrageous predictions are incorrect.

Among the issues that I will discuss are methods of program assessment, the magnitude of genetic influences, the optimum type of program, the dose of exercise needed to obtain maximum benefit, quality of life issues, the influence of age and lifestyle upon both programming and response, opportunity cost as a significant element in program compliance, and the potential of programs to contain health care costs.

Program Assessment: Process or Outcome?

Evaluation is an essential process in refining exercise and lifestyle programs, but unfortunately the tools needed for this purpose are still in their infancy. The traditional approach is to look at process when a program is first introduced and to test outcome responses later.

Activity as the Process Variable

In terms of the basic model of physical activity, fitness, and health underlying this conference, the measure of process is plainly physical activity. We might examine the average level of physical activity achieved in the targeted community, or we might note the proportion of the population who meet some minimum health objective in terms of their average weekly activity. In the case of a work-site program, activity could be assessed from records of class attendance, and in the case of a communitywide initiative, reliance might be placed on questionnaire responses. The latter are commonly validated against physiological or biomechanical monitors in a subsample of the population or are accepted as giving "reasonable" information because of an association between responses and outcome measures such as body fatness or physical working capacity.

Class attendance seems at first inspection a relatively reliable index of process. An increasing number of major exercise facilities are installing computer terminals where class participants can log the activities they have undertaken at each exercise session. Unfortunately, the sophistication of a modern computer does not compensate for those who forget to log their activities, nor does it allow for participants who overestimate the time they have actually been active. Finally, such indexes cannot assess clinically important possibilities such as a compensating suppression of previous patterns of leisure activity because of class participation or a stimulation of interest in a healthy lifestyle that inspires participation in exercise outside of the facility that is being evaluated.

Physical activity questionnaires vary in complexity from a few very simple questions to detailed activity inventories that require several hours to complete. Testing very similar samples of the North American population, different authors have suggested that the proportion of active adults ranges from 9% to 78% (Shephard, 1986c). This discrepancy suggests that most if not all of the available questionnaires lack validity.

One of the problems limiting further progress is that most epidemiological tools such as pedometers and actometers that are used to verify questionnaires have a very limited reliability and validity. If the individual under evaluation engages in a single standard activity such as steady walking, such meters can provide an index of the number of paces taken per day. But with more diverse activity patterns, the counters may record zero, one, or two for each movement the subject makes.

Oxygen consumption data offer a reasonably valid indication of the intensity of physical activity, provided the subject is able to use a facepiece or mouthpiece while performing the tasks under investigation. But because data are recorded for only a few minutes, subjects may accelerate their pace to impress the observer.

Physical Fitness as the Outcome Variable

With a more mature program, interest turns to outcome. Unfortunately, it seems almost equally difficult to obtain reliable and valid population data on the outcome of fitness and lifestyle programs.

Many physicians and some other health practitioners have been content to note changes of body mass. Such data is not very helpful in evaluating a particular regimen, because any program-related decrease of body fat tends to be confounded with increases of lean tissue.

Changes of skinfold thickness can be assessed fairly readily at a single program site, but because of interobserver differences in skinfold readings, it is difficult to assess the decrease of subcutaneous fat in large-scale, communitywide investigations.

Gains of maximal oxygen intake can be evaluated by direct treadmill testing in small subsamples of a population, but such tests are too costly for large-scale application. Despite repeated efforts to upgrade field tests such as the Canadian Home Fitness Test, there is still no reliable and unequivocal field measure of aerobic fitness.

Challenge One. The first challenge to future investigators is thus to develop reliable, valid, and internationally standardized methods of measuring both process (the adoption of physical activity) and physiological outcomes (the optimization of body composition and increase of aerobic fitness) in large samples of the population.

Magnitude of Genetic Effect

P.O. Åstrand (1967) suggested in the first conference of this series that those who wish to excel in either athletic competition or its physiological correlates such as aerobic fitness must choose their parents wisely. The magnitude of the genetic contribution to the exercise and health interaction is an important issue, not only for the sport scientist but also for the health practitioner. If Åstrand was correct in his deliberately provocative statement, the major emphasis of health promotion should shift from exercise programming to genetic counseling!

Despite the careful research of exercise geneticists such as Claude Bouchard (1990), we are far from resolving this problem. Estimates of the relative contributions of environment and inheritance, and their interactions, to the various components of fitness and lifestyle seem inherently unstable. Within just a few years one investigator has published almost diametrically opposed estimates of inherited effects (see Shephard, 1982, for examples).

In the past, reliance has been placed on indirect approaches to the assessment of heritability, comparing fitness levels in relatives of varying closeness. However, such analyses presuppose, without any strong justification, that methodological error, initial fitness status, environmental influences, and even conspiracies to outwit rigid experimental conditions are independent of the closeness of familial relationships.

Hope is now pinned on the human genome project. As the entire DNA sequence in human chromosomes becomes identified, it may prove possible to tease out the particular gene combinations that contribute to human activity, fitness, and health and to assess those responses that are more susceptible to environment than to genotype. One continuing obstacle to progress will be the complexity of the genotype responsible for fitness phenotypes.

Challenge Two. The second challenge to investigators is thus to obtain stable and consistent estimates of the relative extent to which habitual activity patterns, inherent levels of fitness, and the response to training programs are determined by genetic rather than environmental influences. Where possible, demonstrated genetic influences should also be linked to specific gene configurations.

The Optimum Program

To obtain any postulated health benefits, target populations must be offered fitness and lifestyle programs that are optimal in both type and rigor.

Early exercise scientists worked in relative isolation from those concerned with other facets of lifestyle, offering strictly fitness and physical activity programs, usually of the aerobic type. But in recent years, the trend has been to offer a package of lifestyle initiatives, including diet and obesity clinics, smoking withdrawal programs, treatment for alcoholism and drug dependency, and stress relief. Commonly, individual clients can select those items most appealing to them.

The rationale for a broadening of program content is often pragmatic rather than scientific. All of the lifestyle initiatives are regarded as necessary in a given community. It is thus perceived as cheaper and administratively more effective to combine programs in a single facility under a single coordinator.

However, there remains a need to check the extent to which the various health behaviors are mutually reinforcing, using sophisticated techniques of behavioral modeling. It is often argued that exercise helps smoking withdrawal, but in practice there seems remarkably little evidence to support this hypothesis. Future studies need to distinguish any enhancement of smoking withdrawal by endurance-type activities from a possible adverse response to participation in sports where the primary motive seems increased social contact, competition, risk, or vertiginous stimulation. Likewise, theoretical reasons can be advanced as to why an increase of physical activity might help the reduction of body fat, conserving lean tissue, but there remains a need for careful studies of changes in resting metabolic rate and body composition, comparing dieters with those who engage in combined exercise and diet therapy.

Challenge Three. The third challenge to investigators is thus to establish whether there are favorable or unfavorable interactions between exercise and other possible components of a multifaceted lifestyle program, setting such information within the context of modern behavioral theory.

Dose–Response Relationship

The dose of exercise that is recommended must be sufficiently rigorous to offer effective therapy, but not so intense or sustained that it provokes cardiovascular emergencies, musculoskeletal injuries, or psychological discouragement in those who are unable to fulfill the required prescription.

Given that many national and regional governments have been encouraging an increase of physical activity for almost 30 years, it is remarkable that there is still little agreement on the relationship between exercise dose and resultant health benefit. Both the American College of Sports Medicine (1990) and Fitness Canada (O'Brien-Jewett, 1990) have recently shifted their focus away from the traditional recommendation of very intensive aerobic effort to more moderate but sustained bouts of physical activity as part of a general search for "wellness."

However, we still do not know whether there is a minimum training threshold, or whether benefits show a linear or a probit-type relationship to increased doses of exercise. Much more work on the mechanisms of health benefit is needed before we can resolve this question and make a definitive recommendation of exercise dose to the general public.

If the program objective is to control body mass, can we simply apply the law of the conservation of energy, assuming that exercise programs of equal total energy demand will achieve equal results? Or will program response be influenced by differences in the relative metabolism of carbohydrate and fat, differential suppression or stimulation of appetite, differences in postexercise stimulation of metabolism, and compensatory metabolic reactions to a negative energy balance?

If the intent is to develop aerobic fitness, it is reasonably well established that the rate of training response varies in some manner with the intensity of conditioning, considered in relation to the individual's initial level of fitness. But most investigators have wanted to publish their results within 12 weeks. It thus remains unclear whether an equal response can be achieved more safely and with a higher compliance rate if a more moderate regimen is pursued for a longer period per session over a longer total period of time.

If the intent of the program is to relieve stress and anxiety, even less is known about an appropriate intensity of effort. Is there a need for the vigorous effort likely to induce a secretion of endorphins and neurogenic amines? Is there a need to increase arousal by proprioceptive stimulation, or is it preferable to engage in gentle, relaxing activity in an agreeable environment?

Unfortunately for the investigator, a wide variety of therapeutic benefits are sought from exercise, and it is unlikely that all demand the same type of regimen. There are also many possible combinations of intensity, frequency, duration, and type of activity program with such demographic variables as the age, sex, and initial fitness of the participants. Resolution of the dose–response question thus becomes a complex multifactorial problem. It is unclear whether a definitive experiment could ever be organized. This would call for a large subject pool that was prepared to conform closely to individually prescribed patterns of exercise for a long period. Investigators would have to be willing to monitor the progress of each participant for an equally long time, revising prescriptions upward regularly to sustain the intensity of training.

Challenge Four. Investigators thus face a major challenge to determine the average dose–response relationship for the various therapeutic benefits sought from exercise. They must further evaluate variations of response, testing subjects of both sexes at various ages and in various initial levels of health. A definitive experiment would involve assembling a large pool of volunteers who were willing to be assigned randomly to one of a variety of exercise regimens. The experiment also would present the challenge of sustaining the enthusiasm of such volunteers over a period of several years.

Quality of Life Issues

The cross-sectional data of Paffenbarger and associates (1986) suggest that regular endurance activity leading to a weekly energy expenditure of about 8 MJ will extend lifespan. The gain is about 2 years if exercise is begun at age 35, but it decreases to about 0.4 years if the program is not begun until age 75. Although the added longevity is a useful practical reward, cynics have objected that much of the additional 2 years must be spent in the mechanics of jogging. If such activity is enjoyed, the time that is allocated to the program will be seen as rewarding, rather than as a hardship. But if the exerciser regards jogging as an unpleasant duty, then the added lifespan may be valued no more than a few extra weeks that could have been won by living in the surgical ward of a hospital.

It is here that the assessment of quality of life becomes a major issue. Typically, a 35-year-old person may live for a further 45 years. During nine of those years the individual suffers from partial dependency and during the final year he or she becomes almost totally dependent. Irrespective of their age, many people claim that exercise makes them feel better. Let us make an arbitrary supposition that the exercise-related improvement in quality of life as a middle-aged adult is 10%. Then for the period from 35 to 70 years of age there is a 35 × 10% or a 3.5 year gain in quality-adjusted years of life (QAY). During the period when others are becoming partially dependent, the active individual may show a 30% advantage over a sedentary person, equivalent to 9 × 30%, or another 2.7 year gain in QAY, and during the final year of life this advantage may rise to 50%, equivalent to a further 0.5 year gain in QAY. Rather than the calendar gain of 2 years, the total advantage of the active person over a sedentary contemporary is thus 2 + 3.5 + 2.7 + 0.5, or 8.7 QAY.

The numbers indicate the potential importance of the quality of life issue, but unfortunately we have as yet no reliable data on the average "quality" that people assign to various states of health. Moreover, although there is a little evidence to suggest that dependency is reduced and life quality is enhanced by habitual physical activity (Shephard & Montelpare, 1988), the extent of this benefit still requires much more careful quantitation.

Challenge Five. Investigators should thus establish the quality that large samples of the population assign to various states of health and should then determine the likelihood that selected patterns of activity will increase the proportion of individuals attaining a higher quality of life at various ages. In particular, there is an urgent need to explore how far regular physical activity maintains cardiovascular function, muscular strength, and flexibility, thus reducing the likelihood of partial or total dependency in old age.

Influence of Age and Lifestyle on Response

The Growing Child

In children, perhaps the most important unanswered question of the exercise scientist is whether participation in a required program of physical activity at school has a positive or a negative influence on exercise habits and other facets of lifestyle as an adult. Many physical educators continue to press for required daily school programs of physical education. One justification for this demand is that children currently show a decrease of aerobic power (expressed per kilogram of body mass) over the period of school attendance (Bailey, 1974). This apparent change has been interpreted as a deterioration of fitness, although it is not seen if data are expressed as a quadratic function of standing height. Investigators therefore still need to resolve the vexing theoretical question as to how measures of aerobic fitness should be standardized for interindividual differences in body size (Shephard, 1982).

There is some evidence that preexisting exercise habits have a positive influence on current exercise behavior (Godin & Shephard, 1990). But there is also a great deal of anecdotal material suggesting that many adults recall with loathing the physical education they received as children and stop all physical activity as soon as they escape from the school's exercise requirement (Ilmarinen & Rutenfranz, 1980).

A third unresolved issue is whether adolescent activity can induce gains that cannot be duplicated if the program is initiated at a later age.

Challenge Six. There thus remains a need to decide the appropriate method of standardizing response variables in a growing child, to determine whether the gains realized from training as an adolescent can be attained equally well by initiating exercise at an older age, and whether participation in required school exercise programs has a positive or a negative effect on exercise habits and other facets of personal lifestyle as an adult.

Responses of the Elderly

There continue to be occasional reports suggesting that the aging of biological functions such as aerobic power is greatly slowed by regular exercise (Kasch, Wallace, Van Camp, & Verity, 1988). It is also claimed that active individuals with a healthy myocardium can compensate for an age-related decrease of peak heart rate by an increase of cardiac stroke volume (Weisfeldt, Gerstenblith, & Lakatta, 1985). Such findings probably arise because study participants have superimposed a slow training response upon a largely unaltered intrinsic rate of aging. Nevertheless, the issue of a potential retardation of aging is of sufficient importance to merit careful examination in populations that are known to have maintained habitual activity for many years (Kavanagh, Mertens, Matosevic, Shephard, & Evans, 1989).

Another important and unresolved issue is the relative magnitude of the training response in young and old individuals. Factors such as a slowing of protein synthesis might suggest that conditioning would proceed more slowly in an old person, but in many older individuals this disadvantage is probably offset by a low initial level of fitness (Shephard, 1987, 1990).

Finally, many older people have concerns about the safety of exercising, and there is a need to confirm the observation of Vuori, Suurnäkki, and Suurnäkki (1982) that the relative risk of exercising is less at an age of 50 to 69 years than at 40 to 49 years.

Challenge Seven. Longitudinal studies should thus compare the rate of aging between sedentary individuals and athletes who maintain a constant pattern of moderate physical activity. The relative risks and the relative response to training should also be compared between young and elderly people.

Lifestyle Influences

It is generally assumed that therapeutic benefits will be realized from an enhancement of physical activity, independently of the presence or absence of other risk factors. However, this is not necessarily the case. For example, heavy smokers may be at an increased relative risk of a cardiac catastrophe if they decide to undertake vigorous exercise, and obese individuals may have a higher relative risk of hyperthermia if they exercise in warm conditions.

Challenge Eight. Future investigations should thus examine interactions between exercise response and other features of lifestyle, looking for potential negative as well as positive interactions.

Opportunity Cost as the Key to Compliance

One of the major challenges to the whole concept of exercise therapy is, "Those who know but don't do..." (Fitness Ontario, 1981). The participation rate, even in well-conceived fitness and lifestyle programs, is disappointingly low.

Existing research has established that lack of time is the common excuse for poor compliance with exercise programs (Shephard, 1986a, 1986b). Paradoxically, a simple time inventory suggests that most individuals have 3 to 4 hours of free time per day. But most adults seem unwilling to invest such free time in travel to and from an exercise facility and in pursuing the activity itself. The *opportunity cost* of exercising, in their view, is too high. There is a need to explore what evaluation potential exercisers place upon their free time, to determine whether this differs between those who exercise and those who do not. There is also a need to examine how such costs might be changed by the use of work site rather than community facilities, by altering the amenities associated with a facility, or by incorporating the recommended exercise into everyday active living.

Challenge Nine. Future investigations should thus explore the issue of opportunity cost as a primary barrier to exercise participation, looking at ways in which this cost might be modified.

Containment of Health Care Costs

One of the major hopes of governments is that the support of health promotional programs will contribute to containment of escalating medical costs.

Several short-term studies from Canada and the United States have supported such a suggestion (Shephard, 1989), but given the rapid reduction of medical expenditures observed in these studies, the reasons for the response have been less obvious. Possibly, an improvement of mood has led to a better perceived health and thus a reduced demand for medical services. It has yet to be shown whether such savings continue and increase if the individual continues in an exercise program.

There is also a need to answer several criticisms of economic analyses made by health economists. There remains a need to clarify how much of the enormous cost of treating conditions such as cardiovascular disease is attributable to unwarranted treatment in the final few weeks of a patient's life. Further, irrespective of the age at which most of the cost is incurred, there is a need to document the assumption that current nonparticipants who begin an exercise program will show health benefits equal to those of current participants, that benefits will persist after appropriate discounting of postulated savings, and that any immediate reductions in medical costs will not be offset by longer survival and a resultant need for greater pension payments (Shephard, 1992).

Challenge Ten. The final challenge is thus to complete a much more sophisticated and exhaustive economic analysis that will define the economic effect of enhanced physical activity. Given the importance that government currently attaches to a containment of medical expenditures, this is perhaps the most pressing of future research challenges. Assuming we can demonstrate that exercise programs are a cost-effective method of improving health, such programs will gain much-needed public and governmental support.

References

American College of Sports Medicine. (1990). The recommended quantity and quality of exercise for developing and maintaining cardiorespiratory and muscular fitness in healthy adults. *Medicine and Science in Sports and Exercise,* **22,** 265-274.

Åstrand, P.O. (1967). Concluding remarks. *Canadian Medical Association Journal,* **96,** 907-911.

Bailey, D.A. (1974). Exercise, fitness, and physical education for the growing child. In W.A.R. Orban (Ed.), *Proceedings of National Conference on Fitness and Health* (pp. 13-22). Ottawa: Health & Welfare, Canada.

Bouchard, C. (1990). Discussion: Heredity, fitness, and health. In C. Bouchard, R.J. Shephard, T. Stephens, J. Sutton, & B. McPherson (Eds.), *Exercise, fitness, and health* (pp. 147-154). Champaign, IL: Human Kinetics.

Fitness Ontario. (1981). *Those who know but don't do.* Toronto: Ontario Ministry of Culture and Recreation.

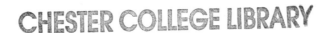

Godin, G., & Shephard, R.J. (1990). Use of attitude–behavior models in exercise promotion. *Sports Medicine*, **10**, 103-121.

Ilmarinen, J., & Rutenfranz, J. (1980). Longitudinal studies of the changes in habitual activity of schoolchildren and working adolescents. In K. Berg & B.O. Eriksson (Eds.), *Children and exercise IX* (pp. 149-159). Baltimore: University Park.

Kasch, F.W., Wallace, J.P., Van Camp, S., & Verity, L. (1988). A longitudinal study of cardiovascular stability in active men aged 45 to 65 years. *Physician and Sportsmedicine*, **16**(1), 117-126.

Kavanagh, T., Mertens, D.J., Matosevic, V., Shephard, R.J., & Evans, B. (1989). Health and aging of Masters athletes. *Clinical Sports Medicine*, **1**, 72-88.

O'Brien-Jewett, B. (1990, February). A framework for active living and health. Paper presented at Commonwealth and International Conference on Physical Education, Sport, Health, Dance, Recreation, and Leisure, Auckland, New Zealand.

Paffenbarger, R., Hyde, R.T., Wing, A.L., & Hsieh, C.C. (1986). Physical activity, all-cause mortality, and longevity of college athletes. *New England Journal of Medicine*, **314**, 605-613.

Shephard, R.J. (1982). *Physical activity and growth*. Chicago: Year Book.

Shephard, R.J. (1986a). *Economic benefits of enhanced fitness*. Champaign, IL: Human Kinetics.

Shephard, R.J. (1986b). *Fitness and health in industry*. Basel, Switzerland: S. Karger A.G.

Shephard, R.J. (1986c). *Fitness of a nation: Lessons from the Canada Fitness Survey*. Basel, Switzerland: S. Karger A.G.

Shephard, R.J. (1987). *Physical activity and aging*. London: Croom Helm.

Shephard, R.J. (1989). Current perspectives on the economics of fitness and sport with particular reference to work-site programs. *Sports Medicine*, **7**, 286-309.

Shephard, R.J. (1990). Exercise for the frail elderly. *Sports Training, Medicine, and Rehabilitation*, **1**, 263-267.

Shephard, R.J. (1992). A critical analysis of work-site fitness programs and their postulated economic benefits. *Medicine and Science in Sports*, **24**, 354-370.

Shephard, R.J., & Montelpare, W. (1988). Geriatric benefits of exercise as an adult. *Journal of Gerontology: Medical Sciences*, **43**, M86-M90.

Vuori, I., Suurnäkki, L., & Suurnäkki, T. (1982). Risks of sudden cardiovascular death (SCVD) in exercise. *Medicine and Science in Sports and Exercise*, **14**, 114-115.

Weisfeldt, M.L., Gerstenblith, G., & Lakatta, E.G. (1985). Alterations in circulatory function. In R. Andres, E.L. Bierman, & W.R. Hazzard (Eds.), *Principles of geriatric medicine* (pp. 248-279). New York: McGraw-Hill.

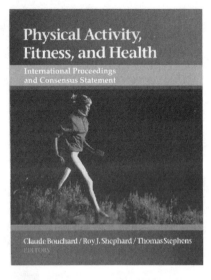
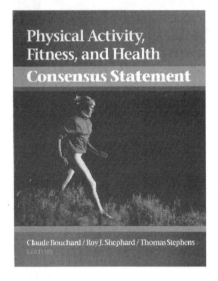